A Pound of Prevention:
The Case for Universal Maternity Care
in the U.S.

D1717197

A Pound of Prevention : The Case for Universal Maternity Care in the U.S.

Edited by
Jonathan B. Kotch, MD, MPH
Craig H. Blakely, PhD
Sarah S. Brown, MSPH
Frank Y. Wong, PhD

American Public Health Association
1015 Fifteenth Street, NW
Washington, DC 20005

American Public Health Association
1015 Fifteenth Street, NW
Washington, DC 20005

William H. McBeath, MD, MPH
Executive Director

The opinions expressed in this publication are the editors' and do not
necessarily represent the views or official policies of the Association or
of the Bureau of Maternal and Child Health.

ISBN 0–87553–206–3

2M2/92

Printed in the United States of America

Design: Ingrid Gehle
Typesetting: Unicorn Graphics, Washington, DC
Set in: Stone Serif
Printing and Binding: Victor Graphics, Baltimore, MD

Contents

This volume represents the collaborative efforts of a large number of individuals, each of whom has devoted a considerable portion of his or her life's work to bettering the delivery of and access to health care services for women and children in the United States. The acceleration since the early 1980s of the larger maternal and child health (MCH) movement, despite (or perhaps because of) the constraints imposed by recent administrations in Washington, has truly fueled this effort.

The book evolved from some early discussions among the volume editors and Jeff Taylor, a colleague with the Michigan Department of Public Health. The book first took on a formal existence in the summer of 1989, when Vince Hutchins of the Bureau of Maternal and Child Health provided crucial resources to convene in Washington, DC, the chapter authors who had been recruited to date. Woody Kessell and Ellen Hutchins, also from the Bureau, joined us for those initial discussions and contributed considerably to our early planning. From that meeting emerged the prospectus with which we hoped to attract a publisher.

That barrier was scaled when the American Public Health Association (APHA), recognizing the growing importance of maternal and infant health in the larger context of the debate over the future shape of America's health care system, agreed to publish the volume. The editors and authors gratefully acknowledge the encouragement and support of APHA and Jaclyn Alexander, the Director of Publications. Chapter writing began in earnest in the summer of 1990.

Each of the authors has made considerable contributions to the field in the past. Each has been a pleasure to work with and gave generously of both time and wisdom to this project. We hope that you, the reader, find their contributions to this volume another significant addition to a critical literature.

Several others have played key roles in the production of the manuscript. Karla Gratehouse orchestrated some of the travel plans to the initial meeting and transcribed the meeting tapes. Janet Thurman was solely responsible for assembling work from the chapter authors, transferring files to a common software package, maintaining calendars, and, in general, lending a sense of sanity to the process. Debby Thompson provided word processing assistance, and Lisa Halperin handled some of the graphics work. Lewis Margolis contributed to the introduction and several chapters. Plaudits for suggesting the most "mellifluous" book title go to William S. Davidson II. Cecil Sheps and Dorothy Lane reviewed an early draft of chapters in the spring of 1990. Their insights regarding the flow of chapters and the content were greatly appreciated and should be reflected in the final product. Finally, we must acknowledge the countless hours invested by Nancy McQuistion in providing technical writing and editorial assistance to early and final drafts of chapters.

This book is dedicated to the women and children of America in hope that our efforts will contribute in some small way to improving their access to the quality health care they deserve.

Jonathan Kotch
Craig Blakely
Sarah Brown
Frankie Wong
September 1991

Contributors

Sheila Avruch, MBA
Human Resources Division
US General Accounting Office
Washington, DC

Rosemary Barber-Madden, EdD
Center for Population and Family Health
Faculty of Medicine of Columbia University
New York, New York

Craig H. Blakely, PhD, MPH
Public Policy Resources Laboratory
Texas A&M University
College Station, Texas

Sarah S. Brown, MSPH
Institute of Medicine
National Academy of Sciences
Washington, DC

Ezra C. Davidson, MD
Department of Ob/Gyn
King-Drew Medical Center
Los Angeles, California

James G. Emshoff, PhD
Department of Psychology
Georgia State University
Atlanta, Georgia

Samuel S. Flint, PhD
Department of Child Health Care Finance and
   Organization
American Academy of Pediatrics
Elk Grove Village, Illinois

Rachel B. Gold, MPA
Alan Guttmacher Institute
Washington, DC

Robert L. Goldenberg, MD
Department of Ob/Gyn
School of Medicine
University of Alabama at Birmingham
Birmingham, Alabama

Rae K. Grad, PhD
National Commission to Prevent Infant
   Mortality
Washington, DC

Arden S. Handler, DrPH
School of Public Health
University of Illinois at Chicago
Chicago, Illinois

Ian T. Hill, MPA, MSW
Maternal and Child Health Division
Health Systems Research, Inc.
Washington, DC

Charles J. Homer, MD
Harvard Medical School and Children's
   Hospital
Boston, Massachusetts

Lynne Hudson, MPH
State Health Data and Policy Analysis
Texas Department of Health
Austin, Texas

Charles D. Johnson, PhD
Public Policy Resources Laboratory
Texas A&M University
College Station, Texas

Joan F. Kennelly, BSN, MPH
Center for Health Services and Research
University of Illinois at Chicago
Chicago, Illinois

Lorraine V. Klerman, DrPH
Department of Epidemiology and Public
   Health
School of Medicine
Yale University
New Haven, Connecticut

Jonathan B. Kotch, MD, MPH
Department of Maternal and Child Health
School of Public Health
University of North Carolina
Chapel Hill, North Carolina

Debra J. Lipson
Health Policy Consultant
Washington, DC

Jeffrey P. Mayer, PhD
School of Public Health
St. Louis University Medical Center
St. Louis, Missouri

C. Arden Miller, MD
Department of Maternal and Child Health
School of Public Health
University of North Carolina
Chapel Hill, North Carolina

Nigel Paneth, MD, MPH
Program in Epidemiology
College of Human Medicine
Michigan State University
East Lansing, Michigan

Janet D. Perloff, PhD
University Center for Policy Research
State University of New York at Albany
Albany, New York

Adrienne Puches
Health Policy Consultant
Washington, DC

George M. Ryan, MD, MPH
Department of Ob/Gyn
University of Tennessee
Memphis, Tennessee

Donald W. Schiff, MD
University of Colorado School of Medicine
  and Denver Children's Hospital
Denver, Colorado

Sarah H. Scholle, MPH
Department of Health Policy and
  Management
School of Hygiene and Public Health
Johns Hopkins University
Baltimore, Maryland

Paul H. Wise, MD, MPH
Joint Program in Neonatalogy
Harvard Medical School
Boston, Massachusetts

Frank Y. Wong, PhD
Department of Psychology
Hofstra University
Hempstead, New York

Policy for Maternal and Infant Health: Where We Stand

C. Arden Miller, MD

The United States separates itself from all other industrialized nations and from much of the developing world in important matters of maternal and infant health policy. No other advanced nation provides so little help and so few incentives for mothers and infants to participate in essential social supports and health services. No other advanced nation places such a large unsupported burden on families and such a small one on society for protecting the health and well-being of childbearing women and their infants.[1] As this volume persuasively argues, new attention must be focused on issues of equity and social justice, on a redefinition of national self-interest, and on the directions of a changing health policy.

During the 1980s important indicators of maternal and infant health in the United States faltered, prompting uncertain prospects for a vigorous and productive rising generation of young people.[2] The weight of the evidence confirms that infants, children, and childbearing women have indeed suffered under recent policies. Trends that worsened in the mid- and late 1980s, sometimes for particularly vulnerable population subgroups, include use of prenatal care, low birthweight, infant mortality rates, and immunization status. Measles, predicted in the late 1970s to be eradicable, is resurfacing in multiple outbreaks, often among preschool-aged children. Reported cases of pertussis and mumps are on the increase. Homicide is the most common cause of death from injury for children under 1 year of age. Overall US rates of childhood death from injuries declined in the late 1970s but increased again in the mid-1980s for some events in some age groups, while rates were declining in most other industrialized countries.[3] Families with children make up one third of the nation's homeless population, and in parts of the country they constitute the majority.[4] Child abuse and neglect have increased beyond any suspicion of reporting artifact. Because of fiscally forced staff cutbacks, many cases are not thoroughly investigated, which leads to underreporting of abuse. Data sources for other health indicators—such as iron deficiency anemia, growth stunting, and lead poisoning—have diminished in the past decade to the extent that careful monitoring cannot be easily accomplished. What data sources still exist would have to be observed for a long time to generate enough data points to draw definitive conclusions.

No quick fixes exist for these numerous problems facing mothers and children in this country. If we are to improve the quality of life for young families, both the government and the public at large must adopt new ways of thinking about health care for women and children. An important first step, as this book conclusively documents, is universal access to maternity and infant health services. This goal has been achieved by numerous other developed and developing countries, many of which spend less of their gross national product on health care than the United States while achieving better infant survival records.

INTERNATIONAL CONTEXT

Partly to illuminate pathways for reform in the United States, a 1987 study reviewed perinatal care in 10 Western European countries that have better records of infant survival than the United States has (Belgium, Denmark, Federal Republic of Germany, France, Ireland, Netherlands, Norway, Spain, Switzerland, and United Kingdom). Only countries with a component of pluralism in their medical care delivery systems were selected for study; excluded were those with state-controlled monopolies of medical care according to definitions advanced by a committee of the World Health Organization.[5] Two of the study countries (Ireland and Spain) have low per capita income and high unemployment rates.

The medical organization and content of perinatal care among the study countries are remarkable more for diversity than consistency. Each country has developed a style of care derived from its own traditions. For example, among study countries, the average number of prenatal visits for uncomplicated pregnancies varies between 4 and 14 and cesarean section rates range from 4.9% to 13.2%; the highest rate is only slightly more than half the current US rate for cesarean sections.

Although the medical content of maternity care differs among study countries, two impressive consistencies prevail. The first is universality of participation. Very few pregnant women fail to become involved in early prenatal care. Policies that promote participation include universal eligibility for all services without means testing and without out-of-pocket payments. Study countries also make impressive efforts to overcome language and culture barriers. Immigration from former colonies and migration in search of employment render the populations of several of the study countries less homogeneous than they sometimes are presumed to be. Participation in health care services is high among the foreign-born populations; their health indicators adhere closely to the national norms in the nation of residence, unlike indicators for racial and ethnic subgroups in the United States.

The second consistent feature of perinatal care among the study countries is the extensive array of social supports and income benefits associated with pregnancy and childbearing: paid absences from employment for clinic visits, paid maternity leaves, birthing bonuses, family allowances, transportation privileges, housing benefits, assured day care, job protection, and home visiting by workers who counsel, instruct, arrange follow-up medical appointments, and even help with the shopping and housework. These benefits vary among study countries but are extensive and internally consistent—without means testing—for all women and families in each country. Arrangements for these benefits are ordinarily made at the first prenatal visit, providing a powerful incentive for early attendance to confirm pregnancy and enroll in the sequence of comprehensive health and social benefits.

Income transfer and tax benefit programs in the United States are much more limited than in other industrialized nations and differ from their foreign counterparts in three important respects.[6] The first is the prevalence in other countries of benefits that are either (1) universal and not means tested (eg, as children's allowances), or (2) based on social insurance principles that include all families with an employment history. US programs, on the other hand, are welfare oriented, directed only toward families that qualify according to income and other criteria.

ALLEVIATING POVERTY

The second difference pertains to rates of participation. In other countries the orientation is to include poor families with infants and children in social benefit programs. In those countries, 99% of families defined as poor according to the US poverty line receive some kind of income support.[6] In the United States, on the other hand, the welfare orientation is to exclude as many poor families as possible. At the time of the comparative study (1979 to 1981—even before the welfare retrenchments that came after 1981),[7] 27% of all poor families with children in this country received no public income support. Participation in benefits such as the Special Supplemental Food Program for Women, Infants, and Children (WIC); Early and Periodic Screening, Diagnosis, and Treatment (EPSDT); and Food Stamps is seldom more than 40% of those who are eligible. Several studies have shown that such low rates of coverage are often the result of administrative and procedural obstacles, not an absence of need. For example, a recent study of Medicaid certification, which includes EPSDT, revealed that among 17 southern states 43.9% of all applications for Medicaid were denied and that less than 23% of the denials were related to excess income.[8] Two thirds of denials were attributed to failure to comply with a procedural requirement.[8]

The third difference between benefit programs in the United States and other countries relates to adequacy of support. The United States provides the least income support per family of any of the study countries and has the widest gap between average income of poor families and the poverty line. The United States distributes about 0.5% of its gross domestic product as income transfers to families with infants and children, about half the amount the other countries provide. As a result, although tax and cash transfer benefits in the United States reduce the pretransfer poverty level by about 17%, the reduction is twice as much in other countries.[6]

PRINCIPLES AND LESSONS FOR THE FUTURE

The international experience just summarized, along with the rich lessons of our own domestic history—much of which is covered in this volume—suggests at least the following ideas for reforming policies that govern the health care provided young children and pregnant women.

1. Acknowledging health care as a right. Many years ago, rumors circulated that Wilbur Cohen, former secretary of the US Department of Health, Education, and Welfare, had predicted that the chaos resulting from Medicaid would compel the nation to move quickly toward a program of universal compulsory health insurance. Unfortunately, Cohen underestimated our capacity to endure chaos. Formulations that protect a presumed right to health care are not as conspicuous now as they were 10 years ago. Attempts to extend the social insurance principle, which is already well established for the elderly, to include all childbearing women, infants, and children are opposed by proponents of incrementalism and cost containment; that opposition perpetuates an exclusionary, means-tested approach to services.

2. Emphasizing organized community-based health services. Conventional medical care is sufficient for many people, but more extensive services are required to protect and promote maternal and infant health, particularly among low-income and high-risk populations. An adequate system of care for women and infants must ensure universal participation in a set of basic health services and must also link those services to a broad array of ancillary and supportive care services, such as nutritional and educational services and psychosocial supports and counseling. Simply removing the financial barrier to existing mainstream medical services is not sufficient (see chapters 8 and 10). Neither is item-by-item financing that rarely covers the nonmedical services judged by most analysts to be an essential part of comprehensive care. Managed care, formulated around the needs of middle-class families enjoying employment-related benefits, shows little more promise. Up-front financing must be available to develop community services that assure outreach efforts, case management, and access to comprehensive programs of care.

Accumulated evidence shows that public clinics in particular address the complex medical and social problems of poor people more adequately than private providers do.[9] Medical care is presumably adequate in all settings, but only the clinics provide WIC, transportation, home visiting, organized programs to promote cessation of smoking and substance abuse, and related ancillary services. Between 1986 and

1988 the infant mortality rate in North Carolina for Medicaid women served in health department clinics (partially financed through Title V of the Social Security Act) was 11 deaths per 1000 live births. For the same period, Medicaid women served by other providers—largely private-practicing physicians—had a rate of 15.3.[10] Similar findings comparing pregnancy outcomes in different provider systems were reported by Michigan,[11] North Carolina,[9] and Tennessee.[12] Similar, unpublished findings were communicated from Kentucky and South Carolina.

Despite such evidence, current trends in health care financing do not include the expansion of community health services. Many other countries rely on neighborhood public health clinics to assure participation in routine preventive care, parallel to and interactive with the network of practitioners, hospitals, and other providers who serve childbearing women and infants when they are ill or indisposed. Such systems exist in some places in the United States, but this approach to health care has yet to be incorporated into national policy. If our society neglects this simple lesson, childbearing will become medicalized to the neglect of simple, low-cost preventive care and related social supports.

Conventional medical care is sufficient for many people, but more extensive services are required to protect and promote maternal and infant health . . .

3. Recognizing the limits of Medicaid. Advocates of expanding existing maternity care programs have focused on pushing Medicaid eligibility levels up the income scale, thus adding enormously to the burden of understaffed and underfunded welfare agencies. One particularly unfortunate consequence of this trend is that funds previously earmarked for community-based preventive health services in maternal and child health have been diverted in some states to help pay hospital bills for newly eligible maternity patients. Hospitals have rejoiced at the reduction in uncompensated care, but testimonials from local health departments from North Carolina to California detail struggles to provide prenatal care for increasing numbers of Medicaid and uninsured women and despair that agency funds have been cut with the uncertain expectation that Medicaid reimbursement will make up the difference.

Practitioners' widespread denial of services to Medicaid enrollees is often attributed to low levels of compensation and to red tape. Those deterrents are real, but so is the frustration that attends practitioners' efforts to cope with complex biosocial problems by means of nothing more than conventional office-based resources. Although conventional medical care meets the needs of most people most of the time, such care fails to meet many of the most pressing health needs of people who are suffering from chronic or disabling disease and various deprivations. Organized comprehensive community programs are required.

4. Providing adequate funds. The most troublesome obstacle in the way of progress toward an enlightened policy for maternal and infant health is the national debt. Although popular sentiment regarding the need for new public initiatives is growing, our capacity to finance such initiatives is seriously constrained by an annual deficit of $150 billion to $200 billion and a requirement to achieve budgetary balance by 1993. The nation's cautionary stance on social spending has been fortified by a strategy that spends 28% of the federal budget on the military establishment, accumulating a debt burden that forecloses other initiatives. Breaking the stalemate will necessitate increasing taxes, which most analysts advocate and nearly all politicians deny, and recognizing that enormous military expenditures fail to protect national security in the sense of providing health, education, and economic viability for many people.

MODELS FOR REFORM

These key themes provide the basis for significant restructuring of health care for children and childbearing women in the United States. A long history of expressed dissatisfaction with the status of maternity and infant health exists in this country. The means are now available for defining precisely what we hope to achieve in this arena and for controlling the ways in which those expectations can be met. Chapter 15 of this volume presents one particularly appealing proposal for reform. It is consistent philosophically with at least three other possible approaches, none of which is alien to our national traditions.

The first approach would establish a universal national health care financing system that might be age specific, possibly in the fashion of Medicare. This system would discontinue the means-tested reimbursement system (Medicaid) that links health care to welfare agencies and allows extensive state-level discretion regarding the scope of implementation. Public financing of maternity and infant health care would institutionalize standards that include both outcome and selected process measures. The standards, based on the Surgeon General's Year 2000 Health Objectives for the Nation and the Model Standards for Preventive Health Services,[13,14] could be incorporated into block grants. Federally qualified health insurance plans could then be required to meet these standards. Adopting even a few outcome standards could have a profound effect on our ability to achieve greater equity of care and on the rationing of resources.

The second approach would require dramatically strengthening the public health infrastructure at the local level. Community health care providers would monitor trends in maternal and infant health and would have the means to intervene by rendering appropriate services either directly or through contracts with other providers. The infrastructure would require federal financing, and standards and accountability would be consistently implemented between federal government and the various state health agencies.

Under this scheme, direct federal health service operations at the community level would be invoked (1) when problems such as inaccessibility or unavailability of care are so severe that they do not yield to state action and/or (2) when a state is persistently derelict in complying with national performance standards. Such federally supported community health services of the future could learn from results of similar efforts in the 1960s, when federal sponsorship of organized ambulatory care at the community level—bypassing state and local health departments—had the effect of weakening the very agencies that were required to widely institutionalize the most beneficial demonstration programs.[15] Strengthening the public health infrastructure is not intended to supplant office-based care by practitioners for the many people for whom that system works. It would instead benefit those people who require case finding, outreach, and a constellation of services that few office-based practitioners can muster.

The third initiative would link health care to a range of existing social benefit programs that are known to work but reach only a small proportion of eligible families. Well-established programs such as Head Start, Aid for Families With Dependent Children, Food Stamps, and WIC have proved effective in improving health and relieving poverty. These programs currently serve only 15% to 45% of eligible families. Although we can aspire to a future in which an expanded list of promising social benefit programs such as paid maternity leaves, assured access to infant day care, and housing benefits is universally available, we must in the meantime fully implement existing programs and policies.

People may ask if perhaps these approaches rely excessively on the weakest part of our health care system—the public health infrastructure. Skeptics should look carefully at the best public models, just as we tend to look to the best private models. The best public health models are both commendable and replicable.[16] Our present problems derive largely from the fact that we have starved public health while lavishly financing every other part of the health care system. Even so, strong public health services are not an absolute answer to improved maternal and infant health. Income transfers, housing, day care, supervised recreation, family planning, and sexuality education are all legitimate and desirable approaches. But, to be successful, every feasible approach must include a strong public health component.

In short, the time has come for maternal and infant health to be recognized as a necessary and legitimate priority for social action. Along with other vulnerable populations, pregnant women and infants deserve publicly guaranteed health benefits, broadly defined to include a rich mix of medical and social services.

REFERENCES

1. Kahn AJ, Kamermann SB. *Income Transfers for Families with Children: An Eight Country Study.* Philadelphia, Pa: Temple University; 1983.
2. Miller CA, Fine A, Adams-Taylor S. *Monitoring Children's Health: Key Indicators.* 2nd ed. Washington, DC: APHA; 1989.
3. Williams BC, Kotch JB. Excess injury mortality among children in the United States: comparison of recent international statistics. *Pediatrics.* 1990;86(suppl 6, pt 2):1067–1073.
4. Children's Defense Fund. *The State of America's Children 1991.* Washington, DC: Children's Defense Fund; 1991.
5. Miller CA. *Maternal Health and Infant Survival.* Washington, DC: National Center for Clinical Infant Programs; 1987.
6. Smeeding TM, Torrey BB. Poor children in rich countries. *Science.* 1988;242:873–877.
7. Congressional Budget Office. *Major Legislation Changes in Human Resource Programs Since January 1981.* Washington, DC: APHA; 1983.
8. Shuptrine SC, Grant VC. *Study of the AFDC/Medicaid Eligibility Process in the Southern States.* Washington, DC: Southern Governors Association; 1988.
9. Buescher PA, Smith C, Holliday JL, Levine RH. Source of prenatal care and infant birthweight: the case of a North Carolina county. *Am J Obstet Gynecol.* 1987;156:204–210.
10. Buescher P. Data provided from Division of Statistics and Information Services, Department of Environment, Health, and Natural Resources. Raleigh, NC: NC State Health Department; 1990.
11. Schwethelm B, Margolis LH, Miller C, Smith S. Risk status and pregnancy outcome among Medicaid recipients. *Am J Prev Med.* 1989;5:157–163.
12. Piper JM, Ray WA, Griffin MR. Effects of Medicaid eligibility expansion on prenatal care and pregnancy outcome in Tennessee. *JAMA.* 1990;264:2219–2223.
13. Public Health Service. *Healthy People 2000: National Health Promotion and Disease Prevention Objectives.* Washington, DC: U.S. Government Printing Office; 1991.
14. Model Standards Work Group. *Healthy Communities 2000: Model Standards.* 3rd ed. Washington, DC: APHA; 1991.
15. Lemann N. The unfinished war. *The Atlantic.* 1988;262:53–68, and 1989;263:37–56.
16. Miller CA, Moos M-K. *Local Health Departments: Fifteen Case Studies.* Washington, DC: APHA; 1981.

Section 1

Introduction

History and Overview

The preface provided a sense of urgency about maternal and child health care reform and briefly assessed the state of maternal and child health in the United States relative to other countries. Section 1 provides a critical orientation to the focus of the volume that follows. The history of the movement to establish universal access to maternity care is outlined and the social context within which this movement has arisen is presented.

In the volume introduction, Jonathan Kotch provides the central thesis of the volume—that we must provide comprehensive care for our pregnant women and young children to bolster the health of the country now and in the future. He discusses the need for policy change and outlines the recent history of legislation that has directly affected maternal and child health services. A brief discussion of four major policy options facing legislators today—retain current policies, implement a national health insurance program, institute a national health service, or implement Universal Maternity Care—leads to the conclusion that Universal Maternity Care is the most logical step to take at this time. This theme is developed in more detail in the book's concluding chapter.

Paul Wise's chapter presents the case for policy change in this arena. Leaving a detailed discussion of the medical consequences of inadequate access to maternal and infant health care to later chapters, Wise instills a sense of the social injustices that are inextricably linked to inadequate health care in the United States. He argues that an advanced society such as ours must take on additional responsibilities for the health care of its population, with special attention to the most vulnerable among us.

History and Overview

Jonathan B. Kotch, MD, MPH

The 1990s will be the decade in which the United States takes the next giant step toward improving the health and well-being of its people. Wilbur Cohen, former secretary of Health, Education, and Welfare, observed that major social reform in this country occurs every 30 years, beginning (give or take a year) with the Food and Drug Act of 1906. In 1935, the United States, during no less an economic catastrophe than the Great Depression, legislated the most comprehensive social program in its history: the Social Security Act. Thirty years later, amendments to the Social Security Act created Medicare and Medicaid. By 1995, we can expect no less than Universal Maternity Care (UMC), guaranteeing access to maternal and infant health services without regard to geography, health status, ability to pay, or other attributes.

The United States has lagged far behind Western Europe in promulgating social insurance programs, letting states address pressing social issues with innovative, if limited, responses. The Children's Bureau, established in 1912, oversaw the administration of the Sheppard-Towner Act, which provided federal funds to states that elected to establish maternal and child hygiene stations. Before those services had spread to all 48 states, Congress, afraid of bolshevism on the one hand and the American Medical Association on the other, failed to reauthorize the grant-in-aid program. Nevertheless, discussion and debate about the relationship of a national health program to maternal and child health (MCH) continued in the meetings and final report of the Committee on the Costs of Medical Care in 1927.

Although recommendations for a national health insurance scheme were deleted from the Social Security Act of 1935, grants-in-aid for MCH were preserved in Title V. No significant amendments to Title V were made until the early 1960s, when interest in reducing mental retardation led to the establishment of such special programs as the Maternity and Infant Care (1963) and Children and Youth (1965) projects. Continuing advocacy for a federal role in the financing of medical care found expression in the community and neighborhood health center movement during the War on Poverty and culminated in the passage of Medicare and Medicaid in 1965. Although interest in a national program of maternal and infant health services has continued to percolate, no progress toward a truly universal system of health care for mothers and children has occurred in the past half-century.

One bright spot in the otherwise fallow period between 1935 and 1963 offers an important precedent for UMC. The Emergency Maternity and Infant Care (EMIC) program provided absolutely free maternity and infant health services to the civilian wives of enlisted servicemen during World War II. Considered by Congress to be a necessary part of the war effort, the program was responsible for a number of innovations that are taken for granted today: universal coverage without a means test of any kind, fixed payments for a minimum prescribed package of prenatal services, mandatory assignment of physician fees, inclusion of social workers on the health consultant team, standards of care for maternity wards and nurseries, and accurate cost accounting for hospitals. At its peak, EMIC paid in full for the maternity and infant health care for one of every seven infants born in the United States. By 1947, however, this precedent-setting program had gone the way of Rosie the Riveter.

A variety of reports and studies[1-5] in the 1960s and 1970s outlined the major principles of MCH services and provided the basis for several unsuccessful legislative initiatives. In the second session of the 94th Congress (1976), New York Senator Jacob Javits and New York Representative James Scheuer sponsored a national health insurance act for mothers and children, which, although inadequate in certain key areas such as prevention, addressed many essential features of a universal maternal and infant health program.[6] President Carter's Child Health Assurance Plan in 1978 sought to enhance preventive services for children and facilitate continuity of care in the context of the Medicaid program.[7]

Among many innovative proposals recently under consideration are two from the American Academy of Pediatrics (AAP). One, the Child Health Incentives Reform Plan, would allow businesses to retain the tax deduction for contributions to employee health insurance premiums only if children's preventive care is included in their insurance plans.[8] Another, the Children First proposal, advocates the development of employer-based insurance with parallel state-administered private health insurance that covers prevention as well as treatment.[9] Both of these proposals are, unfortunately, too dependent on employment status to serve as models for universal care.

Although none of the proposed national maternal and infant health programs were enacted during the 1980s, two substantial programmatic changes did occur during that period. First, many of the categorical programs administered under Title V of the Social Security Act were dismembered and reorganized into the MCH Block Grant, giving states additional discretion in MCH spending. In our view, this change represented a setback to coherent national maternal and infant health policy because surveillance and reporting requirements were greatly reduced or eliminated. Provisions in the Omnibus Budget Reconciliation Act of 1989 (OBRA 1989), however, have reversed this trend. MCH Block Grant applications must now document status of maternal and infant health in the state and tie the monitoring of programs to the surgeon general's national health objectives for the year 2000.

Second, the 1980s also saw developments in the way health care is financed and coordinated. Specifically, OBRA 1989 brought about an initial disentangling of the health and welfare elements of public assistance by requiring states to provide Medicaid to children under the age of 6 with family incomes below 133% of the poverty level, whether or not they meet the state-determined eligibility criteria for Aid for Families with Dependent Children. Furthermore, states have the option of extending Medicaid eligibility to pregnant women and to children up to the age of 1 year with family incomes below 185% of the poverty level. These changes are critical in that they establish national eligibility criteria for Medicaid reimbursement for MCH services while distancing health care from the onus of being associated with welfare.

... the problem of infant mortality is not "their" problem, but a problem that condemns our nation to present shame and future disaster.

In a further attempt to influence and broaden state determinations of Medicaid eligibility, OBRA 1989 Medicaid amendments require states to finance services for conditions discovered during Early and Periodic Screening, Diagnosis, and Treatment programs even if the state Medicaid program does not specifically cover those services. This mandate opens the door for payment for medical treatment and ancillary health services such as home visitor programs, developmental programs, and others. Finally, state Title V and Medicaid agencies are now expected to increase their efforts toward coordination of programs.

These positive developments have set the stage for UMC. Incremental improvements in Medicaid have prevented the crisis in maternal and infant health documented in this volume from descending to catastrophe by making it possible for states to reverse the decline in federal support for MCH services. Meanwhile, annual political skirmishes over what percentage of poverty or age limit for eligibility was written into that year's bill distracted attention from the fact that health care and health status indicators failed to improve and in some cases continued to decline. The apparent inability of such incremental changes to substantially improve access to care or health status for increasing numbers of poor women and children speaks eloquently for fundamentally changing the way we provide maternal and infant health services.

The call for UMC that began the cascade of events leading to this book was first heard from the newly enfranchised Council on Maternal and Child Health of the National Association for Public Health Policy (NAPHP) in 1982. That same year, the MCH Block Grant shifted more authority for MCH services to the state level and efforts to reform MCH followed suit. Unfortunately, the block grant was accompanied by 18% to 25% cuts in federal support for MCH at a time when states were reeling from the worst recession since the period 1974 to 1975. Ironically, it was the inability of the states to act without federal support that prompted the Southern Governors' Association (SGA) to be the next organization to call for guaranteed access to prenatal care and for the federalization of the Medicaid program.[10]

Since that 1985 SGA report, the Institute of Medicine, the National Commission to Prevent of Infant Mortality, and the American Academy of Pediatrics, to name a few, have one by one joined the UMC bandwagon, albeit each under its own logo.

This book brings together in print for the first time many of the spokespersons for these organizations. Represented here are individuals from professional organizations such as the American Academy of Pediatrics, the American Public Health Association, the American College of Obstetricians and Gynecologists, the Southern Governors' Association, and the National Governors' Association; advocacy groups such as the Children's Defense Fund, the National Association for Public Health Policy, and the Alan Guttmacher Institute; and outstanding health academicians and researchers, whose joint efforts to assure access to maternity and infant care for all continue. We would be remiss if we failed to observe that the seminal idea for this volume occurred among a small group of visionaries who were instrumental in establishing a right to prenatal care in the early 1980s in Michigan. With the assistance of the Bureau of Maternal and Child Health (one of the modern offshoots of the Children's Bureau), the editors and authors convened in Washington, DC, in the summer of 1989 and left with a commitment to contribute as complete an exposition of the UMC idea as possible.

This book is both descriptive and prescriptive, attempting to define and defend UMC. The manifesto by Paul Wise in section 1, articulating the social justice argument for UMC, powerfully reminds us that the problem of infant mortality is not "their" problem, but a problem that condemns our nation to present shame and future disaster. The succeeding chapters are organized into sections by theme. Section 2 describes and offers evidence for the efficacy of the most conspicuous pieces of the maternal and infant health care cycle. These chapters provide the basis for a common understanding of what is included in medical care during pregnancy and childhood (both routine and special care), and in nonmedical prenatal services such as nutrition, social support, and substance abuse services. Section 3, a needs assessment, documents the fact that many American women, infants, and young children do not obtain necessary preventive and primary care services because systematic barriers have been created in the way such services are organized and paid for. The section concludes with problems inherent in private health insurance coverage for working Americans during this period of shifting labor markets, decreasing real income for young families, and rising health care costs.

Section 4 introduces some of the federal, state, and local interim solutions that have mushroomed across the country. Ironically, the success of some of these efforts does not bode well for the future. In the first place, local successes, which are the result of unique circumstances, may not be generalizable to other settings. Second, despite the remarkable variety of state-by-state solutions collectively referred to as Medicaid enhancements, adverse trends in access to prenatal care have yet to be reversed.

Section 5 introduces the UMC proposal, first by describing the continuum of services for women and children commonly understood to be "comprehensive," then by addressing the problem of ensuring that participants in a universal system providing such services receive those services at an acceptable level of quality, and finally by listing the principles of UMC and comparing UMC with other national health care proposals according to a policy analysis matrix. By the time readers reach that point, we hope they will be persuaded that specific maternal and infant health services are known to be effective, that growing segments of the population are finding it increasingly difficult to obtain such services, and that public and private efforts thus far, although exciting, have been inadequate.

... the logic of providing quality health care for pregnant women and children has an imperative all its own.

We have proposed a specific solution to the problem of inadequate access to maternal and infant health services that requires a significant departure from the way doctors and patients currently do business. Other proposals have been put forward as well. None of them, including UMC, will by itself solve the health problems of pregnant women and children. Additional initiatives—such as affordable and accessible day care, enhanced public educational services, jobs that pay wages sufficient to support young families, and decent, available housing—will also be required. But the logic of providing quality health care for pregnant women and children has an imperative all its own. In many ways, good health is a prerequisite for enjoying the benefits of quality education, affordable housing, and an adequate job. And in health care, there is no better way to begin building a just system of services than at the beginning.

REFERENCES

1. Select Panel for the Promotion of Child Health. *Better Health for Our Children: A National Strategy.* Washington, DC: Public Health Service; 1981. US Dept of Health and Human Services publication No. (PHS) 79-55071.
2. Wallace HM. National planning for the health care of mothers and children. In: Wallace H, Gold EM, Oglesby AC, eds. *Maternal and Child Health Practices.* New York, NY: John Wiley & Sons; 1982.
3. Silver GA. *Child Health: America's Future.* Germantown, Md: Aspen Systems Corp; 1978.
4. Wallace HM, Miller CA. A national health program for infants, children, and youth in the United States, I: some characteristics. *Health Care Manage Rev.* 1978; 3:11–27.
5. Marmour TR. Children and national health insurance. In: Harvard Child Health Project Task Force. *Developing a Better Health Care System for Children.* Cambridge, Mass: Ballinger Publishing Co; 1977.
6. North AF. National health insurance for mothers and children. *Am J Dis Child.* 1977; 131:17–20.
7. Berkelhamer JE, Noyes EJ, Chen RT. Child health policy—an overview of Federal involvement. *Adv Pediatr.* 1982; 29:211–228.
8. Chafee JH. Insuring the health of children. *Business and Health.* 1985; 5–8.
9. American Academy of Pediatrics. *An Overview of the AAP Access to Care Legislative Proposal.* Elk Grove, Ill: American Academy of Pediatrics, 1989.
10. Southern Regional Task Force on Infant Mortality. *Interim Report.* Washington, DC: Southern Governors' Association; 1985.

CHAPTER 1

The Social Context of Maternal and Child Health Care Reform

Paul H. Wise, MD, MPH

Like all reform, the struggle for universal maternity and infant health services is defined by the perception of need, the perception of a societal capacity to respond, and a vision of justice. Social forces have shaped need by transforming traditional mechanisms by which children have been provided with the necessities of life. Although societal capacity to address this arena of health is commonly viewed as strictly a technical issue, it is heavily influenced by social perceptions of government efficacy and the availability of public resources. Evolving concepts of justice define the legitimacy of the public guarantee to health services and therefore frame the moral basis for advocating access to those services.

THE SOCIAL DETERMINANTS OF NEED

The Crisis of Providing for Children

As the 1980s came to an end, the United States was confronted with a worrisome paradox: despite the largest economic expansion in the nation's history, the relative economic position of children had never been worse. That these two phenomena could coincide suggests that important structural changes have occurred in the means by which society funnels its assets to children.

In 1960, approximately one in four children younger than 18 were living in families with reported incomes lower than the officially designated poverty level (approximately three times the income needed to meet a federal estimate of minimal nutritional subsistence).[1] By the mid-1960s poverty among children had begun to fall, and it reached a low point of approximately 14% in 1974, where it remained for the rest of the decade (Fig 1-1). However, during the 1980s an alarming increase in childhood poverty occurred; the rate stabilized at more than 22% by 1983. Despite the boom years of the mid- and late 1980s, the poverty rate for children remained a startling 20.6% in 1987, a level from which it has since fallen only slightly.[2]

Evidence proves that the most vulnerable children have fared the worst during this period. Although the median family income of

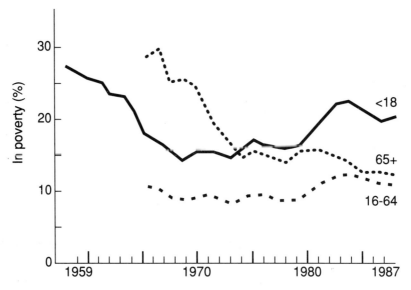

Fig. 1-1.—Trends in the proportion of population living below the poverty line by selected age groups: 1959–1987.

White children has regained the losses experienced in the early 1980s, the family incomes of Black and Hispanic children have continued to fall.[3] Between 1979 and 1987 the median family income of Black children fell from $16 704 to $15 005 (in constant 1987 dollars). The comparable decline for Hispanic children was from $22 011 to $17 962. Almost half of all Black children and more than a third of Hispanic children currently live in poverty.

The fundamental challenge of these recent trends in childhood poverty is underscored by the contrasting experience of other segments of American society in the same period. In the mid-1960s the elderly suffered from higher poverty rates than children. However, by the mid-1970s, the rate for the elderly fell below that for children and continued its overall decline, concurrent with significant increases in the rate for children.[2] Thus, during the 1980s the childhood poverty rate rose by 37% while the rate among the elderly fell a dramatic 49%. When noncash benefits such as Medicare are included, the divergence of fortunes is even more profound.[4]

The disturbing rise in childhood poverty has been met by a series of misperceptions about its causes and, therefore, its challenge to social policy. Perhaps the most serious myth has developed regarding the relative concentration of child poverty in the inner city, in what is commonly labeled the underclass. Although the desperate needs of inner-city youth should never be discounted, most poor children in the United States do not live in the ghettos of large urban centers. Rather, almost a third of poor children live in rural areas and another 28% in suburban communities.[5] Fewer than 1 in 10 poor children live in census tracts in the 100 largest American cities in which poverty affects more than half their neighbors.

The danger in portraying the recent decline in the social position of children as having occurred in only highly concentrated areas of the inner city is that the profound structural changes these trends imply may be minimized. At the heart of this complex social experience have been the dynamic state of the American family and the failure of public policy to respond.

The Changing Capacity of the Family

A central principle of American society has always been that the primary provider for children is the family. Familial responsibility for children's well-being, including health, continues to lie at the heart of current social policies. However, at different periods in American history the family's capacity to provide for children has been strained by powerful changes in family structure and economic opportunity. Such strains emerged dramatically in the past decade, shaped increasingly by alterations in parental relationships and the economic prospects of young families in the United States.

Changing family structure. In general, a family with two parents present is more likely to be able to generate sufficient income to keep a child out of poverty than is a single-parent household, most of which are headed by women. In 1960, approximately 88% of children younger than 18 were living in two-parent families and 9% in single-parent families. By 1988, 73% were living in two-parent families and a full 25% in single-parent households (Table 1-1).[6] The most dramatic increase in single-parent households has occurred in mother-only families. After increasing more than 270% between 1960 and 1988, mother-headed households are now the family setting for more than 21% of all children.[7] Father-only households also rose dramatically in that period, but this form of household is still less than 5% of all households with children.

These figures suggest that more children live in single-parent families in the United States than in any other developed country for which comparable data are available.[8] (Table 7) For example, in Japan approximately 6% of children live in single-parent households. Although the number of single-parent households has grown in all ethnic and social groups, Black and Hispanic children are most likely to be living in a single-parent family. In 1988, 16% of White children, 27% of Hispanic children, and 51% of Black children were living in mother-only families.[7]

Although the causes of this shift to single-parent families are complex and have defied easy explanation, a major factor has been the dramatic rise in divorce in the United States (Fig 1-2). After doubling between 1960 and 1975, the rate of divorce in the United States began to

Like all reform, the struggle for universal maternity . . . services is defined by the perception of need, . . . a societal capacity to respond, and a vision of justice.

TABLE 1-1
Distribution of US Children Under 18 Years of Age by Family Living Arrangements, 1981 and 1988

Living Arrangement	1981		1988	
	Number*	%	Number*	%
Both biological parents	42.6	67	38.0	60
Mother only	11.6	18	13.5	21
Father only	0.9	2	1.8	3
Mother-stepfather	4.5	7	5.1	8
Father-stepmother	1.0	2	1.8	3
Adoptive parents	1.1	2	1.1	2
Grandparents or other relatives	0.9	2	1.5	2
Foster parents, other nonrelatives, or group quarters	0.5	1	0.4	1

SOURCE: Reference 3, Table 19.
* In millions.

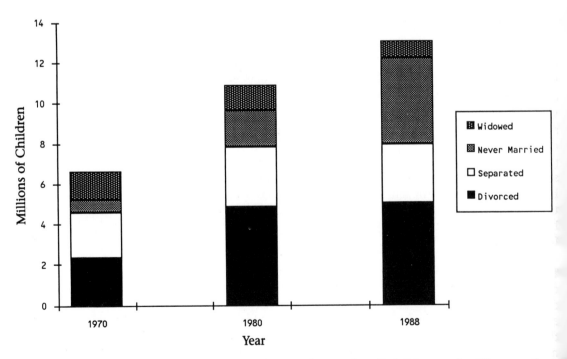

Fig. 1-2.—Distribution of causes for maternal marital status for all children under 18 years of age living with their mothers only.

plateau in the second half of the 1970s and remained relatively stable through the 1980s. Currently, approximately half of all marriages end in divorce and 1 in 50 children confront parental divorce each year.[9]

In addition to marital disruption, the birth of children to unmarried women has also had a profound impact on the social well-being of children. In 1970, less than 10% of all children living in female-headed households were born to unmarried women. By 1988, this percentage had risen by some 678% to represent almost a third of all children living in female-headed households.[3] (Table 21) In 1950, less than 5% of all births were to unmarried women; by 1986, 25% were. For Blacks, 61% of all births were to unmarried women.[10]

The rise in the percentage of births occurring among unmarried women has been due to both a striking decline in the rate at which women marry and the declining birth rate among married women, rather than to increased likelihood that unmarried women are going to give birth. On the contrary, particularly for Black women, the rise in the proportion of unmarried births has emerged in the face of a falling rate of birth among the unmarried. Focusing only on the fertility of unmarried women can obscure a more complex group of determinants: economic trends, the changing role of women in American society, and the deteriorating earning prospects of young males in many areas of the United States.[11, 12]

In aggregate, these trends have had an important impact on the capacity of families to provide for their children. In 1987 the median income for female-headed households was $9838; for all families, $29 892; and for two-parent families, $35 423.[3] (Table 42), 13 Fifty-five percent of all female-headed families and 66% of female-headed families with children younger than 6 had incomes below federal poverty standards. Although the number of female-headed households has increased steadily in the past two decades, the likelihood that they are poor has remained fairly stable, hovering at approximately 50% in the same period. Therefore, the steadily rising contribution of female-headed households to the childhood poverty rate has been primarily the result of the increasing frequency of children living in female-headed households rather than of rising poverty rates among such families.[3] (Table 47), 5

Providing for children in two-parent families. Although the increase in the number of poor, female-headed households has prompted concerns about the feminization of poverty in the United States, it is equally important to recognize that the greatest contributing factor to the recent increase in childhood poverty has been the worsening economic plight of families with two parents at home. Unlike the fairly stable poverty rate among single-parent families, poverty among two-parent families tends to be more variable. During the 1960s, poverty among two-parent families fell dramatically from more than 20% to approximately 8%, where it remained throughout the 1970s.[2] In the

Almost half of all Black children and more than a third of Hispanic children currently live in poverty.

early 1980s, however, the poverty rate among two-parent families rose significantly. By 1983 approximately one of every seven children in a two-parent family lived in poverty. Since 1983, the poverty rate among two-parent families has stabilized at levels significantly higher than those of the 1970s.

... the eroding capacity of the family to provide for children and the inadequacy of the state's response have together created a crisis in providing for American children ...

Although employment rates play an important role in determining poverty in two-parent families, parental employment is no guarantee that a child will not grow up in poverty. Most two-parent families living in poverty are poor even though at least one of the parents is working. Indeed, Bane and Ellwood, using March 1988 Current Population Survey data, documented that among all poor families with two nonelderly, healthy parents at home, 91% had some income from parental employment.[5] Almost half of all such families had at least one parent who was employed in a full-time position for the whole year. This point suggests that relatively high poverty rates for two-parent families may persist even in the face of relatively low unemployment rates.

This worsening in the economic condition of the traditional two-parent family with children appears to be based on significant structural shifts in the nature of the American economy and the resulting stagnation of wages in the face of ongoing inflation. Indeed, it has been suggested that the rate of poverty among two-parent families closely follows the median income of year-round, full-time, male workers.[5] It is significant that this figure (adjusted for inflation) fell between 1979 and 1987.

Traditional two-parent families with fathers earning at the lower end of the wage scale may live perilously close to poverty. Between 1979 and 1986, poverty rates for two-parent families in which the father was younger than 25 rose from 10.5% to 21.5%. For married men younger than 30 who have children, the real median income fell an alarming 16% between 1973 and 1986 and the poverty rate more than doubled.[2, 14] For such men who never completed high school, the median income fell a full 32%, from $17 239 to $11 770, in the same period. Their counterparts with high school diplomas fared only slightly better: their median income fell by 22%.

Ninety percent of this decline in the real income of all young, married fathers with children has been due to reductions in real hourly wage rates. This point is particularly evident when one considers the major decline in the value of the minimum wage in the past two decades. During the 1980s a full-time worker receiving the minimum wage of $3.35 earned only 75% of the poverty level for a family of four. A family of four with one parent working full-time and another half-time earned some $2000 less than the official poverty line.[5] The declining earning power of young men has meant that the young American family has had increasing difficulty achieving the material well-being that has traditionally defined the image of young family life in America. Young families are at increased risk of living in or near poverty.

Women in the work force and child care. Among the many changes in the status of women in American society has been a dramatic increase in the participation of women in the work force. Although the causes are complex, this trend has been, in some measure, a response to the growing number of woman-headed households and the dwindling capacity of men to support their families without the assistance of their spouses.

By the late 1980s, less than a third of all American children lived in two-parent families with a working father and a homemaker mother.[3] (Table 29) In 1986, some 38 million children—a full 60% of all children— had mothers in the labor force. By far the most common living arrangement (42%) has become the two-parent family in which both parents participate in the labor force. Of the single women who care for one quarter of all children in the United States, 67% are in the labor force. Employment has become the rule even for women with extremely young children. Fifty-two percent of all married women with children younger than 1 year report participation in the labor force; 72% of Black married mothers with infants at home are labor force members.[15] Among single mothers with children younger than 1, 45% are in the labor force.

. . . children have suffered from more serious deprivation than they do now, but rarely have they been so disproportionately deprived in relation to the rest of society.

Clearly, the increased earnings associated with growing maternal employment have significantly enhanced the capacity of families to provide for their children. However, this enhancement has been significantly offset by the falling earning power of young fathers. For young, two-parent families, the portion of income from the father's earnings fell from 77% to 67% between 1973 and 1986.[14] In the end, the dramatic increase in maternal employment contributed significantly to young family incomes but could not completely compensate for the major decline in male earning power. The real median family income for all young, two-parent families fell by 4% in the same period, versus a 16% decline in young males' earnings.

The growth in maternal employment has also dramatically altered child care arrangements in American families. Census data for the years 1984 to 1985 revealed that the primary child care arrangement for 24% of children younger than 5 with working mothers was a day care center or preschool.[16] Another 22% were cared for by a nonrelative in the provider's home and 15% by a relative in the relative's home. Thirty-one percent were cared for by a relative or father in the child's home. Forty-six percent of all infants with working mothers were cared for by nonfamily members, 37% outside the child's home. Projections clearly indicate that this trend in nonparental care, particularly in nonrelative day care settings, will continue to increase in the 1990s.[17]

The Changing Role of the State

For children, the primary alternative to the family for societal resources is the state. This role acknowledges the collective interest in ensuring minimal standards of subsistence to children after familial provision has failed. In earlier times, this communal responsibility for children took the form of local charity or informal care-giving relationships. However, although these informal arrangements persist, much of this communal responsibility for children has shifted to governmental processes and institutions. Often viewed as a system of last resort, or a safety net, these state programs have come to represent a critical mechanism of providing for a growing portion of America's children.

The increasingly strained capacity of the family to provide resources to children necessarily focuses attention on the adequacy of the state's response to children's needs. This issue is difficult to address, in part because of the complex and deeply fragmented nature of state programs as well as the fractious ideologic controversies that surround the public discussion about them. Nevertheless, certain objective indicators frame the scope of the state's commitment and provide insight into the extent to which state programs compensate for the deterioration of the economic well-being of the young American family.

The nature of the state's response. Most industrialized countries provide the major portion of assistance to poor families through generally available social insurance programs like social security. In the United States, however, most benefits provided to poor families are funneled through means-tested welfare programs, in which eligibility is restricted to categorically defined groups based on income and family structure.[8] Approximately 70% of all state assistance to poor families with children in the United States is provided through such means-tested programs. In Canada, approximately half of all state assistance to poor families is means tested, whereas in the Federal Republic of Germany the figure is near 10%. Although this major distinction in how resources are transferred is rooted in differing administrative and bureaucratic histories, it also reflects far-reaching differences in the social perception of the legitimacy and scope of the family's claim to societal resources.

In the United States a constrained view has predominated, taking form in the structure of means-tested government programs to assist families in poverty. The primary mechanism for transferring income to poor families with children is Aid for Families with Dependent Children (AFDC), which in most areas of the country represents the core of the welfare program. For the most part, states establish their own eligibility and benefit levels within broad federal limitations. Traditionally, children and their primary caretaker are eligible when their family income and assets fall below a specified level and when the father is absent, incapacitated, unemployed despite seeking work, or deceased. Recent changes at the federal level have eased eligibility criteria to allow entry to a broader range of families with a father at home. Another vehicle for transferring income to families in need has occurred through tax mechanisms, particularly the earned income tax credit, which reduces the tax burden on families that have low, albeit some, income.[18]

The primary pathway whereby the state provides health insurance to poor families (Medicaid) is intricately linked with AFDC. Eligibility for Medicaid has historically depended chiefly on eligibility for AFDC. Although this tight relationship has been eased somewhat, it has nevertheless meant that the state's providing health insurance has been means tested and that the state's interest in access to health care has been tied to poverty.

... full AFDC benefits do not bring the income of ... families to the official poverty level.

Other state programs for poor families are not only means tested but also are constrained in the character of the resource to be transferred. Unlike AFDC, which involves cash payments, many state programs restrict benefits to highly selective areas of family need. The Food Stamp program provides families that meet designated income standards with coupons exchangeable for food. Head Start, a comprehensive educational program for preschool children, is confined to low-income children. The School Lunch program provides meals to children in school who meet family income criteria. The Special Supplemental Food Program for Women, Infants, and Children (WIC) requires both low income and designation of "nutritional risk" for program entry. Here, benefits are highly restricted, taking the form of specified foods deemed especially nutritious for pregnant and lactating women and young children. In general, the state response to families in need has been through categoric, means-tested programs the benefits of which are largely restricted to precise areas of provision.

The level of the state's response. The level as well as the nature of the state's response defines its adequacy. Here, with few exceptions, the record is disturbing. Between 1980 and 1987, despite the enormous growth in the number of poor families with children, the actual number of children served by the AFDC program remained relatively constant.[3] Furthermore, real AFDC expenditures during this period fell from $17.2 billion to $16.4 billion (constant 1987 dollars). Perhaps most troubling has been the erosion of the monthly AFDC payment in the past two decades. In 1970 the average monthly payment to AFDC families was $471. However, the persistent failure to increase AFDC benefits in accordance with inflation meant that by 1987 this amount had fallen to $361, a decline of some 23%.[3]

In addition to the effects of inflation, AFDC eligibility and benefit levels continue to vary considerably by state. In some states, income eligibility standards are so low that they exclude families earning less than half the official poverty level. Benefits also vary enormously, ranging from more than $500 per month to less than $120 per month.[3] However, in virtually all areas, full AFDC benefits do not bring the income of beneficiary families to the official poverty level.[19] Of the one quarter of all children in the United States who are classified as poor before receiving government payments, only one fifth will be raised out of poverty by these funds. More than half of the poor children in the United States will remain poor despite government support. The rest of poor children—approximately one quarter—receive no government support.[3] In 1975, 73% of all poor children received AFDC payments. In 1987 this figure had dropped to 56%.[3]

With the federal budget now topping $1 trillion, resources are hardly limited; they are merely competitive.

Other government programs for young families of particular interest to the health community have also fared poorly. Despite the widespread growth of hunger in the United States,[20] participation in the Food Stamp program fell by nearly 14% during the 1980s.[3] The average benefit level remained virtually constant over the same period. Since 1980 the number of lunches served by the School Lunch program has fallen by some 2 million, largely in response to a funding decline of some 25%.[3]

There have been some significant successes in expanding programs that address the growing needs of young families with children. WIC funding rose during the 1980s, although it still serves only about half of all eligible women and children.[3, 21] Head Start funding, after a decade of only slight growth, has recently received significant increases. Although coordinated child care legislation remains in flux, a broadened, more highly integrated approach to funding child care is likely to emerge in the early 1990s.

Despite the expansion of these selected programs, the overall record of recent state responses to the eroding capacity of families to provide for children in the United States appears to have been severely inadequate. This inadequacy becomes even more apparent when assessed in relation to the state's response to the needs of the elderly, another segment of the population for which traditional mechanisms of provision had deteriorated. In 1960, state spending on the elderly was approximately three times greater than spending on children.[22] Expenditures for both the elderly and children grew substantially during the next two decades so that by 1980 the ratio remained at about the 1960 level. However, the 1980s witnessed significant reductions in major programs that primarily affect young families with children, while programs for the elderly continued to expand. Currently, for every $1 the federal government spends on children, it spends approximately $10 on the elderly.

It is common for this divergence in state commitments to be featured in arguments that pit the needs of the elderly against those of the young. Clearly, the elderly and children have far more in common than their role in conflict and policy debate. This purported generational strife has somewhat obscured the lessons we might deduce about society's capacity to foster the cause of children. The recent experience of the elderly is significantly compelling testimony to the power of public action to improve the life conditions of a significant portion of American society.

The central premise of this discussion is that the eroding capacity of the family to provide for children and the inadequacy of the state's response have together created a crisis in providing for American children and that this crisis is a critical context in which to deliberate public guarantees of health care for childbearing women and children. The evolving service base of the American economy and the changing structure of families have significantly reduced the traditional role of the family as an institution that provides children with the essentials of life.

CONFRONTING THE CRISIS OF PROVISION: PERCEPTIONS OF SOCIETAL CAPACITY

However, public policies concerned with the well-being of children have not kept pace with this expanded privation. The result is a mismatch of need and service of historic proportions; children have suffered from more serious deprivation than they do now, but rarely have they been so disproportionately deprived in relation to the rest of society. This relative deprivation has become so profound and so well documented that the public examination of it has cast a harsh light on the very nature of the public commitment to the well-being of children in the United States. Although the central elements of this public debate are complex and extend far beyond the scope of this discussion, they may indeed prove relevant to the development of the social strategies and political will necessary to adopt an expanded public commitment to health services for women and children.

Arguments over the relative adequacy of public resources devoted to women's and children's needs will likely continue for some time to come. However, regardless of whether public resources are adequate, questions about the state's capacity to respond to these needs have also emerged at the forefront of public debate. This concern about societal capacity to address social problems tends to take two forms: questions of expense and questions of efficacy. The former are usually discussed in terms of what society can "afford" and the latter in terms of what "works."

Too often the issue of whether our society can afford greater expenditures on childbearing women and children is framed by notions of a newly arrived age of limited societal resources. With the federal budget now topping $1 trillion, resources are hardly limited; they are merely competitive. As always, it is how women's and children's interests will compete in a contentious political environment that will determine the measure of resources allocated to their needs.

The issue of what society can afford is difficult to address. Decisions about affordability are closely related to questions of value and the perception of costs associated with not acting. However, questions about the capacity of our society to absorb the cost of expanded programs for childbearing women and children are circumvented somewhat by invoking comparisons of scale: programs for pregnant women and children are relatively inexpensive versus other major societal expenditures, particularly military expenditures. For example, the recent widely hailed $500 million expansion in the Head Start program is similar in cost to one B-2 bomber. Other concerns may also be relevant in this context, including the relatively low tax rates and societal expenditures on maternity and children's health services in the United States versus other industrialized countries.[23]

A second component of the societal capacity issue is related to the perceived efficacy of state action to achieve desired goals. Here, broad judgments regarding the utility of "social engineering" may be coupled with specific concerns related to the functioning of specific public programs. Human service programs, particularly those with roots in the War on Poverty, have been harshly attacked as ineffective or, worse, as responsible for magnifying poverty and human suffering.[24]

These assaults on the efficacy of state interventions undermine advocacy arguments for expanded access to these programs.[25] This inherent tension has compelled advocates of a broader public commitment to human services to make counterarguments, carefully documenting the efficacy of a variety of human service programs.[26] Even questions regarding the utility of basic medical care have required cogent response.[27] Moreover, the need to document efficacy has led to a wave of complex program evaluations and demonstration efforts, often involving interventions the efficacy of which was likely to have been deemed self-evident in prior years.

CHILDREN, FAMILIES, AND CLAIMS TO SOCIAL JUSTICE

The great tragedy of children in America is that their claim to justice is inherently tied to that of their parents. Social concern for children is framed by the fact that their access to societal resources depends on the legitimacy of their parents' claim. This linkage is derived from the long-standing belief in the primacy of familial responsibility in caring for children. A clear tension develops, however, when families cannot provide adequately for their children, because concern for the well-being of children clashes then with traditional attachments to familial autonomy and responsibility. What emerges is confused public policy, through which resources are directed to children only when complex bureaucratic mechanisms judge legitimate the parental claim to resources. Programmatically, children may be considered truly needy, but if their parents refuse to seek work, they may be deemed ineligible for state funds. Politically, voters may be concerned for poor children but may hesitate to support expanded welfare funding because of their misgivings about the parental actions that allowed these children to become poor in the first place because these funds are, in effect, used to support the parents as much as the children.

Elevating the Claims of Children: A Double-edged Sword

This tension between the needs of children and the worthiness of their parents has set in motion a long history of efforts by reformers and child advocates to reframe the debate. The primary response has been an attempt to uncouple the claims of children and then elevate them above those of their parents, because it is generally acknowledged that the case for allocating resources to children may be far more compelling than a case based on the needs of their parents. Services for homeless children may have far more political currency than services for their homeless young fathers.

This elevation of the children's claim for justice has taken root in several central justifications for expanded state programs for children: children as innocents, children as legacy, and children as investment. Although elevating children's claim to resources as a basis for policy has resulted in important improvements in the state's commitment to children, it may, if not carefully amended to fit the changing social determinants of children's well-being in the United States, have untoward effects that in the end could prove decidedly counterproductive to the interests of children and a broader progressive agenda.

Children as innocents. Because childhood is defined by innocence, the suffering of children is cast almost reflexively as inherently unjust. No child, regardless of what he or she has done in life, deserves to be impoverished; no newborn deserves to be born addicted to cocaine; and no infant deserves to go hungry. The public embrace of childhood innocence represents a fundamental basis for all child advocacy and is a central mechanism for elevating the claim of children above that of their parents.

However, innocence may ultimately prove to be a less than fruitful basis for public advocacy, because the responsibility for the suffering of children is assigned to noninnocents, usually the parents. Children are often portrayed as innocent victims, an image that is a true but troubling basis for advocacy. If, for example, in the advocating for improved services for newborns exposed to cocaine in utero these children are portrayed as innocent victims, then virtually by definition their mothers are cast as assailants. This dynamic has contributed to a spate of criminal actions against women for using illegal substances in pregnancy, a trend that virtually all child advocates view as counterproductive.

Children as legacy. The elevation of the children's claim for justice has also taken hold in the notion of children as legacy—that is, the strong current in American public opinion that is concerned for the well-being of children in relation to the future of our society. The notion that children are our future is indeed compelling and touches a strong chord to mobilize public concern for the current needs of children. However, it can also be problematic. If children are our future, their parents are our present. A reliance on children as legacy to mobilize resources generates a logic that tends to write off young adults, including young women, as a lost cause. Again, such a policy dynamic may not serve the best interests of children who are poor mostly because of the deteriorating economic position of their parents.

Children as investment. The third justification that elevates the children's claim is children as investment. Here, arguments for improved services for children are based on the need to have a vibrant work force in the future to better advance our national status in an increasingly competitive world economy. This argument has clearly played a large role in the recommendations from the business community for increased services to children. However, like legacy arguments, this approach shifts concern away from the claims of those who are already in the work force. It calls for state action to remedy what is partly the result of the inadequacy of current industrial policies and wage scales to keep families with children out of poverty. Moreover, this human investment approach can at times confine the social claims of children to the indifferent requirements of the national economy.

Given the problems inherent in elevating the children's claim above that of parents, why, then, is it still the core of much of the current advocacy for children's issues? Although the answer to this question is complex and deeply rooted in the great turn-of-the-century reformist impulses, it undoubtedly lies in the desperate nature of the recent struggles to provide children with what they need. Particularly in the past decade, the ferocity of political battles over human service programs—many of which are fought merely to protect existing programs rather than to expand funding—has required the use of all advocacy arguments that possess significant political currency. In this light, it must be acknowledged that the elevation of the children's claim has generated important public support for many recent policy successes that, in turn, are providing very real and direct services to large numbers of children in need.

Yet few suggest that these successes are adequate. As the struggle to confront our crisis of providing for children continues into the 1990s and the 21st century, the uncritical acceptance of current child advocacy positions may require urgent review. Child advocacy policies must be reformulated to incorporate more fully the needs of parents into a common social agenda. A common ground must be found in which the political currency of children's issues is interwoven with social strategies that attend to the needs of young adults and young families.

Social Trends, Health Care, and the Construction of Common Agendas

The need for a common agenda in the face of major social forces that are endangering the life chances of children seems particularly relevant to constructing an expanded children's health policy. Including maternity care with proposals for young children's health is an important step that recognizes that the health of infants and young children depends heavily on access to a range of services provided in the prenatal period. However, the political basis for including maternity care is, in practice, the extension of the children's claim to include the fetus. This concern for birth outcome per se must by definition involve the needs of mothers. However, in general, this concern for mothers is concentrated by policy on their health only to the extent that it affects that of newborns. It remains unclear how proposals directed at prenatal and child health care are linked conceptually and politically to broader programs for enhanced access to health care for all Americans. To argue for enhanced prenatal care services without a purposeful strategy to advance the cause of enhanced access to health services for all women regardless of childbearing status is to cling to an isolated elevation of the children's claim and a rejection of a shared agenda.

... policy should reflect the family-based approach of the clinical world.

The political prospects of isolated and shared health agendas may differ significantly; accordingly, each strategy may assume different levels of priority at different times. This discussion often takes root in the tension between incremental and more universal health care strategies. What is nevertheless more fundamental is that these programs, whether incremental or universal, further a truly common agenda. Incremental policies can be pursued in a framework expressly dedicated to reaching some form of universal system. On the other hand, a universal proposal must be crafted to meet the quite specific needs of children, who by definition would represent only a small portion of all those served by such a broad-based program.

The dramatic social changes of the past three decades have defined the need for a universal maternity and infant care program in the United States. But they have also defined the need for such a program to extend beyond this one arena of provision. The crisis of providing for children has emerged from profound structural changes in the American economy and the American family.

This complex network of causes places new burdens on proposals for expanded state action. Both the nature of the problem and the character of the moral debate demand that advocacy for children's programs respect, if not serve, the parents' claims to justice. This imperative is generated less from moral logic than from the front lines of providing service to children. Indeed, recognition that policy should reflect the family-based approach of the clinical world seems long overdue. However, the struggle to fashion such a common social agenda will require considerable disciplinary self-reflection and a broader revisioning of the course of maternal and infant health policy in the United States. More fundamental still will be the interweaving of diverse political constituencies into a common effort that will best ensure that justice for children is not rendered hollow by the deteriorating social position of their parents.

1. Orshansky M. How poverty is measured. *Monthly Labor Rev.* 1969; 34:41–44.
2. US Dept of Commerce. Bureau of the Census. Money, income, and poverty status of families and persons in the US. *Current Population Reports.* Series P-60. Washington, DC: US Govt Printing Office; various years.
3. US House of Representatives. *US Children and Their Families: Current Conditions and Recent Trends, 1989.* Washington, DC: US Govt Printing Office; 1989.
4. Smeeding T. Noncash benefits and poverty. *Policy Stud J.* 1982; 10:499–509.
5. Bane MJ, Ellwood DT. One fifth of the nation's children: why are they poor? *Science.* 1989; 245:1047–1053.
6. US Dept of Commerce. Bureau of the Census. *Statistical Abstract of the United States, 1988.* Washington, DC: US Govt Printing Office; 1988: Table 69.
7. US Dept of Commerce. Bureau of the Census. Marital status and living arrangements. *Current Population Reports.* Series P-20. Washington, DC: US Govt Printing Office; 1988.
8. US Dept of Commerce. Bureau of the Census. *Children's Well-being: An International Comparison.* Washington, DC: US Govt Printing Office; 1988.
9. National Center for Health Statistics. Advance report of final divorce statistics, 1987. *Monthly Vital Statistics Report.* 1989; 39.
10. National Center for Health Statistics. *Monthly Vital Statistics Report.* Various years.
11. Ellwood DT. *Poor Support.* New York, NY: Basic Books; 1988.
12. Wilson WJ. *The Truly Disadvantaged.* Chicago, Ill: University of Chicago Press; 1987.
13. US Dept of Commerce. Bureau of the Census. Money, income, and poverty status of families and persons in the US. *Current Population Reports.* Series P-60. Washington, DC: US Govt Printing Office; 1989.
14. Johnson CM, Sum AM, Weill JB. *Vanishing Dreams: The Growing Economic Plight of Young Families.* Washington, DC: Children's Defense Fund; 1988.
15. US Bureau of Labor Statistics. *Marital and Family Characteristics of the Labor Force from the March 1988 Current Population Survey.* Washington, DC: US Govt Printing Office; 1988.
16. US Dept of Commerce. Bureau of the Census. Who's minding the kids? child care arrangements: winter 1984-5. *Current Population Reports.* Series P-70. Washington, DC: US Govt Printing Office; 1987.
17. Hofferth SL, Phillips DA. Child care in the United States, 1970 to 1995. *J Marriage Fam.* 1987; 49:559–571.
18. Lerman RI. Child support policies. In: Cottingham PH, Ellwood DT, eds. *Welfare Policy for the 1990's.* Cambridge, Mass: Harvard University Press; 1989:225–230.
19. Hughes D, Johnson K, Rosenbaum S, Liu J. *The Health of America's Children.* Washington, DC: Children's Defense Fund; 1989:Table 4.34B:153.
20. Physicians' Task Force on Hunger. *Hunger in America.* Boston, Mass: Harvard University Press; 1986.
21. US Dept of Agriculture. *Estimation of Eligibility for the WIC Programs.* Washington, DC: US Govt Printing Office; 1987.
22. Preston SH. Children and the elderly: divergent paths for America's dependents. *Demography.* 1984; 21:435–457.

23. O'Higgins M. The allocation of public resources to children and the elderly in OECD countries. In Palmer JL, Smeeding T, Boyle BB, eds. *The Vulnerable.* Washington, DC: Urban Institute Press; 1988.
24. Murray C. *Losing Ground.* New York, NY: Basic Books; 1986.
25. Wise PH. Poverty, technology, and recent trends in the United States infant mortality rate. *Paediatr Perinat Epidemiol.* 1990; 4:390–401.
26. Schorr LB, Schorr D. *Within Our Reach: Breaking the Cycle of Disadvantage.* New York, NY: Anchor Press; 1988.
27. Starfield B. *The Effectiveness of Medical Care: Validating Clinical Wisdom.* Baltimore, Md: The Johns Hopkins University Press; 1985.

Section 2

Maternity and Infant Care: Definitions and Approaches

Conventional images of maternal and infant health care begin with medical care, or "what doctors do." To define what we mean by maternal and infant health care, we too begin with the medical components, the foundation of the comprehensive package of services this volume advocates.

Robert Goldenberg begins the section with a review of evidence for the efficacy of medical care during pregnancy. Despite the inadequacies of access to services extant in our current health care system (see Section 3), it remains important to remember the enormous gains in both maternal and infant health that have been made in this century, many of which may be attributed to medical supervision, especially of pregnancies at risk and of seriously ill newborns. Nigel Paneth documents the contribution of neonatal intensive care to the steep declines in infant mortality in the late 1960s and 1970s, but he observes that regionalization of perinatal care remains unrealized and increasingly threatened.

The health benefits of routine medical care of pregnant women and their infants, while accepted by us and by most observers, are more difficult to prove, as Charles Homer explains in his chapter. Nevertheless, there is evidence for both short- and long-term benefits of "augmented" prenatal care and for some components of routine pediatric health supervision.

The final chapter in this section, by Jeffrey Mayer, James Emshoff, and Sheila Avruch, reviews some key nonmedical components of comprehensive prenatal care that are increasingly recognized as important for many pregnant women and infants—namely, smoking cessation, substance abuse services, nutrition services, and home visiting. Fortunately, there is evidence that these services can be effective; they are essential to the Universal Maternity Care program proposed in this volume and to any comprehensive system of care aimed at preventing low birthweight and infant mortality.

CHAPTER 2

Prenatal Care and Pregnancy Outcome

Robert L. Goldenberg, MD

Before the modern era, the journey through pregnancy and infancy was frequently hazardous. Although it is difficult even today to measure pregnancy-associated mortality and morbidity in many areas of the world with any confidence, statistics available from the United States and northern Europe before 1900 suggest that maternal mortality associated with pregnancy ranged from 10 to 100 deaths per 1000 births and that infant mortality averaged about 150 deaths per 1000 births.[1] Similar mortality rates are seen in underdeveloped countries today. In developed countries, however, even those with a relatively low standard of living, maternal mortality is extremely rare (in the range of 0.1 to 0.2 deaths per 1000 births) and infant mortality is in the range of 5 to 15 deaths per 1000 births—a 95% to 99% reduction from both sets of mortality rates seen only 90 years before.[2]

The frequency and change in frequency over time of various types of maternal and infant morbidity are much more difficult to determine. Population-based rates of short-term infant morbidity that do not lead to death or handicap (such as respiratory distress, infections, and trauma) are rarely reported. The rates of long-term morbidity, usually defined as neurologic or orthopedic handicap, are reported more frequently but often are of limited value in determining population-based statistics. For example, in contrast to the legal requirements to report maternal and infant deaths, there are no universal reporting requirements for conditions such as mental retardation and cerebral palsy. In addition, the definition of these conditions, unlike the definition of death, is not uniform and differs from place to place and time to time. For these reasons, most health workers measure and report death, not morbidity, as the major outcome of concern related to pregnancy.

Where long-term morbidity has been measured, there is little evidence of change in the rates over time. For example, the prevalence of cerebral palsy has remained 2 to 3 per 1000 children in virtually all populations that have been studied for the past 40 years.[3,4] Although cerebral palsy is more common in preterm infants and in infants who suffered intrauterine asphyxia or perinatal infection, it is unclear whether pregnancy-related medical care can reduce the prevalence of this condition.[5,6]

Mental retardation is much harder to define, and changes in rates over time are more difficult to document. What is clear, however, is that much of the retardation, especially the less severe types, is related to the child's home environment rather than to pregnancy per se. The more severe types of retardation are more frequently associated with a prenatal or perinatal condition or event, but the extent to which the prevalence of mental retardation may be reduced by providing appropriate prenatal care is also unclear.[7] Many authorities suspect that procedures such as rubella immunization, screening for and treating congenital syphilis, and monitoring prenatal populations for risk of growth retardation and asphyxia have reduced the prevalence of moderate to severe mental retardation in children. Certainly, prenatal screening for Down's syndrome, neural tube defects, and other major anomalies followed by termination of pregnancy has had significant impact on the prevalence of severe mental retardation.[8]

FACTORS RELATED TO IMPROVEMENT IN PREGNANCY OUTCOME

Although many factors are related to the improvement in pregnancy outcome in this century—including positive changes in the standard of living, nutrition, sanitation, and the availability of effective contraceptives—much of the reduction in both maternal and infant mortality is associated with improvements in medical care. In this century, the major factors resulting in reduced maternal, fetal, and infant mortality are associated with improved outcomes of infectious disease.[1] For example, through a combination of improved diagnostic capabilities, antibiotic therapy, immunizations, and improved aseptic surgical technique, infectious disease has been reduced substantially as a major cause of maternal mortality.

Hemorrhage, a second major cause of maternal death, has been minimized by improved blood-banking techniques and the widespread availability of blood products. The third major pregnancy-associated killer has been and still is preeclampsia. This systemic vascular disease of still-unknown origin is associated with maternal death due to stroke, hemorrhage, kidney, liver, lung, and heart failure as well as with fetal and infant death due to asphyxia, placental separation, and premature delivery. Although the origin of preeclampsia remains obscure, improvements in medical care have substantially reduced maternal, fetal, and infant mortality and short-term morbidity associated with this condition and its complications.

Major improvements in medical care have also resulted in diminished maternal, fetal, and infant mortality and morbidity previously associated with a host of other conditions. Maternal diabetes and Rh disease are examples of conditions in which advances in medical care have led to substantial improvements in pregnancy outcome. Improvements in surgical technique and anesthesia have also led to improved outcome.

The current mortality and short-term morbidity associated with pregnancy is, therefore, but a small residual of the potential poor outcomes that would occur without modern medical care, and infant mortality and morbidity rates in the United States and other industrialized countries should be viewed in that context. Currently, in most industrialized and many developing countries, about 10 infants die per 1000 live births; the range runs from 5 to 6 per 1000 births in Japan and Sweden to about 20 per 1000 births in Cuba and Eastern Europe. Most Western European countries and others such as Israel have rates between Japan's 5 per 1000 and the United States' 10 per 1000 live births.[2] In all of these countries, about 25% of the infant deaths are associated with congenital anomalies. Because the causes of most of those anomalies are unknown and advances in prevention and treatment have been slow, nearly all infant deaths associated with anomalies are unpreventable except through early discovery and abortion.

Because of the great improvement in outcome in most other situations that previously led to infant mortality—such as asphyxia, trauma, Rh disease, and infection—most infant deaths not associated with anomalies have in recent years been associated with preterm delivery. Although infant mortality has decreased by nearly two thirds in the past 20 years, with much of the improvement in survival of low birthweight (LBW) infants, preterm delivery remains the major problem today. For example, in Alabama in recent years, 50% to 60% of all neonatal deaths occurred in preterm infants weighing between 500 and 1000 grams; furthermore, in most studies preterm delivery alone accounts for 70% to 85% of all neonatal deaths.[9,10]

Problems such as infection, asphyxia, birth trauma, and meconium aspiration still cause some fetal and neonatal deaths, though they are no longer statistically major factors in the mortality rates. It has become clear, however, that life style or maternal behavioral characteristics play a major role in pregnancy outcome. A low prepregnancy weight or failure to gain a reasonable amount of weight in pregnancy, smoking, and alcohol and drug abuse together are the major predictors of both intrauterine growth retardation and preterm delivery; they now clearly account for the major portion of preventable mortality and morbidity.[11,12]

The primary reason why the United States compares poorly with other industrialized nations in infant mortality statistics is that the number of preterm or LBW infants born here is excessive. On a weight-for-weight basis, preterm infants born in the United States actually have higher survival rates than all others reported.[13] Yet preterm delivery rates in the United States have not changed measurably in the past 30 years. Whether this fact reflects the ineffectiveness of all prevention and treatment measures (eg, prenatal care, nutrition programs, and tocolytics) or whether decreases in rates caused by these treatment measures are offset by increases due to factors such as poverty and increased alcohol and drug abuse is unknown.

What part of the mortality and morbidity currently associated with pregnancy can be eliminated? If improvement is possible, how can it

FACTORS CURRENTLY ASSOCIATED WITH POOR PREGNANCY OUTCOME

31

be achieved? The difference in infant mortality between the United States and those countries with the lowest mortality (Sweden and Japan) is in the range of 4 deaths per 1000 live births. Nearly all of this difference is due to increases in very low birthweight births. When mortality is analyzed by birthweight and cause of death, it becomes obvious that the room for improvement in term births is relatively small.[14] Half of these deaths are associated with lethal anomalies and generally are unpreventable.

Most of the remainder of US infant mortality is associated with fetal growth retardation, hypertension, and asphyxia. Practices such as better screening, ensuring that high-risk patients receive prenatal care, and careful follow-up of high-risk patients have the potential, especially among poor women, to reduce the fetal death rate by several per 1000 and the neonatal death rate by 1 or 2 deaths per 1000 births.[14] Providing medical care and ensuring that all infants receive that care in the first year of life should reduce overall postneonatal mortality by about 1 death per 1000. In certain high-risk groups and especially in Black infants, the improvement in mortality promises to be even greater.

The biggest potential for improvement in infant mortality and morbidity, however, would be a reduction in the rate of preterm delivery.[15] Although there has been no conclusive demonstration of the ability of medical care to reduce the rate of preterm delivery, women who receive prenatal care seem to experience fewer premature births. More important, women who are in a system of medical care at the time of a preterm birth have higher fetal and neonatal survival rates than do those who are not in a system of care. Our estimates in Alabama suggest that transferring mothers who are about to deliver preterm infants to the appropriate level of care had the potential of reducing neonatal mortality by about 20%.[14]

PRENATAL CARE AND PREGNANCY OUTCOME

The potential benefits of prenatal care can be better visualized in light of the preceding discussion. Essentially, prenatal care has three major components (see chapter 13). The first is risk assessment or screening for correctable causes of morbidity or mortality. Based on this screening, the second major component consists of treating medical conditions or reducing discovered risk where appropriate. The third major component of prenatal care is education, with two goals in mind: (1) to reduce risk (ie, encourage pregnant women to gain a reasonable amount of weight, refrain from risk-enhancing behaviors, etc), and (2) to provide general information about pregnancy, medical care, infant feeding, and related issues.

Risk assessment is the most visible component of prenatal care.[15] It is a continual process, beginning in the preconception period and continuing through labor and delivery and even afterward. The addition of hundreds of screening tests to routine prenatal care has been suggested by various advocates over the years. Although screening can be done for virtually any known risk factor, common sense and (more recently) cost-benefit analysis have tended to limit the screening to modifiable conditions that are likely to have an adverse effect on the pregnancy. The type and timing of screening vary depending on the population being screened and the conditions screened for. For example, screening for tuberculosis may be appropriate in a poor inner-city or immigrant population or among those with acquired immunodeficiency syndrome, but not in others. Similarly, screening for sickle cell disease is appropriate in certain racial groups but not in others. Because preeclampsia is a disease of middle to late pregnancy, screening for it early in pregnancy makes little sense.

Screening for a condition carries with it an obligation to do something if the screen is positive. Appropriate responses to the full range of positive screens requires the availability of a wide array of interventions, including further diagnostic tests and treatments. For example, if screening is done for maternal alcohol or drug use, it is reasonable to expect the provider to offer referral if the response is positive. Similarly, if providers screen for infectious diseases such as gonorrhea and syphilis, treatment should be available.

The biggest potential for improvement in infant mortality and morbidity would be a reduction in the rate of preterm delivery.

Whether to screen for human immunodeficiency virus (HIV) is a more difficult decision, because no curative treatment is available. Abortion is the only option providers can offer a woman diagnosed as HIV positive early in pregnancy. Graded levels of risk and graded response to risk should be established. For certain conditions, (eg, Rh disease with fetal compromise), a full-scale high-technology approach may be necessary to achieve a satisfactory outcome; for others (eg, gestational diabetes), prescribing an appropriate diet may be sufficient.

The current visit schedule and visit content of prenatal care developed empirically. Little evidence suggests that this package or its specific components achieve the best results possible.[16] For example, the current schedule of visits evolved in the early 1900s because of concern about diagnosing and treating preeclampsia, a late pregnancy complication. Thus the visit schedule is heavily weighted toward the last 2 months of pregnancy.[17] As new screening tests were added, they were performed at an appropriate time in the prenatal period.

The entire prenatal care package, however, has never been tested for efficacy. In fact, there is a strong—but unvalidated—belief that the mere involvement of pregnant women in prenatal care has value in improving pregnancy outcome. It seems more likely, however, that the sum total of the preventive measures, risk screening, treatments, and education, together with the medical care provided during labor, delivery, and the postpartum period explains the current low mortality rates in the countries where modern prenatal care is now available.

There is little doubt, for example, that screening for diabetes and then treating it has substantially lowered perinatal mortality associated with this disease. So has screening for and treating syphilis. Rh disease has been virtually eliminated by the use of a combination of prenatal and postpartum $Rh_o(D)$immune globulin. In addition, antibody screening and treating of Rh-sensitized women and their newborns have lowered mortality rates as well. Outcomes for sickle cell disease, which were formerly very poor, now approach those of the general population because of prenatal blood transfusions. Indeed, a very long list of screening and treatment combinations that lead to improved outcomes could be generated.

The major reason why prenatal care has been criticized is that there is no evidence suggesting that it substantially reduces the incidence of preterm delivery, the current major cause of perinatal mortality.[18,19] Because prenatal care has not yet been able to achieve this goal, some authorities tend to question the value of prenatal care in general. This attitude is unreasonable. If it were possible to evaluate differences in outcomes between women who received adequate prenatal care compared to those who received no prenatal care (if such a comparison could ethically be conducted), the value of prenatal care would be obvious.

Perhaps too much is expected of prenatal care. Preterm birth is related to a multitude of factors, most of them poorly understood. To a significant degree this problem is associated with poor socioeconomic status. It would be extremely beneficial if prenatal care could overcome the difficulties associated with a lifetime of deprivation and unhealthy behaviors, but that is simply too much to expect.

RECOMMENDA-TIONS OF THE PANEL ON THE CONTENT OF PRENATAL CARE

In 1986 the National Institutes of Health (NIH) and the Public Health Service convened its Expert Panel on the Content of Prenatal Care to make recommendations concerning the content of and the visit schedules for prenatal care. The report of the panel, after a lengthy investigative process, was published in 1989.[16] Perhaps the most obvious finding was that little specific science supports the system of prenatal care as it stands now. However, when individual components were evaluated and a "new" system was designed from the components that seemed to have merit, the new system looked more or less like the one currently in place. The panel's major finding was that factors such as life style, unhealthy behavior, and substance abuse contribute to an inordinate amount of the perinatal mortality and morbidity and that the best hope in improving outcomes now seems to be reducing risk associated with life style and substance abuse.

The NIH panel also recommended a slight shift in visits from the old system, which was heavily weighted toward the end of pregnancy, to a system in which more of the visits are early in pregnancy so that risk-associated behavior can be screened for and an attempt made to reduce it. Although the panel had little evidence to call on, it felt that a prepregnancy visit for risk screening and education about the effect of life style on pregnancy outcome would be useful.

In addition to this "preconception visit," the panel suggested that more emphasis be placed on life style education directed toward decreased smoking, alcohol use, and drug use. In healthy low-risk women, the panel felt that the number of late pregnancy visits could be reduced without adding substantial risk. High-risk women, on the other hand, would receive additional targeted visits aimed at reducing their risk or improving the outcome associated with their risk factor.

The value of prenatal care as a whole, or even of its components, is difficult to determine. Firm recommendations on the subject are equally difficult to make. Clearly, much has been accomplished through the current system of care. From the baseline in which no care existed, more than 99% of maternal mortality and 95% of perinatal mortality has been eliminated. Nevertheless, we continue to strive for even more impressive results.

Poverty and its associated drug, alcohol, and tobacco abuse and the high rates of LBW births are the major factors responsible for the United States' excess mortality.

It may be too much, however, to hope that the United States will match the rate of infant mortality that has been achieved in more egalitarian societies simply by providing more or better medical care. Poverty and its associated drug, alcohol, and tobacco abuse, and the high rates of LBW births are the major factors responsible for the United States' excess mortality. To eliminate the excess mortality without eradicating the socioeconomic causes may simply be beyond the capability of any medical care system, no matter how good or comprehensive.

REFERENCES

1. McKeown T. *The Modern Rise of Population*. New York, NY: Academic Press; 1976.
2. US Department of Health and Human Services. Proceedings of the International Collaborative Effort on Perinatal and Infant Mortality. vol II. Hyattsville, Md: National Center for Health Statistics; 1988. Publication No. Ph588-1252-1.
3. Paneth N, Kiely J. The frequency of cerebral palsy: a review of population studies in industralized nations since 1950. In: Stanley F, Alberman ED, eds. *The Epidemiology of the Cerebral Palsies*. Clinics in Developmental Medicine No 87. Oxford: Blackwell Scientific Publications; 1984.
4. Pharoah POD, Cooke T, Rosenbloom L, Cooke RWI. Trends in birth prevalence of cerebral palsy. *Arch Dis Child.* 1987; 62:379–384.
5. Niswander K, Henson G, Elbourne D, et al. Adverse outcome of pregnancy and the quality of obstetric care. *Lancet.* 1984; 2:827–831.
6. McDonald AD. Cerebral palsy in children of very low birthweight. *Arch Dis Child.* 1963; 38:579–588.
7. Hagberg B, Hagberg G, Lewerth A, Lindberg U. Mild mental retardation in Swedish school children. *Acta Paediatr Scand.* 1981; 70:441–444
8. Windham GC, Edmonds LD. Current trends in the incidence of neural tube defects. *Pediatrics.* 1982; 70:333–337.
9. McCormick MC. The contribution of low birthweight to infant mortality and childhood morbidity. *N Engl J Med.* 1985; 312:82–90.

10. Goldenberg RL, Humphrey JL, Hale CB, Wayne JB. Neonatal mortality in Alabama 1970–1980: an analysis of birthweight and race specific neonatal mortality rates. *Am J Obstet Gynecol.* 1983; 145:545–552.
11. Wen, SW, Goldenberg RL, Cutter G, Hoffman HJ, Cliver SP. Intrauterine growth retardation and preterm delivery: risk factors in an indigent population. *Am J Obstet Gynecol.* 1989; 162:213–218.
12. Miller CM, Meritt TA. *Fetal Growth in Humans.* Chicago, Ill: Year Book Medical Publishers; 1979.
13. Guyer B, Wallach L, Rosen S. Birth-weight-standardized neonatal mortality rates and the prevention of low birth weight: how does Massachusetts compare with Sweden? *N Eng J Med.* 1982; 306:1230–1233.
14. Goldenberg RL, Humphrey JL, Hale CB, et al. Neonatal deaths in Alabama, II: policy and research implications derived from a comparison of birth-weight specific state and medical center neonatal mortality rates. *Am J Obstet Gynecol.* 1983; 146:450–458.
15. Selwyn BJ. The accuracy of obstetric risk assessment instruments for predicting mortality, low birthweight, and preterm birth. In: Merkatz IR, et al., eds. *New Perspectives on Prenatal Care.* New York, NY: Elsevier Science Publishing Company; 1990:39–65.
16. *Caring for our Future: The Content of Prenatal Care. A Report of the Public Health Service Expert Panel on the Content of Prenatal Care.* Washington, DC: US Dept of Health and Human Services; 1989.
17. Thompson JE, Walsh LV, Merkatz IR. The history of prenatal care: cultural, social, and medical contexts. In: Merkatz IR, Thompson JE, eds. *New Perspectives on Prenatal Care.* New York, NY: Elsevier Science Publishing Company; 1990:9–30.
18. King JF, Grant A, Keirse MJNC, Chalmers I. Beta-mimetics in preterm labour: an overview of the randomized controlled trials. *Br J Obstet Gynaecol.* 1988; 95:211–222.
19. Goldenberg RL, Davis RO, Copper RL, Corliss DK, Andrews JB, Carpenter AH. The Alabama preterm birth prevention project. *Obstet Gynecol.* 1990; 75:933–939.

CHAPTER 3

Benefits of Preventive Health Care for Pregnant Women and Infants

Charles J. Homer, MD, MPH

The health condition of women and children poses a key paradox about the well-being of these population groups. Although women and children are healthier today than at any time in our nation's past, health disparities between the economically more and less advantaged remain at least as great as and perhaps greater than in the past.[1] The health status of infants in our nation also suffers in comparison with that of infants in other, comparably developed nations such as Japan and Sweden. The existence of such disparities in large part spurs the drive toward universal maternity care that is articulated in this book.

This chapter addresses the extent to which more universal provision of preventive care services can be expected to improve the health status of women and children in general, and of disadvantaged women and children in particular. I argue that a significant number of specific prenatal and infant preventive interventions have been demonstrated effective in improving health and reducing disease; that the global effectiveness of prenatal care in reducing the risk of low birthweight (LBW) delivery has been demonstrated; but that the global effectiveness of well-child services has not yet been shown as clearly. I also argue that the greatest health benefits will be obtained not only by providing access for disadvantaged women and children to the basic health services now received by more affluent women and children, but also by providing comprehensive services and special health care delivery systems for this population.

HISTORICAL CONTEXT

The historical improvement in the health status of women and children is easily documented. Maternal mortality has decreased from more than 600 deaths per 100 000 live births in the early 20th century to approximately 19 per 100 000 in 1970 and then to 6.6 per 100 000 in 1987.[2] Infant mortality has also plummeted. A 1908 study in New York City revealed a rate of 170 deaths per 1000 live births, compared with only 47 per 1000 in 1940 and 9.9 per 1000 in 1988.[2,3] Birthweight-specific neonatal mortality among infants born weighing

37

between 1000 and 1499 grams decreased from 527.4 per 1000 in 1960 to 186.5 per 1000 in 1980.[4] Deaths due to acute infectious illness in childhood have plummeted as well, due both to prevention of infections such as measles and polio and to treatment of conditions such as acute gastroenteritis. Deaths among children younger than 18 from gastrointestinal disease declined from 1.1 per 100 000 in 1975 to 0.4 per 100 000 in 1984.[5]

Mortality for children with severe chronic conditions such as sickle cell disease and cystic fibrosis has also diminished dramatically; 80% of these children now survive into adulthood.[6] Medical therapy from conception through the period of organogenesis among women with preexisting diabetes mellitus can reduce the risk of delivering an infant with a major congenital anomaly by 70% or more.[7]

Unfortunately, the social disparities in health status and health care use are just as easily documented. The infant mortality rate for Black infants is twice the rate of White infants: 17.6 deaths per 1000 live births among Blacks versus 8.5 deaths per 1000 live births among Whites.[8] Diarrheal deaths, although rare, demonstrate the same racial disparity; they occur primarily in the South among disadvantaged Black infants and children. The death rate from gastroenteritis is four times greater for Black children than for White children (32.2 vs 8.2 per 100 000).[9] Death rates and hospitalization rates for asthma, the most common chronic illness among children, also show profound socioeconomic differences.[10,11] Recent outbreaks of measles in New York, Chicago, Los Angeles, and Houston have been concentrated in inner-city, minority communities where immunization rates remain very low. The US infant mortality rate is twice as high as that of the nations with the lowest rates; the US rate of 10 deaths per 1000 live births places it 21st on the list of national infant mortality rates—with a rate nearly twice that of Japan.[8]

DEFINITION OF PREVENTIVE SERVICES

Health care services can be crudely divided into (1) the treatment of known conditions and (2) promotion of health or early identification and amelioration of occult (ie, hidden) disease. Improvements in health status of women and children have resulted from advances in both these areas. The reduction in birthweight-specific mortality rates typifies the benefits of therapeutic medicine. For example, the reduction in mortality due to respiratory distress syndrome in very low birthweight infants has been largely influenced by improvements in the use of ventilators and our general ability to deliver very intensive care. Immunizations, on the other hand, are a prime example of the health benefits of prevention. Through the use of polio vaccine, we have reduced the number of cases of paralytic polio from the more than 18 300 that occurred in 1954 to the 5 cases that were reported in the United States in 1987.[12]

The important policy distinction between therapeutic medicine and preventive medicine is that the recommendations for both content and schedule of preventive maneuvers are determined by health care providers and, in the case of maternal and infant care, are recommended for the entire population. Services are not sought out and received on the basis of symptoms that have developed and been perceived. Because all encounters with medical care entail some risk and cost, these characteristics of preventive care place a special burden on policymakers and providers to carefully assess the benefits of such care. The remainder of this chapter assesses the identified benefits of preventive health services for pregnant women (prenatal care) and infants (well-child care).

The effectiveness of preventive health services for pregnant women can be evaluated both as a whole and as the sum of its component parts. Goldenberg (see chapter 2) lists several specific examples of effective prenatal interventions, such as the use of $Rh_o(D)$ immune globulin for Rh disease, and screening and treatment for syphilis. This chapter focuses on the global assessment of prenatal care services.

PREVENTIVE HEALTH SERVICES FOR PREGNANT WOMEN

The goal of prenatal care is the best possible health of both the mother and the infant. The Expert Panel on the Content of Prenatal Care specified in 1989 that the objectives of prenatal care are "to promote the health and well-being of the pregnant woman, the fetus, the infant, and the family up to one year after the infant's birth."[13] Despite these broadly articulated goals and objectives, prenatal care is usually assessed only by examining infant perinatal health outcomes—birthweight and neonatal mortality.

Although birthweight as an outcome is constrained and neglects other important potential outcomes of prenatal care, it is nevertheless of central importance as a predictor of infant health outcomes. Birthweight is the strongest single predictor of risk of neonatal mortality. Small infants are also at increased risk of both medical and developmental disability.[14] The care of small infants is expensive, both at the time of their birth and afterward, because of their increased medical and developmental morbidity.[14] Approximately 6.7% of infants born in the United States weigh less than 2500 grams.[15] Some two thirds of deaths within the first 28 days after birth occur among infants whose birthweight is lower than this arbitrary 2500-gram cutoff.[14]

The content of prenatal care consists of risk assessment, treatment of identified conditions, and education (see chapters 2 and 13). Despite the broad array and complexity of services encompassed in these activities, studies considering the global effectiveness of prenatal care most often use summary measures of the adequacy of care. Such measures consist of categorizing prenatal care as adequate, inadequate, or intermediate depending on the trimester during which it began and on the number of visits to a health care provider (adjusted for the duration of the pregnancy).[16]

The literature on the effectiveness of prenatal care with respect to birth outcomes has been thoroughly reviewed.[14,15] Reports from both the Institute of Medicine (IOM) and the Office of Technology Assessment (OTA) of the US Congress conclude that participating in a package of prenatal services along the lines currently recommended by the American College of Obstetricians and Gynecologists significantly lowers the risk of delivering an LBW infant.[17] These guidelines call for prenatal care to begin as early as feasible in the first trimester and continue every 4 weeks until the 28th week of pregnancy, every 2 weeks thereafter until the 36th week, and weekly therafter.

> *... total health expenditures for the short- and long-term care of infants would be reduced by $3.38 for each $1 spent on prenatal care.*

The IOM report estimates that improving prenatal care from inadequate to adequate would reduce LBW rates by approximately 10% to 15%. Approximately one third (31.8%) of women who delivered live infants in 1985 obtained nonadequate care (intermediate care, 23.9%; inadequate care, 7.9%).[14] The OTA report calculated that a switch from late or no prenatal care to first-trimester care would result in at least a 4% to 8% reduction in the LBW rate for those who had previously received late or no care.[15]

Cost-Effectiveness

Both the IOM and the OTA reports buttressed their findings about the benefits of prenatal care with estimates of its cost-effectiveness. The IOM report concluded that if prenatal care was effective in reducing LBW rates from 11.5% to 9% in high-risk populations, total health expenditures for the short- and long-term care of infants would be reduced by $3.38 for each $1 spent on prenatal care.[14] The OTA cost analysis concluded that reductions in health care costs resulting from reductions in LBW rates would likely be "at least as great" as the additional cost required to extend Medicaid coverage to all women in poverty at the time of the OTA report.[15]

Who Receives Care?

It has been demonstrated that many specific components of prenatal care and the intervention as a whole have a positive effect on maternal and infant health. The overall impact of these services also results in cost savings. Despite such research findings, however, significant barriers still stand in the way of appropriate use of prenatal services. Some 59% of pregnant women on Medicaid and more than two thirds (67%) of women without health insurance fail to receive adequate prenatal care.[18] Of pregnant women who experience no medical complications, 64% of both Medicaid recipients and uninsured women obtain less than adequate care, whereas only 19% of women with private health insurance receive such limited services.[18] Thus the first step in improving outcomes must be to improve access to the existing array of prenatal services.[19] (See chapter 6 for a more complete discussion of evidence on the current need for prenatal care services.)

Role of Comprehensive Care

Improving access, however, is not likely in itself to achieve the greatest benefit that preventive health services can offer socioeconomically disadvantaged pregnant women. When built into a basic system of care, several types of services have produced better outcomes than access to the basic system alone. For example, Buescher demonstrated that poor women served by a multidisciplinary, multiservice prenatal care program experienced better pregnancy outcomes than socioeconomically comparable women who were served through the traditional health care system of private practitioners.[20]

Home visiting is another type of comprehensive intervention component that is broadly geared toward improving maternal and infant health outcomes.[21-23] Home visiting provides both education and emotional support for pregnant women and mothers of young children. Such programs usually target women who are at risk of encountering adverse infant health outcomes by virtue of their disadvantaged socioeconomic conditions. Many home visiting programs begin in the prenatal period and continue at weekly to monthly intervals. The visitors themselves may be laypersons or professionals, are either paid or volunteer, and undergo a variety of training activities. Several home visiting programs have demonstrated reductions in LBW, mostly among the highest risk groups;[24] improved participation in prenatal care; improved home environments for infant development;[25] decreased child abuse and neglect;[26] and improved subsequent maternal education and employment.[27]

Not all such programs have been successful in meeting their objectives. The General Accounting Office (GAO) reviewed home visiting programs (see chapter 5) and identified several factors necessary for them to work well: adequate planning and specification of objectives, secure funding, adequate training and supervision of outreach workers, and integration of home visiting services into the broader networks of social and health care services.[23]

WELL-CHILD CARE

The purposes of providing preventive care to ostensibly well children are to reduce premature mortality, prevent or reduce functional limitations due to physical or mental illness, and promote the social functioning of the individual throughout the life span.[28] The success of preventive health services for children has been relatively difficult to assess because of the fortunate rarity of premature mortality and the difficulty in measuring other outcomes.

Like prenatal care, well-child care services consist of both risk assessment activities (history, physical examination, and laboratory tests) and physical and psychosocial interventions (eg, immunizations and anticipatory guidance). Over time, experts have agreed on recommending more visits in the first 6 months of life (at 2 weeks, and at 2, 4, and

6 months), fewer visits in the second 6 months (at 9 and 12 months), and less frequent visits thereafter.[29,30]

The effectiveness of well-child services can be assessed by gauging the effectiveness both of the individual components and of the services as a whole. Few of the specific activities that constitute well-child care have been carefully studied. However, two interventions—newborn screening and immunizations—have been unequivocally demonstrated as effective. One that remains unproved—anticipatory guidance for injury prevention—indicates the difficulty in establishing the utility of such interventions. More extensive reviews of the effectiveness of specific well-child interventions are available.[27,30,31]

Newborn Screening

One component of well-child services is the screening of newborns for a variety of metabolic or other medical conditions. The most widely screened conditions are phenylketonuria and congenital hypothyroidism. Both of these conditions, when left untreated, result in mental retardation. Both are easily treatable when detected, the former with diet and the latter with medication. The efficacy, effectiveness, and cost-effectiveness of screening for these conditions have been documented. Indeed, screening all infants for these two conditions results in health care savings of $3.2 million per 100 000 infants screened.[15] Screening for a number of other conditions, including sickle cell disease, cystic fibrosis, maple syrup urine disease, and others, is also either under consideration or already done in a number of states. The efficacy of screening and early prophylactic treatment with penicillin in reducing the risk of sepsis and sudden death among children with sickle cell disease has also been demonstrated.[31]

Immunizations

Immunization against a variety of infectious diseases in the first 2 years of life clearly reduces the risk of contracting these conditions. Children are now vaccinated for diphtheria, pertussis, tetanus, polio, measles, mumps, rubella, and hemophilus influenza type b bacterial disease. Some aspects of vaccine use remain controversial: the complications due to pertussis vaccine, the use of inactive versus live polio, the efficacy of *Haemophilus influenzae* vaccine and the optimal timing of new conjugate vaccines, and the need for and timing of repeat measles vaccine. Nevertheless, the cost-effectiveness of using them has been demonstrated repeatedly.[32] Specifically, the benefit-to-cost ratio of pertussis vaccination is 11:1; of the measles vaccine, 10:1; and of the polio vaccine, 10:1.[32]

Anticipatory Guidance for Injury Prevention

The well-child visit in pediatric practice consists of an initial or interval history, the physical examination, behavioral and developmental assessment, anticipatory guidance, and, at times, additional tests. Anticipatory guidance involves providing health education, information, or counseling to influence the parents' or child's behavior and thus favorably influence the child's health. Subjects that are considered in anticipatory guidance range from traditional medical guidance (such as avoidance of contact with children with certain communicable diseases) and nutritional advice to suggestions for appropriate behavioral management at specific developmental ages and information about good health behaviors such as avoiding tobacco and alcohol use. Anticipatory guidance is relatively inexpensive and poses little risk.

Medical practitioners traditionally spend relatively little time in such activities. Reisinger and Bires found that pediatricians spent 8.4% of well-child visits on anticipatory guidance and that the percentage diminished with increasing patient age.[33]

Studies evaluating the effectiveness of anticipatory guidance for injury prevention have been reviewed by Bergman et al.[34-36] These reviews indicate that early studies suffered from severe methodologic limitations—primarily nonrandom assignment of experimental and control groups and use of parental self-report in the assessment of outcome (restraint use). Even if the results of these studies were valid, they may not be easily generalized to the population, because they usually relied on either military samples or White, middle-class populations.

The more methodologically sophisticated studies failed to demonstrate a substantial effect due to educational interventions.[37-39] For example, Reisenger and colleagues offered an educational program encouraging the use of car restraints—with written materials, verbal reinforcement, and direct demonstration performed by the physician—to parents who used a pediatric practice during certain time periods.[38] A comparison group, using the same practice at different periods, was not offered the intervention. Use of infant car restraints was assessed by observing parents as they entered the practice parking lot. Reisinger et al did find a significant increase in proper restraint use at 2 months; by 4 months, however, no treatment effect was identified, primarily because of increased use of restraints in the control group.[38] Thus, the findings indicate only that pediatricians can accelerate use of infant restraints by those who are likely to use such restraints eventually anyway.

Whether the limited efficacy of physicians' counseling about using infant restraints can be generalized to all of anticipatory guidance is uncertain. Use of infant restraints requires some expense and repeated individual action. Moreover, as the recent repeal of seat belt laws in Massachusetts indicates, Americans have strong opinions about their right to make their own choices about using seat belts and other restraints when traveling in their own automobiles. The physician may not be viewed as an authority on automobile safety for children. However, strong feelings often exist in families about most aspects of child rearing, such as discipline and diet, and in these areas, physicians' ex-

... the first step in improving outcomes must be to improve access to the existing array of prenatal services.

pertise rests on a much narrower body of evidence. Thus, the impact of physicians' advice on use of infant restraints may accurately reflect the generally limited impact of anticipatory guidance.

The limited efficacy of anticipatory guidance has stimulated the development of alternative approaches to traditional well-child care. Osborne has proposed and piloted the use of group well-child care.[40] One evaluation of the impact of such care on safety behaviors—in particular on the adjusting of maximum hot-water temperature in the home—showed a significant positive effect from this style of care.[41] Thus, the limited efficacy of anticipatory guidance may be overcome by more creative approaches to education and motivation.

Child Health Supervision as a Whole

In contrast to the demonstrated impact of the whole package of prenatal care services, the benefits of the whole package of well-child services (ie, full use of the recommended number of visits and implementation of recommended visit content) have been more difficult to document. Specifically, a variety of studies examining comprehensive care services; Medicaid's Early and Periodic Screening, Diagnosis, and Treatment program; and various care systems and insurance plans have not consistently shown improvements in childhood mortality or morbidity in the populations studied.[28,42–44] Such studies have demonstrated that participation in primary care programs does result in more appropriate use of health care services. Specifically, children participating in model programs tend to have lower emergency room and medical hospital use rates and fewer acute visits in general; they show correspondingly higher use of preventive care and elective corrective surgical procedures.[45]

The lack of consistently positive health-related findings from this research results in large measure from the difficulties in conducting such research. These difficulties include both measuring the exposure to well-child care and selecting and measuring relevant outcomes. In contrast to prenatal care, no widely accepted summary measure of the adequacy of well-child services exists. Moreover, although use of prenatal care services is documented on birth certificates for all pregnancies that result in delivery after 28 weeks, the use of well-child services is not documented populationwide for infants and children.

Measuring the potential outcomes of well-child care is similarly more complex than measuring pregnancy outcome. Although birthweight is not a complete indicator of the potential outcomes of prenatal care, it is universally recognized as important, universally available, and reasonably accurate. No comparable measure exists in infant and child health. Moreover, measuring social and psychological well-being (the areas of greatest contemporary concern) is complex and has been done only in studies with relatively limited numbers of subjects.

Practitioners and experts believe that other health-related benefits may accrue to children and families who receive the full array of well-child health services. These benefits may include increased parental satisfaction, increased ability to cope with subsequent serious childhood illness, and improved access to other social, educational, and specialty health care services. Thus, children who participate more in well-child services may have more appropriate school placements, or their families may make better use of community services than the families of children who participate less. Such hypotheses need to be explored by the pediatric health services research community.

Who Receives Care?

What do we know about who currently receives preventive care services? One imperfect indicator of the adequacy of preventive care services is the completeness of immunizations. National surveys indicate that inner-city children are less likely to be fully immunized than non-inner-city children. For example, 80% of inner-city children aged 1 to 4 years received three or more diphtheria-pertussis-tetanus immunizations versus 90% of non-inner-city children. Similarly, Black and Hispanic children are less likely to be fully immunized than White children (75% versus 89%).[15] Such patterns are a likely major cause of the current large measles outbreaks in these inner-city, minority communities.

Survey data confirm this general pattern of diminished use of preventive services by the poor and the uninsured. More than one third (37%) of poor children younger than 5 have no physician visits in a given year, a pattern incompatible with the recommendations of the American Academy of Pediatrics. Only 16% of nonpoor children fail to visit a physician in a year. By contrast, 53% of uninsured children and 40% of Medicaid children younger than 5 have no physician visit in a given year.[46] Review of Medicaid claims data also confirms this pattern of inadequate use: 30% of continuously enrolled California Medicaid children younger than 1 year receive no preventive visits in a given year.[47]

The first step in improving health care for disadvantaged children is to improve access to the basic array of currently recommended health care services.

Comprehensive Services

The greatest possible improvement in child health will result from use of preventive health care services if comprehensive services are also provided along with basic services. A number of additional health care services may be indicated. These additions or modifications may be as subtle as changing the emphasis of the provider visits from the traditional medical screening to affirming parental and child strengths. They might also include group sessions, providing multiple service

Practitioners and experts believe that other health-related benefits may accrue to children and families who receive the full array of well-child health services.

programs in one setting (including nutritional, developmental, psychological, and educational services), and home visiting programs.[22,40,48] Some studies support the advantages of each of these approaches, particularly with high-risk populations.

The caveats by the GAO that have been noted in reference to home visiting programs will likely be applicable to all comprehensive programs; that is, such programs should be carefully administered, include relevant populations, and be integrated with other services including regular medical services.

CONCLUSIONS

Health care provides substantial health benefits for women and children. Such care can be crudely divided into treating known conditions and promoting health or early identification of occult disease. The benefits of the former type of care are easier to document. The benefits of the latter have been extensively examined both for pregnant women and well children. Despite major limitations in the quality of the evidence, data suggest that participating in a package of early and comprehensive prenatal care services significantly reduces the risk of adverse pregnancy outcome, principally LBW.

Neonatal screening for metabolic disorders and immunizations significantly improves child health outcomes. Other components of well-child care are likely to confer benefits, but most of these benefits have yet to be well documented by research.

The poor, minorities, and the uninsured use recommended preventive services substantially less. The first step in addressing the health care needs of the women and children of this nation is to eliminate barriers to the use of currently recommended services. Additional benefits will likely accrue from further development, implementation, and integration of additional health care services such as home visiting into the expanded system of comprehensive care.

REFERENCES

1. Wise PH, Meyers A. Poverty and child health. *Pediatr Clin North Am.* 1988;35:1169–1187.
2. Wegman ME. Annual summary of vital statistics—1988. *Pediatrics.* 1989;84:943–956.
3. Heaten CE. Fifty years of progress in obstetrics and gynecology. *NY State J Med.* 1951;51:83–85.
4. Buehler JW, Strauss LT, Hogue CJR, Smith JC. Birthweight specific causes of infant mortality, US 1960–1980. *Public Health Rep.* 1987; 102:162–171.
5. Hoekelman RA, Pless IB. Decline in mortality among young Americans during the 20th century: prospects for realizing national mortality reduction goals for 1990. *Pediatrics.* 1988;82:587–595.
6. Gortmaker SL. Demography of chronic childhood diseases. In: Hobbs

N, Perrin JM, eds. *Issues in the Care of Children with Chronic Illness.* San Francisco, Calif: Jossey-Bass; 1985:827–863.

7. Braveman P, Showstack J, Browner W, et al. Evaluation of outcomes of pregnancy in diabetic women: epidemiologic considerations and recommended indicators. *Diabetes Care.* 1988;11:281–287.
8. Wegman ME. Annual summary of vital statistics—1989. *Pediatrics.* 1990;86:835–847.
9. Ho MS, Glass RI, Pinsky PF, et al. Diarrheal deaths in American children—are they preventable? *JAMA.* 1988;260:3281–3285.
10. Weiss KB, Wagener DK. Changing patterns of asthma mortality: identifying target populations at high risk. *JAMA.* 1990;264:1683–1687.
11. Wissow LS, Gittelsohn AM, Szklo M, et. al. Poverty, race, and hospitalization for childhood asthma. *Am J Public Health.* 1988;78:777–782.
12. US Centers for Disease Control. Summary of notifiable diseases, United States, 1987. *MMWR.* 1988;36:1–59.
13. Expert Panel on the Content of Prenatal Care. *The Content of Prenatal Care.* Washington, DC: US Govt Printing Office; 1989.
14. Committee to Study the Prevention of Low Birthweight. *Preventing Low Birth Weight.* Washington, DC: National Academy Press; 1985.
15. US Congress, Office of Technology Assessment. *Healthy Children: Investing in the Future.* Washington, DC: US Govt Printing Office; 1988. OTA H-345.
16. Kessner DM, ed. *Contrasts in Health Status,* vol 1: *Infant Death: An Analysis by Maternal Risk and Health Care.* Washington, DC: Institute of Medicine, National Academy of Sciences; 1973.
17. American College of Obstetricians and Gynecologists. *Standards for Obstetric and Gynecologic Services,* 6th ed. Washington, DC; 1985.
18. US General Accounting Office. *Prenatal Care: Medicaid Recipients and Uninsured Women Obtain Insufficient Care.* Washington, DC: US Govt Printing Office; 1987. GAO/HRD-87-137.
19. Brown S, ed. *Prenatal Care: Reaching Mothers, Reaching Infants.* Washington, DC: Committee to Study Outreach for Prenatal Care, National Academy Press; 1989.
20. Buescher PA, Smith C, Holliday JL, Levine RH. Source of prenatal care and infant birth weight: the case of a North Carolina county. *Am J Obstet Gynecol.* 1987;156:204–210.
21. Chapman J, Siegel E, Cross A. Home visitors and child health: analysis of selected programs. *Pediatrics.* 1990;85:1059–1068.
22. Olds DL, Kitzman H. Can home visitation improve the health of women and children at environmental risk? *Pediatrics.* 1990; 86:108–116.
23. US General Accounting Office. Home Visiting: A Promising Early Intervention Strategy for At-risk Families. Washington, DC: US Govt Printing Office; 1990. GAO/HRD-90-83.
24. Olds DL, Henderson CR, Tatelbaum R, Chamberlin R. Improving the delivery of prenatal care and outcomes of pregnancy: a randomized trial of nurse home visitation. *Pediatrics.* 1986;77:16–28.
25. Barnard KE, Magyary D, Sumner G, et al. Prevention of parenting alteration for women with low social support. *Psychiatry.* 1985; 51:248–253.
26. Olds DL, Henderson CR, Chamberlin R, Tatelbaum R. Preventing child abuse and neglect: a randomized trial of nurse home visitation. *Pediatrics.* 1986;78:65–78.
27. Olds DL, Henderson CR, Tatelbaum R, Chamberlin R. Improving the life course development of socially disadvantaged mothers: a randomized trial of nurse home visiting. *Am J Public Health.* 1988; 78:1436–1445.
28. Homer C. Evaluation of the evidence on the effectiveness of well child care for children. Background Paper for US Congress, OTA; 1987. Available through National Technical Information Service.

29. Strain JE. AAP periodicity guidelines: a framework for educating patients. *Pediatrics.* 1983;74 (suppl):924–927.
30. American Academy of Pediatrics. *Guidelines for Health Supervision.* Elk Grove Village, Ill: AAP; 1985.
31. Gaston MH, Venton JI, Woods G, et al. Prophylaxis with oral penicillin in children with sickle cell anemia. *N Engl J Med.* 1986; 314:1593–1599.
32. Hinman AH. Public health considerations. In: Plotkin SA, Mortimer EA, eds. *Vaccines.* Philadelphia, Pa: WB Saunders; 1988:587–611.
33. Reisinger KS, Bires JA. Anticipatory guidance in pediatric practice. *Pediatrics.* 1980;66:889–892.
34. Bergman AB. Use of education in preventing injuries. *Pediatr Clin North Am.* 1982;29:331–338.
35. Pless IB. Accident prevention and health education: back to the drawing board? *Pediatrics.* 1978;62:431–435.
36. Christophersen ER. Accident prevention in primary care. *Pediatr Clin North Am.* 1986;33:925–933.
37. Miller JR, Pless IB. Child automobile restraints: evaluation of health education. *Pediatrics.* 1977;59:907–911.
38. Reisinger KS, Williams AF, Wells JK, John CE, Roberts TR, Podgainy HJ. Effects of pediatricians' counseling on infant restraint use. *Pediatrics.* 1981;67:201–206.
39. Reisinger KS, Williams AF. Evaluation of programs designed to increase the protection of infants in cars. *Pediatrics.* 1978;62:280–287.
40. Osborn L, Wooley FR. Use of groups in well child care. *Pediatrics.* 1981; 67:701–706.
41. Thomas KA, Hassanein RS, Christopherson ER. Evaluation of group well child care for improving burn prevention in the home. *Pediatrics.* 1984;74:879–882.
42. Hoekelman RM. An appraisal of the effectiveness of child health supervision. *Curr Opin Pediatr.* 1989;1:146–156.
43. Casey P, Sharp M, Loda F. Child health supervision for children under 2 years of age: a review of its content and effectiveness. *J Pediatr* 1978; 95:1–9.
44. Shaddish WR. A review and critique of controlled studies of the effectiveness of preventive child health care. *Health Policy Q.* 1982;2:24–52.
45. Alpert JJ, Robertson LS, Kosa JK, Heagarty MC, Haggerty RJ. Delivery of health care for children: report of an experiment. *Pediatrics.* 1976; 57:917–930.
46. Wood DL, Hayward RA, Corey CR, Freeman HE, Shapiro ME. Access to medical care for children and adolescents in the United States. *Pediatrics.* 1990;86:666–673.
47. Fleming GV, Yudkowsky BK, Ellwood MR, Adams K, Sredl KM. *Preventive Health Care for Medicaid Children: Related Factors and Costs.* Elk Grove Village, Ill: American Academy of Pediatrics; 1990.
48. Casey PH, Whitt JK. Effect of the pediatrician on the mother-infant relationship. *Pediatrics.* 1980;65:815–820.

CHAPTER 4

The Role of Neonatal Intensive Care in Lowering Infant Mortality

Nigel Paneth, MD, MPH

The medical profession has long recognized that some newborns need more labor-intensive forms of care than others need. At the turn of the century, care of newborns generally fell under the discipline of obstetrics; the earliest organized hospital units devoted to newborn care were developed by obstetricians such as Tarnier[1] and Budin[2] in France. These units were among the first examples of specialized care in hospitals and thus were organizational forerunners of coronary care units, burn units, and the like.

The primary concern of these early specialized care units was care of premature infants; particular attention was paid to maintaining body temperature. The central technological focus was on developing effective incubators, the earliest versions of which were the warming tubs constructed in Russia and France in the mid-19th century.[3] Nutritional support, the other great difficulty in prematures, was handled by skilled nurses using meticulous feeding techniques.

In the United States, the first hospital unit for the care of premature infants was developed by Hess in the 1920s.[4] The first academically based unit, which included a vigorous component of research in newborn nutrition and metabolism, was developed by Dr. Harry Gordon at New York Hospital in the 1930s. By this time, pediatrics had developed as a separate medical discipline—the American Academy of Pediatrics (AAP) was organized in 1930—and had gradually adopted responsibility for the care of newborns.

Parallel to these conventional models of care, Martin Cooney, a German-born practitioner and student of Budin, ran freestanding premature care units at Coney Island, NY, and Atlantic City, NJ, that were financed by paid admission to see the tiny infants through windows. Cooney's infants, some of whom were exhibited at the New York World's Fair of 1939, experienced mortality rates at least as low as

HISTORICAL OVERVIEW

49

those of similar infants cared for in hospitals.[5] Established pediatricians often referred infants to Cooney for care.

Developments in newborn care in the first decades after World War II were erratic at best. Major setbacks were encountered when the introduction of oxygen was found to be associated with retrolental fibroplasia (a frequently blinding eye condition),[6] and sulfonamides and chloramphenicol (antibiotics introduced into nurseries to control infection) were shown to increase mortality or morbidity.[7,8] For a time in the 1950s the withholding of early feeding was thought advisable in prematures[9]; some authorities thought it had adverse consequences.[10]

... substantially lower mortality occurs in infants born in full-scale neonatal intensive care units ...

Neonatal intensive care can be said to have begun in earnest in the late 1960s, when increasing successes were achieved in mechanical ventilation of infants with respiratory problems. These techniques proved to be valuable in treating both premature infants and asphyxiated term infants. The 1971 paper by Gregory et al describing the application of constant distending pressure to the lungs to prevent alveolar collapse in prematures with respiratory distress syndrome is often cited as a landmark in this development.[11]

At about the same time, the pediatric and obstetric subspecialties focusing on high-risk mothers and neonates were formally established. The sub-board in maternal-fetal medicine of the American College of Obstetricians and Gynecologists was organized in 1972, and the corresponding sub-board of the AAP, titled neonatology-perinatology, was formed the following year.

With increasing frequency, high-volume hospital obstetric departments have created special units and clinics, staffed by maternal-fetal medicine subspecialists (sometimes referred to as perinatologists) to care for women with especially complicated pregnancies and labors. The most medically sophisticated programs now are joint obstetrics-pediatrics ventures with two intensive care units—perinatal for the mother and neonatal for the baby. Since 1983 the obstetric standards of care for mothers in hospitals and the corresponding pediatric standards of care for newborns, formerly separate documents, have been combined in a report written jointly by the two specialty organizations.[12]

The evolution of neonatal intensive care was not an isolated development; many other forms of intensive care in hospitals began at about the same time, including coronary care units. In the United States, the Great Society programs of the 1960s played a major role in fostering these developments. But although the will to do more to alleviate human suffering may have been part of the ethos of the time, it was the Medicare and Medicaid legislation, which provided infusions of capital to hospitals and medical providers, that allowed these programs to be developed. Similarly, the premature centers (important forerunners of newborn intensive care units) established in New York City by Leona

Baumgartner, Helen Wallace, and Jean Pakter in the late 1940s and early 1950s could not have been established without construction funds from the Hill-Burton legislation of 1946.[13]

Regional organization of neonatal intensive care services has been given high priority by providers and state regulatory agencies. Both groups agree that services need to be differentiated by level of technology and expertise and in correspondence to the health needs of mothers and babies. In the United States, three levels of neonatal hospital care are usually recognized: level 1, care for normal or mildly ill newborns; level 2, care for infants at moderate risk, usually limited to those born in the same hospital; and level 3, care at regional centers that provide the most complex care and receive sick infants transported from other hospitals.[14] Some states, such as Michigan, recognize only two levels of care, bypassing the intermediate (level 2) category.

Assessing the Effect of Neonatal Intensive Care

A useful formulation for evaluating any health care service is the triad proposed by Sackett:[15]
- Efficacy—can it work?
- Effectiveness—does it work?
- Efficiency—is it worth doing?

In the pages that follow, each of these questions is applied to the issue of neonatal intensive care and its impact on infant and neonatal mortality. A comprehensive assessment of the efficiency of neonatal intensive care would necessarily include a weighing of the importance of patterns of handicap, not just patterns of survival. However, a complete review of that complex area is beyond the scope of this discussion.

Evidence of Efficacy

The efficacy of an intervention is best assessed by randomized trial, although most health care services, including those intended for neonates, have not been subjected to such an assessment. In 1981, however, Sinclair et al provided a list of components of neonatal care that had been subjected to randomized trial,[16] and the National Perinatal Epidemiology Research Unit at Oxford University now maintains a continuously updated computer file of such trials.[17] Among those components are the timing, manner, and content of early feeding and fluid therapy, phototherapy for jaundice, maintenance of thermoneutrality, and a wide variety of respiratory therapies and maneuvers.

Although many of these trials have demonstrated the efficacy of specific neonatal therapies, their focus has been narrow and, consequently, they have not been influential in demonstrating the efficacy of newborn intensive care. Neonatologists have instead justified expansion of their services by pointing to the sharp decline in mortality for

51

low birthweight (LBW) infants that has occurred in hospitals providing neonatal intensive care.[18]

Epidemiologists are generally skeptical of historical trends alone as evidence for the efficacy of medical care, but two features of neonatal mortality in LBW infants make this evidence more compelling than usual. First, before the new technological developments in care, hospital mortality for LBW infants had been stable for decades. Stewart Clifford, in reviewing mortality at the Boston Lying-in Hospital from 1943 to 1963, observed that "the death rate for the premature infant has been practically unchanged for the entire 21 years."[19]

Second, among LBW infants mortality is relatively independent of the social and demographic factors that so profoundly affect overall neonatal mortality.[20] It appears that factors such as race, maternal age, family income, and maternal education influence neonatal mortality by altering the birthweight distribution, whereas for a given birthweight, the influence of these factors on mortality is negligible or, in some cases, the opposite of the effect on neonatal mortality overall. For example, US Black infants have lower mean birthweight, higher incidence of LBW, and higher overall neonatal mortality, but lower mortality for LBW infants than US Whites.[21]

Table 4-1, reproduced from a report on neonatal intensive care from the congressional Office of Technology Assessment (OTA), presents mortality rates for very low birthweight (VLBW) infants cared for in neonatal intensive care units during the period 1961 to 1985. These data, pooled from many hospitals, indicate a consistent decline in

TABLE 4-1
Inborn Neonatal Mortality Rates for Very Low Birthweight Infants
(Pooled Institutional Data)

| | Birthweight, grams | | | |
| | ≤1000 | | 1001–1500 | |
Year of Birth	Deaths/Births	Rate†	Deaths/Births	Rate†
1961–1965	185/197	939	142/274	518
1966–1970	381/443	860*	212/567	374*
1971–1975	209/274	763*	54/253	213*
1976–1980	458/818	560*	284/1611	176
1981–1985	243/467	520	186/1879	99*

* Significantly different from preceding 5-year rate (*P*<0.01).
† Rate = deaths per 1000 live births.
SOURCE: US Congress. *Neonatal Intensive Care for Low Birthweight Infants: Costs and Effectiveness.* Health Technology Case Study 38. Washington, DC: Office of Technology Assessment; December 1987 OTA-HCS-38.

mortality in each half-decade over the past 25 years. For infants who weighed less than 1000 grams at birth, mortality has been reduced by 45% in the interval; for infants weighing 1001 to 1500 grams, mortality has declined a remarkable 81%.

These figures provide strong prima facie evidence that neonatal intensive care is a powerful and beneficial technology. However, data from level 3 care units alone cannot indicate the effectiveness of the technology in the nation as a whole.

Evidence of Effectiveness

Addressing the question of whether a health care service actually influences mortality or morbidity in the population requires a research strategy that deals with whole populations, not just selected patient subsets admitted to level 3 care hospitals or enrolled in randomized trials. Such population-based studies have been performed as components of neonatal intensive care assessments, and they form the core of evidence that these programs affect newborn survival positively.

An important indication that advances in perinatal care are particularly effective derives from neonatal mortality time trends for all births in the United States. The sharpest reductions in postneonatal mortality, a parameter influenced primarily by hygiene and nutrition, took place earlier in the century. By contrast, the largest recorded proportional decline in neonatal mortality of this century took place in the 1960s and the 1970s. The view that this sudden decline in neonatal mortality was related to perinatal medical care has been supported by analyses that assess the decline in relation to birthweight, the major risk factor for neonatal mortality. In 1978, Kleinman et al examined vital data from several states that linked infant death certificates with the corresponding birth certificates.[22] They demonstrated that mortality *at a given birthweight*, a parameter found to be stable in the United States during the decade from 1950 to 1960,[23] had declined substantially between 1969 and 1975. The authors tentatively concluded that advances in perinatal care may have accounted for this new demographic phenomenon.

Similarly, Lee et al, using the method of indirect standardization for birthweight (because birth-death certificate linkage was not then available for the entire United States), showed that weight-specific mortality had started declining substantially in the entire United States in about the mid-1960s.[24] These authors concluded more assertively that perinatal intensive care was most likely responsible for these changes and argued that shifts in the age and parity distribution of mothers could not account for the trend. Their illustration contrasting declines in mortality with stability in birthweight distributions, updated to include more recent national data, is shown in Figure 4-1.

... the largest recorded proportional decline in neonatal mortality of this century took place in the 1960s and the 1970s ...

53

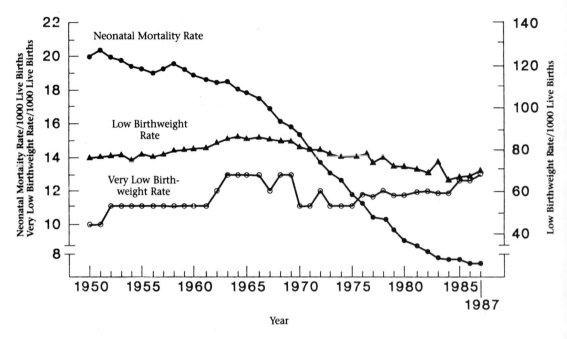

Fig. 4-1.—Decline in mortality versus stability in birthweight, 1950 to 1987. Adapted from Lee et al.[24]

The conclusion of Lee et al that birthweight-specific mortality was declining sharply in the United States overall was confirmed when national birth-death certificate linkage became available in the 1980s. Buehler et al compared 1960 and 1980 US mortality rates for all birthweight groups and found reductions of up to 50%.[25] Substantial improvement in mortality was seen in both normal-weight and LBW newborns.

These improvements in neonatal mortality are not restricted to the United States. Lie et al reported similar findings from Norway between 1967 and 1981.[26] In Norway, 82% of the neonatal mortality decline in the 15-year period was attributable to improvement in mortality at a given birthweight, and 76% of that improvement occurred in infants weighing less than 2500 grams at birth. Pharoah and Alberman have shown that, in the United Kingdom, mortality for LBW infants began to decline in the mid-1960s and continued to decline sharply in the 1970s and 1980s.[27,28]

More direct evidence of the effectiveness of neonatal intensive care in the form of contrasts in weight-specific mortality for LBW infants exposed to different degrees or levels of perinatal care intensiveness emerged in the 1980s. Results of several population-based studies summarized in Table 4-2 confirm that substantially lower mortality occurs in infants born in full-scale neonatal intensive care units.

TABLE 4-2
Population-Based Studies of Newborn Intensive Care

Population	Study Years	Birthweight, Grams	Relative Neonatal Mortality Risk*	
			Level 1	Level 2
Norway[33]	1967–1973	1000–1500	1.26	1.04
New York City[30]	1976–1978	501–2250	1.32	1.37
Franklin county, Ohio[29]	1977–1979	501–1250	1.25	—
Iowa[34]	1978	<1500	1.10	1.08
Louisiana, Ohio, Tennessee, Washington[31]	1978-1979	750–1500	1.27	1.42
State of Washington[35]	1980–1983	1000–2000	2.24†	1.93†
Netherlands[32]	1983	<1500††	1.62	1.56

* Compared with level 3 hospitals, i.e., those with complete newborn intensive care services.
† Perinatal mortality.
†† And <33 weeks.

The earliest of these studies contrasted figures with those for regions of Norway,[33] classified by the level of personnel, equipment, and care facilities in all delivery services. Lower early neonatal mortality rates were generally found in counties that scored higher on this scale, although the results were inconsistent within weight groups. Control for confounders such as maternal age, illegitimacy, and parity did not vitiate the findings.

A small study in Franklin County, Ohio, was the subject of the first US publication to show systematic mortality differences by level of care, although control for potentially confounding variables was not undertaken.[29] A study of all singleton births of infants weighing 2250 grams or less in New York City between 1976 and 1978 found that mortality was a third higher if birth took place outside a level 3 center.[30] Nineteen potentially confounding variables were individually assessed in the analysis, none of which accounted for higher mortality at level 1 and level 2 units. The findings of this study were confirmed by Gortmaker et al in four states,[31] and by Verloove-Vanhorick et al in an analysis of all VLBW infants born in Holland in 1983.[32]

The consistency of findings is striking; in almost all studies, LBW mortality is sharply higher for infants who were born in hospitals not designated as level 3 centers. The degree of potential confounding that was assessed varied across studies, but all the investigations support OTA's conclusion concerning neonatal care effectiveness: "The disturbing fact is that an extremely premature baby's chances for survival and normal development are in large part determined by where the baby is born."[36(p8)]

... an extremely premature baby's chances for survival and normal development are in large part determined by where the baby is born ...

In several studies, level 2 units had excesses of mortality as large as those of level 1 units, thus raising questions about the value of this intermediate level of care. The development of level 2 care represents a greater investment of resources than level 1, making the lack of improved outcome both surprising and disappointing.

Efficiency

Regionalization of services. The improvement in neonatal mortality achieved by newborn intensive care has been purchased at substantial cost. Hospital charges for the care of infants with respiratory distress syndrome exceed those for kidney transplantation and rival the cost of cardiac and bone marrow transplantation.[36,37] The incremental cost to save an LBW infant has been estimated at $86 000 for infants between 1000 and 1500 grams and at $118 000 beneath that weight.[36]

Regionalization of perinatal care is, in part, an attempt to increase the efficient use of newborn intensive care. Because only certain units are licensed to provide this very expensive service, duplication is avoided and the most is made of human and technical resources. Regionalization rests on a foundation of screening: obstetricians and other providers of prenatal care screen for pregnancies at high risk and refer for delivery at level 3 units; pediatricians screen infants born at level 1 and 2 units and refer to level 3 care those whom they judge are at high risk.

Screening in the perinatal period is thus fundamentally unidirectional; referrals are made from the less technologically sophisticated settings to the level 3 units. A modest exception is the increasingly common practice of referring LBW infants back to their hospitals of origin when their acute respiratory insufficiency is over. Financial barriers to this procedure sometimes preclude it. In Michigan, for example, transferring an infant automatically places the child in a diagnosis related group that reduces the reimbursement the sending hospital can obtain from Medicaid.

Organizers of perinatal care, however, have scarcely considered that considerable saving might be effected by screening for *low* risk. Women at low risk of experiencing a complicated delivery or producing a high-risk infant can be referred to birth locations specifically intended for such deliveries and newborns. Birthing rooms have been provided in many hospitals in recent years, but the costs of care in them are no less than in other parts of the labor and delivery suite.

Neonatal mortality in the United States has declined for normal-weight as well as LBW newborns.[24] However, the few studies comparing mortality rates by level of birth that have looked at normal-weight infants have not found lower mortality in intensive care facilities.[36,37] This finding is in large part due to the already very low mortality rates in normal-weight infants (about 2 to 3 per 1000). It seems, then, that the benefit of intensive care facilities is marginal for the overwhelming majority of births.

A major challenge for the organizers of regionalized perinatal care is the development of levels of care intended specifically for low-risk mothers and infants. This level of care would likely involve the use of certified nurse-midwives as well as family practitioners and obstetricians.[39,40] Such a system would have to rely on careful antenatal and intrapartum screening; the single most important reason to refer a woman to level 3 for delivery would be gestational age of less than 37 weeks.[38] Such a system would require the ready availability of adequate transport for mothers and infants to level 3 facilities.

... considerable saving might be effected by screening for risk ...

Access to care. Accessibility to the population at risk is fundamental to the organization of any regional system of care. Neonatal intensive care has been developed principally in urban hospitals with large, high-risk delivery services, and thus many high-risk infants have immediate access to such care. In addition, the relatively short distances between hospitals in urban areas would seem to allow for frequent transfer of mothers and infants.

Nevertheless, maternal referral for delivery in level 3 units was found to be surprisingly rare in New York City, although infant transfer from level 1 units was common.[41] The most impressive evidence of systematic referral of mothers for delivery of high-risk infants comes from rural areas such as Iowa.[34] This paradox may be a result of the concern, which is felt more strongly in rural areas, that infant transfer is a dangerous procedure for a fragile infant. Thus, efficient infant transport, a traditional strength of perinatal regionalization in New York City,[42] may have actually served to reduce maternal referral for delivery.

It is not easy to monitor the movement of mothers and babies across levels of care. Birth certificates and other sources of data available on the entire population have not usually recorded information on maternal and infant transport. Information on these key indicators of regionalization has generally been obtained from lists maintained by individual hospitals. An exception is New York City, where one agency accounted for the large majority of infant transports and maintained an excellent data collection system.[42] The 1989 revised US standard birth certificate (recommended for adoption by states, but not required) records whether the infant was transported to another hospital. Time will tell how many states will adopt this recommendation and whether hospital staff will regularly enter this new information on the birth certificate. Also unclear is how many infant transfers take place after the birth certificate is filed, which in many states must, by law, be within 48 hours of birth.

Maternal transport and referral are even more difficult to ascertain because mothers may be transferred to level 3 units from outpatient settings as well as from hospitals. No hospital record of transfers exist in such cases, and perhaps as a result the 1989 birth certificate revision does not recommend recording maternal transfers.

In the absence of data on maternal and infant transfers, proxy indicators have been suggested to measure the effectiveness of a regional screening and referral process. The following three indicators should be determined for level 3 units:

- The proportion of infants weighing <1500 grams in a region born in level 3 units.
- The proportion of all deaths in a region taking place in level 3 units.
- The proportion of all infants born outside level 3 units who die in level 3 units.

The use of these indicators is predicated on the assumption that certain categories of infants, such as VLBW and dying infants, ought to be cared for in level 3 units. There are obvious exceptions to this rule, such as infants too immature or malformed to survive, but in general, the presence of large numbers of VLBW infants or of infant deaths in hospitals without facilities to care for them is a sign that access to appropriate care is limited.

For a state or region, the proportion of VLBW births taking place in level 3 centers is a key indicator of regionalization, particularly in relation to the proportion of *all* births taking place in level 3 units.[43] This proportion is tabulated in Table 4-3 for several regions of the United States and for one European nation for which such data could be obtained. To better clarify the role of regionalization efforts in concentrating high-risk infants in regional centers, I have also tabulated, where available, the ratio of the percentage of VLBW births in regional centers to the percentage of all births in regional centers. This concentration ratio gives some sense of whether the percentage of VLBW infants born in regional centers simply reflects the size of the hospital rather than efforts specifically aimed at getting high-risk mothers to give birth there.[44] Substantial variation can be seen in the success of different regions of the United States in providing neonatal intensive care to VLBW infants from birth. Inasmuch as several predominantly rural states such as Michigan, Indiana, and Iowa have been able to assure level 3 delivery for 70% or so of their VLBW infants, a national goal of delivering two thirds of all VLBW infants in level 3 care centers seems reasonable.

Another useful exercise in assessing regionalization is examining the places of birth and death of infants who die in the neonatal period. For

TABLE 4-3
Concentration of Very Low Birthweight Births in Regional Centers

Region	Year	% VLBW	Concentration Ratio
Michigan	1986–1988	76	1.8
North Central Illinois	1985–1986	75	2.8
Indiana	1987	73	1.5
Washington	1980–1983	68	2.8
Iowa	1987	65	3.8
Alabama	1980	56	1.8
Tennessee	1978–79	45	...
Washington	1978–79	45	...
Louisiana	1978–79	39	...
New York City	1983	43	1.2
New York City	1976–78	36	1.1
Netherlands	1983	36	4.0
Iowa	1983	34	5.3
Ohio	1978–79	26	...

SOURCE: Paneth N, Rip M. *Perinatal Regionalization in Michigan.* Unpublished report to the Michigan Task Force on Perinatal Regionalization, 1990.

deaths relatively close to the time of birth, discordant locations for the two events virtually guarantee that the infant was transferred, rather than discharged from one hospital and readmitted for another illness to another hospital. Thus, for the subpopulation of infants who die, one can assess whether they were transported. A large number of deaths after the first few hours of life (transfer is unlikely to confer benefit if death occurs soon after birth) with place of birth and death at level 1 or 2 indicates that little transferring of very sick infants is being done. This method of assessment showed that in New York City level 1 units used infant transport extensively but level 2 units did not.[41]

The problem of neurodevelopmental outcome. Few observers of the functioning of a modern neonatal intensive care unit can avoid disquieting thoughts about the eventual quality of life of infants who undergo such extreme measures to ensure their survival. In the words of one keen observer of the newborn scene, "With each decrease in birthweight for which a significant increase in survival is achieved, the angst regarding outcome reemerges."[45(p1767)]

Some recent reviews have concluded that rates of neurodevelopmental handicap are either stable or dropping for infants who survive newborn intensive care.[45,46] The authors of these reviews do, however, express caution in two areas. First, infants weighing 501 to 750 grams are only now surviving in substantial numbers, and their eventual outcome remains uncertain. Second, most studies of outcome are restricted to infants; the challenges of school performance have been much less studied, and existing evidence points to a substantial excess of learning disability and poor school performance in VLBW children.

Not all studies of handicap rates in VLBW survivors account for the changing pattern of survival itself, a consideration that was emphasized a decade ago.[47] The net effect of newborn intensive care on rates of handicap in the population must be calculated by assessing the handicap rate among all live births rather than just among survivors. Doing so accounts for the increase in the population at risk due to increased survival itself. The optimism of some studies is based on the observation that survivors appear not to have experienced an increased rate of handicap, but the fact is that survivors of, for example, birthweight of less than 1000 grams, are several times more common than before. Even with a fixed rate of handicap, the result is a net increase in infants with handicap in the population.

... population rates of childhood cerebral palsy have recently been on the increase, with much of the rise attributable to spastic diplegia in premature infants.

In fact, there is evidence from several parts of the world that population rates of childhood cerebral palsy have recently been on the increase, with much of the rise attributable to spastic diplegia in premature infants.[48,49] Although this rise must be acknowledged and its consequences planned for by providing appropriate services, it is not an indictment of neonatal intensive care. It has been shown that for each infant with a handicap who would have died in the absence of neonatal intensive care, many more infants free of handicap have been added to the population.[48,50] A realistic assessment of the benefits and hazards[51] of newborn intensive care recognizes both the accomplishments and limitations of this extraordinary new form of medical technology.

The achievements of neonatal intensive care must always be viewed in the larger context of maternal and infant care. Our ability to offer expensive, cutting-edge technological support to 1-kilogram infants of homeless mothers contrasts sadly with our inability (or unwillingness) to provide housing for their mothers. Prematurity, the prime determinant of the need for intensive care services, flourishes in conditions of poverty and familial dislocation. Ignorance of the precise causes of prematurity does not absolve us from the societal responsibility to alter the abysmal circumstances under which too many of our women labor and into which too many of our infants are born.

REFERENCES

1. Tarnier CS, Chantrevil G. *Physiologie et Hygiene de la Premier Enfance: Considerees Surtout de la Point de Vue de l'Allimentation.* Paris: H. Lauwereyns; 1882.
2. Budin P. *Le Nourisson.* Paris: Octave Doin; 1900.

3. Cone TE. The first published report of an incubator for use in the care of the premature infant. *Am J Dis Child.* 1981;135:658–660.
4. Hess JH. Premature infants. *JAMA.* 1922;79:552–556.
5. Silverman WA. Incubator baby sideshows. *Pediatrics.* 1979; 64:127–141.
6. Silverman W. *Retrolental Fibroplasia: A Modern Parable.* New York, NY: Grune and Stratton; 1980.
7. Silverman WA, Anderson DA, Blanc WA, et al. A difference in mortality rate and incidence of kernicterus among premature infants allotted to two prophylactic antibacterial regimens. *Pediatrics.* 1956;18:614–625.
8. Kent SP, Wideman GL. Prophylactic antibiotic therapy in infants born after premature rupture of membranes. *JAMA.* 1959;171:1199–1203.
9. Smith CA, Yudkin S, Young W, et al. Adjustment of electrolytes and water following premature birth. *Pediatrics.* 1949;3:34–48.
10. Davies PA. Perinatal nutrition of infants of very low birth weight and their later progress. In: Falkner F, Kretchmer N, Rossi E, eds. *Modern Problems of Pediatrics.* vol 14. Basel: Karger; 1975:119–133.
11. Gregory GA, Kitterman JA, Phibbs RH, et al. Treatment of the idiopathic respiratory distress syndrome with continuous positive airway pressure. *N Engl J Med.* 1971;284:1333–1340.
12. American Academy of Pediatrics and American College of Obstetricians and Gynecologists. *Guidelines for Perinatal Care.* Evanston, Ill: American Academy of Pediatrics; 1983.
13. Oppenheimer G. Prematurity as a public health problem: the premature infant centers in New York City and the origins of neonatal intensive care. Unpublished ms.
14. Committee on Perinatal Health. *Toward Improving the Outcome of Pregnancy.* White Plains, NY: National Foundation-March of Dimes; 1976.
15. Sackett DL. On the evaluation of health services. In: Last JM, ed. *Public Health and Preventive Medicine.* 11th ed. New York, NY: Appleton-Century-Crofts; 1980:1800–1823.
16. Sinclair JC, Torrance GW, Boyle MH, et al. Evaluation of neonatal-intensive-care programs. *N Engl J Med.* 1981;305:489–494.
17. National Perinatal Epidemiology Unit. *A Classified Bibliography of Controlled Trials in Perinatal Medicine, 1940–1984.* Oxford: Oxford University Press; 1985.
18. Stewart AL, Reynolds EOR, Lipscomb AP. Outcome for infants of very low birthweight: a survey of the world literature. *Lancet.* 1981; 1:1038–1041.
19. Clifford SH. High risk pregnancy, I: prevention of prematurity the sine qua non for reduction of mental retardation and other neurologic disorders. *N Engl J Med.* 1964;271:243–249.
20. Paneth N, Wallenstein S, Kiely JL, Susser MW. Social class indicators and mortality in low birthweight infants. *Am J Epidemiol.* 1982; 116:364–375.
21. Collins JW Jr., David RJ. Differential survival rates among low birthweight Black and White infants in a tertiary care hospital. *Epidemiology.* 1990;1:16–20.
22. Kleinman JC, Kovar MG, Feldman JJ, Young CA. A comparison of 1960 and 1973–1974 early neonatal mortality in selected states. *Am J Epidemiol.* 1978;108:454–469.
23. National Center for Health Statistics. A Study of Infant Mortality from Linked Records: Comparison of Neonatal Mortality from Two Cohort Studies, United States January to March, 1950 and 1960. Washington, DC: US Dept of Health, Education and Welfare; 1972. Vital and Health Statistics series 20, no 13. (HSM) 72-1056.
24. Lee K-S, Paneth N, Gartner LM, et al. Neonatal mortality: an analysis of the recent improvement in the United States. *Am J Public Health.* 1980;70:15–21.

25. Buehler JW, Kleinman JC, Hogue C, et al. Birth weight-specific infant mortality, United States, 1960 and 1980. *Public Health Rep.* 1987; 102:151–161.
26. Lie RT, Irgens LM, Skjaerven R, et al. Secular changes in early neonatal mortality in Norway, 1967–1981. *Am J Epidemiol.* 1987; 125:1066–1078.
27. Pharoah POD, Alberman ED. Mortality of low birthweight infants in England and Wales 1953–1979. *Arch Dis Child.* 1981;56:86–89.
28. Pharaoh POD, Alberman ED. Annual statistical review. *Arch Dis Child.* 1990;65:147–151.
29. Cordero L, Backes CR, Zuspan FS. Very low birthweight infants. influence of place of birth on survival. *Am J Obstet Gynecol.* 1982; 143:533–537.
30. Paneth N, Kiely JL, Wallenstein S, Marcus M, Parker J, Susser MW. Newborn intensive care and neonatal mortality in low birthweight infants: a population study. *N Engl J Med.* 1982;307:149–155.
31. Gortmaker S, Sobol A, Clark C, et al. The survival of very low birthweight infants by level of hospital of birth: a population study of perinatal systems in four states. *Am J Obstet Gynecol.* 1985; 152:517–524.
32. Verloove-Vanhorick SP, Verwey RA, Ebeling MCA. Mortality in very preterm and very low birthweight infants according to place of birth and level of care. *Pediatrics.* 1988;81:404–411.
33. Bakketeig LS, Hoffman HJ, Sternthal PM. Obstetric service and perinatal mortality in Norway. *Acta Paediatr Scand (Suppl).* 1978;77:3–19.
34. Hein HA. Evaluation of a rural perinatal care system. *Pediatrics.* 1980; 66:540–546.
35. Mayfield JA, Rosenblatt RA, Baldwin L-M, et al. The relationship of obstetrical volume and nursery level to perinatal mortality. *Am J Public Health.* 1990;80:819–823.
36. U.S. Congress, Office of Technology Assessment. *Neonatal Intensive Care for Low Birthweight Infants: Costs and Effectiveness* (Health Technology Case Study 38). Washington, DC: US Congress, Office of Technology Assessment; 1987. Publication no. OTA-HCS-38.
37. Showstack JA, Stone MH, Schroder SA. The role of changing clinical practices in the rising costs of hospital care. *New Eng J Med.* 1985; 313:1201–1207.
38. Paneth N, Kiely JL, Wallenstein S, Susser MW. The choice of place of delivery: effect of hospital level on mortality in all singleton births in New York City. *Am J Dis Child.* 1987;141:60–64.
39. Baruffi G, Dellinger WS, Strobino DM, et al. A study of pregnancy outcomes in a maternity center and a tertiary care hospital. *Am J Public Health.* 1984;74:973–978.
40. Rooks JP, Weatherby NL, Ernst EKM, et al. Outcomes of care in birth centers. The National Birth Center Study. *N Engl J Med.* 1989; 321:1804–1811.
41. Paneth N, Kiely JL, Susser MW. Age at death used to assess the effect of interhospital transport on neonatal mortality. *Pediatrics.* 1984; 73:854–861.
42. Marcus M, Paneth N, Kiely JL, Susser MW. Determinants of interhospital transfer of low birthweight newborns. *Medical Care.* 1988; 24:462–473.
43. Rosenblatt RA, Mayfield JA, Hart LG, et al. Outcomes of regionalized perinatal care in Washington State. *West J Med.* 1988;149:98–102.
44. Lee K-S, Paneth N, Gartner L, Pearlman M. The very low birthweight rate: principal predictor of neonatal mortality in populations. *J Pediatr.* 1980;97:759–764.
45. McCormick MC. Long-term follow-up of infants discharged from neonatal intensive care units. *JAMA.* 1989;261:1767–1772.

46. Grögaard JB, Lindstrom DP, Parker RA, et al. Increased survival rate in very low birthweight infants (1500 grams or less): no association with increased incidence of handicaps. *J Pediatrics*. 1990;117:139–146.
47. Paneth N, Kiely J, Stein AZ, Susser MW. Cerebral palsy and newborn care: III. estimated prevalence rates of cerebral palsy under differing rates of mortality and impairment of low birthweight infants. *Dev Med Child Neurol*. 1981;23:801–807.
48. Hagberg B, Olow I, Von Wendt L. The changing panorama of cerebral palsy in Sweden, V. The birth year period 1979–1982. *Acta Paed Scand*. 1989;78:283–290.
49. Pharaoh POD, Cooke T, Rosenbloom L, et al. Effects of birthweight, gestational age and maternal obstetric history on birth prevalence of cerebral palsy. *Arch Dis Child*. 1987;62:1035–1040.
50. Stanley FJ. The changing face of cerebral palsy? *Dev Med Child Neurol*. 1987;29:263–265.
51. Hagberg B, Hagberg G, Olow I. Gains and hazards of intensive neonatal care: an analysis from Swedish cerebral palsy epidemiology. *Dev Med Child Neurol*. 1982;24:13–19.

CHAPTER 5

Health Promotion in Maternity Care

Jeffrey P. Mayer, PhD
James G. Emshoff, PhD
Sheila Avruch, MBA

Behavioral risks during pregnancy, including smoking, drug and alcohol use, poor nutrition, and delaying or not seeking needed services, are associated with infant mortality and low birthweight (LBW). As appreciation for such risks has deepened, a growing consensus has suggested that prenatal care that does not address these maternal behavioral risks is less effective than comprehensive care that does. As a result, health promotion interventions have been recognized increasingly as essential components of maternity care.[1,2]

Major questions remain, however, concerning how health promotion interventions will be financed and who will provide them. Unlike the more traditional services discussed in other chapters, health promotion services focus on behavioral rather than medical problems and often involve both service systems and personnel outside the mainstream of medical care. This chapter, which reviews research showing that certain approaches to reducing behavioral risks during pregnancy are effective, underscores the importance of incorporating health promotion into universal access plans.

Our review is limited to four areas: smoking cessation, substance abuse, nutrition, and home visiting. We focus on health promotion program models that have been evaluated as effective and on existing gaps and emerging trends in research and practice. For reviews of other health education and social support approaches, refer to Thompson.[3]

SMOKING CESSATION

Despite concern over high rates of smoking among young women of childbearing age, most women know the risks of smoking during pregnancy,[4] and many quit when pregnancy is confirmed.[5-7] However, estimates of smoking during pregnancy are still unacceptably high, ranging from 21% to 32%.[8]

Smoking during pregnancy is most prevalent among teenaged, unmarried, and less educated women. The National Natality Surveys, which were limited to married women, indicate reductions in smoking during

---

The views and opinions expressed herein do not necessarily reflect the position of the US General Accounting Office.

pregnancy in the past two decades. However, the rate of decrease was much less pronounced among teens and less educated women.[5] Data from Missouri[6] and the Behavioral Risk Factor Surveillance System of the Centers for Disease Control,[9] which included both married and unmarried women, indicate that smoking during pregnancy is greatest among young unmarried White women.

Estimates of the proportion of women who quit voluntarily once pregnancy is confirmed range from 16% to 41%,[8] varying with demographic and other factors. Those who do stop quit very early in pregnancy; in the second or third trimester a pregnant woman is much less likely to quit without further prompting. Unfortunately, about 70% to 80% of women who quit for pregnancy relapse after delivery.[10,11]

Those who do quit, whether the effort is self-initiated or prompted by the advice of a health professional, appear to be different from those who continue to smoke. Continuing smokers are more likely to be unmarried, be heavy smokers before pregnancy, have a husband or partner who smokes, believe less strongly that smoking is harmful to the fetus, have greater parity, begin prenatal care later in gestation, have less education, have an unwanted pregnancy, or begin smoking at an earlier age.[6,9-12]

Behavior, Health, and Cost Effects of Interventions

A growing set of studies[13-25] suggests that cessation interventions result in moderate rates of quitting. The internal and external validity of these studies is strong; 11 of the 13 studies employed random assignment and 9 of the 13 verified self-reported smoking status biochemically. Diverse settings were involved, including health maintenance organizations (HMOs), hospital clinics, health departments, clinics of the Special Supplemental Food Program for Women, Infants, and Children (WIC), and private physician offices. Participation in clinic-based studies has been remarkably strong, where typically about 80% of pregnant smokers agree to attend counseling. However, attempts to establish groups outside clinic routines or the home have uniformly resulted in high attrition.[19,24] Most studies have therefore employed a self-help, individualized approach to intervention, including health educator and physician counseling, home correspondence courses, self-help manuals, informational materials, and home visits.

Eleven of the 13 studies reported quit rates. Subjects lost to follow-up were counted as continuing smokers in the present summary following Windsor and Orleans' reanalysis.[26] The intervention group quit rates ranged from 6% to 32% with a mean of 16%. The usual care or control condition quit rates ranged from 2% to 14% with a mean of 6.7%. Variation in quit rates among studies seems attributable to differences in study target groups (eg, low-income participants exhibit lower quit rates) and intervention strengths (eg, incompletely implemented interventions exhibit lower quit rates). In addition, some variation in quit rates is probably due to differences in patient selection criteria; studies excluding women who are light smokers or women who enter care late in gestation are likely to result in lower quit rates.

Five of the 13 studies reported higher birthweights for women in the experimental intervention groups. The birthweight differences ranged from 68 to 150 grams with a mean of 90 grams. The magnitude of the birthweight differences varies consistently with quit rates; studies with a larger difference in quit rates also reported larger birthweight differences.[8] Three studies reported LBW rates, and in each of those studies the experimental groups had lower LBW rates.

Several studies estimated the cost benefit or effectiveness of cessation interventions. Windsor et al[27] reported on a cost-effectiveness analysis of a randomized trial. The multicomponent intervention yielded a cost of $51 per quit, whereas the intermediate and usual care control groups each cost more than twice as much per quit. Ershoff et al[28] reported a cost-benefit analysis of a serialized self-help program implemented at a California HMO. The low cost of the self-help, home-based program ($11.75 per patient) coupled with higher hospitalization costs for infants of control group mothers (average difference of $46 per delivery) yielded a benefit-cost ratio of 2.8:1. The authors indicate that this estimate is conservative because it includes immediate hospitalization costs only, thus excluding long-term childhood morbidity costs. An earlier quasi-experiment at the same HMO yielded a 2:1 ratio, although the intervention consumed more resources because it included nutrition as well as smoking components.[17]

Implications and Future Needs

As publicity has become increasingly devoted to the risks involved, more pregnant women have quit smoking. However, a quarter to a third of all pregnant women continue to smoke. The consequences in terms of mortality, morbidity, quality of life, and dollars are high and avoidable.

It is encouraging that the intervention literature is impressive and growing and that the quality of study design and measurement is high. Results have consistently indicated greater abstinence for intervention groups during the latter months of gestation. Broad implementation of smoking cessation interventions is therefore likely to be cost-effective. Windsor et al[29] estimate that $19 to $38 in preventable excess costs of infant health care could be saved for every $1 invested if smoking cessation methods were applied nationwide to the 350 000 annual public-sector maternity patients who smoke.

Achieving higher quit rates and maintaining cessation after delivery would require more comprehensive interventions. This point is particularly germane in reaching pregnant women who are more resistant to quitting, such as heavy smokers, multiparous women, and women who are not experiencing nausea and other problems early in pregnancy.[20,24,30] Because group interventions outside clinic routines have not been successful in prompting participation, resourceful methods to increase intervention intensity need to be found. Multiple smoking-focused contacts at subsequent maternity clinic visits, telephone and mail-based approaches, home visits, and use of existing community and social support networks are all areas for additional exploration.

Routinizing cessation interventions on a broad scale in understaffed and overcrowded clinics without additional resources, technical assistance, and training can be difficult.[31] Additional effort must be directed toward the issues of financing, staffing, disseminating, and routinizing cessation interventions in maternity care organizations. Despite the demonstrated effectiveness of these interventions, proactive efforts will be required if widespread adoption is to take place.

Because smoking during pregnancy is most prevalent among teens and low-income women, dissemination seems initially more germane for school-based clinics, local health departments, and WIC sites. For higher income women, cessation interventions should become integrated into private practices[32] and workplaces.[33] Fortunately, clinicians have begun to publish reports encouraging adoption of cessation interventions.[34,35] In addition, a handbook describing how to plan, implement, and evaluate smoking cessation interventions for pregnant women has been distributed to providers nationwide.[29]

SUBSTANCE ABUSE

Clinical and research data suggest that maternal use of alcohol and other drugs carries a wide array of deleterious health and social consequences to offspring. These effects have been reviewed by Householder,[36] Jones and Lopez,[37] and Chasnoff,[38] among others.

Estimates of the frequency of heavy drinking among pregnant women range from consumption of three or more drinks per week by 3% of the national population of pregnant women[12] to 45 or more drinks per month by 9% of a smaller, higher risk population.[39] Weiner et al[40] report that 9 percent of a sample of women registering for prenatal care drank heavily. Estimates of the incidence of fetal alcohol syndrome (FAS) in the United States range from zero to 3.1 per 1000 live births.[41]

More than 5 million women of childbearing age currently use an illicit drug.[42] The results of a survey of 36 hospitals[43] indicate that as many as 375 000 children (approximately 11% of all births) are born each year to women who are using illegal drugs. Others have claimed that the 36 hospitals were not representative and that the estimate of incidence was therefore inflated.[44]

The incidence of births to women using drugs other than alcohol appears to be increasing. The analysis of the National Hospital Discharge Survey by the US General Accounting Office (GAO) in 1990 revealed that indications of maternal drug use increased 49.5% between 1986 and 1988.[45] Local and state data sources suggest increases of even greater magnitude. The reported number of cocaine babies in Illinois increased 78% between 1987 and 1988.[46] The percentage of pregnant women who tested positive for cocaine increased from 7% to 58% in Philadelphia between 1984 and 1987.[37] A hospital in Los Angeles reports that the number of newborns diagnosed with intrauterine exposure to cocaine increased from 28 in 1981 to 226 in 1985.[47] Los Angeles County drug-associated fetal deaths increased from 9 in 1985 to 56 in 1987.[48] Some unknown proportion of the reported increases are the result of increased quantity and sophistication of assessment procedures, but enhanced measurement and screening cannot completely explain the observed trends.

Treatment Needs

Current research does not allow an empirical validation of specific service components; most studies globally evaluate multicomponent efforts. Despite a minimal empirical foundation, there is some consensus on the needs to be addressed and the components of an ideal program.[2,49-51] This consensus is echoed by the recent grant announcement of the Office for Substance Abuse Prevention (OSAP).

Some consensus components are designed to affect the health of the mother and baby directly, others are intended to address the comprehensive and interrelated needs of this population in a holistic fashion, and still others are support services designed to increase the likelihood that the preceding services will be received. The combination of these services dictates the use of multiple disciplines and service organizations, which may be linked through a central organization or through the use of consortia and case management. An ideal strategy for delivering comprehensive treatment consists of outreach and referral (including public education and screening), high-risk prenatal and obstetric care, a continuum of drug treatment services (including inpatient, outpatient, and residential services, and aftercare), and broader social services (eg, counseling, job skill training, legal assistance, stress management, and parenting and life skills training). A 1989 survey of 10 model programs showed that many of these components were present.[52]

The capacity of current treatment systems is inadequate. For example, in Detroit, Hutzel Hospital's High Risk Clinic, which serves pregnant addicts, reports a 7- to 8-week waiting period. Many treatment facilities refuse to serve pregnant women because of their special needs. A recent survey of 78 drug treatment programs in New York City indicated that 54% of the programs refused to treat pregnant addicts, 67% denied treatment if the woman was on Medicaid, and 87% denied treatment to pregnant crack addicts on Medicaid. Of those that offered drug treatment, fewer than half offered prenatal care and only 3% offered day care—without which, entering drug treatment is impossible for some mothers.[53]

Although such services are not inexpensive, failure to provide them is a considerably more expensive alternative. The costs of treating drug-exposed children include $30 000 per exposed child for delivery and other health care and $114 000 additional annual costs per child for investigation of abuse and neglect, foster care placement, and special education and development services.[54] Current treatment costs associated with FAS alone have been estimated at $321 million per year.[41] A recent survey of eight cities identified nearly 9000 babies prenatally exposed to illicit drugs in 1989, at an estimated cost of $500 million for care through age 5.[55]

Program Examples

A description of all programs that are serving pregnant addicts is beyond the scope of this chapter. A few projects for which there are at least minimal evaluation data will be described.

The Georgia Addiction, Pregnancy, and Parenting Project reported that counseling and information distributed to patients resulted in significant reductions in alcohol consumption during pregnancy,[56] which in turn resulted in more positive birth outcomes.[57] Rosett et al[39] reported that 65% of chronic drinking mothers recruited into a counseling program at a Boston hospital reduced their drinking by the third trimester. The infants of these positive responders had infants with weight, length, and head circumference similar to those of infants born to women who drank rarely or moderately. In a replication of this study in Sweden,[58] information distribution alone led to a 74% reduction in alcohol consumption, and information distribution plus counseling led to a 78% reduction.

Early intervention with pregnant women who are using cocaine can also produce positive birth outcomes. Quitting cocaine in the early stages of pregnancy has been shown to reduce the risks to the fetus.[59]

Other programs have focused on educating health care professionals. For example, Little and colleagues[60] described a 2-year community education program that included use of media, distribution of materials, and professional education. After the conclusion of the program, more obstetricians indicated that they were asking patients about alcohol use and recommending abstention.

Legal Policy

At least 44 women have been prosecuted on criminal charges as a result of their use of drugs during pregnancy, primarily in the past 2 years.[61] Thirty-three states have existing or pending legislation on drug use during pregnancy. This issue has generated considerable discussion, one result of which was the formation of the Coalition on Alcohol and Drug Dependent Women and Their Children. Established by the National Council on Alcoholism and Drug Dependence, this coalition of 38 organizational members strongly opposes the criminalization of pregnant addicts. At least two members of the coalition, the American Society of Addiction Medicine and the American Academy of Pediatrics, have issued their own position statements opposing the criminalization of prenatal behavior.

The debate over the wisdom of such prosecution may focus on the relative rights of the woman and her fetus. However, a less moral and more practical concern, which takes into consideration the rights of both parties, is the behavioral effect of this practice on the target population. Specifically, pregnant addicts—a difficult population to engage in services under the best of conditions—are further inhibited from seeking treatment by threats of prosecution, involuntary treatment, or loss of custody of living or unborn children.

If a woman does seek treatment, the trust between her and her service provider is threatened in states where such providers must report pregnant substance users on the suspicion of child endangering; providers thus face considerable professional and ethical difficulty with respect to conflicting responsibilities. Treatment programs are no more expensive than incarceration, and their benefits exceed those of incarceration[50] in terms of outcomes for both mothers and infants. A California program, which diverts substance-abusing pregnant women with children to community alternatives, reports a 20% lower recidivism rate than traditional incarceration.[50] A national survey of prosecutions of pregnant addicts revealed discrimination against ethnic minorities as well as against poor and battered women.[61]

Implications and Future Needs

The rising incidence of substance abuse during pregnancy, the many treatment needs of the population, and the inadequacy of current system capacity all argue for the creation of new programs. More rigorous research must be conducted to identify effective program models and components. Various sources have cited the need for a sustainable funding base for such programs, expansion of the OSAP demonstration initiative, creation of multidisciplinary approaches and training, continuing education for professionals, and inclusion of substance abuse treatment in universal access plans.

NUTRITION

Appropriate nutrition during pregnancy can have a positive impact on outcomes, especially for women whose nutrition status is very poor at conception.[2] A variety of factors may influence need for nutrition services. Women who have anemia or diabetes, have had multiple births or a prior infant with neural tube defects, or who are obese or extremely lean may require special diets and counseling.[62] In addition, extremes of age, unmarried status, low education, and low income are predictive of poor weight gain and poor nutrition behavior.

This section reviews evaluations of both WIC and non-WIC community-based nutrition supplementation and education programs.

WIC Evaluations

The two major reviews of WIC evaluations were performed by the GAO[63] and the research team that conducted the National WIC Evaluation (NWE).[64] Although these reviews and other studies found some evidence of WIC effects in improving dietary behavior, weight gain, anemia, and prenatal care adequacy for pregnant women, as well as growth, cognitive development, well-child care, and anemia for infants and children, in this chapter we focus on studies of WIC influence on birthweight and perinatal mortality.

Birthweight. GAO limited its summary to six studies of high methodologic quality and reported "some support, but not conclusive evidence"[63(pii)] of improved birthweight effects of WIC. The average mean birthweight difference (weighted by study sample size) was 30 to 50 grams, with a 16% to 20% reduction in the LBW rate (7.9% vs 9.5%) among women participating in WIC. However, self-selection problems in the studies were emphasized.

The NWE review distinguished between studies that used community controls and those that used Medicaid women or postpartum WIC recipients as controls. The former studies may underestimate WIC effects because control subjects are at lower risk, having not met the financial and health risk criteria necessary for WIC participation. For example, in the Massachusetts[65] and Missouri evaluations[66,67] the approach involved linking WIC and birth certificate data and applying statistical control or matching with the limited demographic variables available. Because those evaluations were probably undercontrolled, they underestimated effects (only 16 to 21 grams).

On the other hand, the studies using Medicaid and postpartum WIC clients as controls probably overestimate effects. The financial criteria for Medicaid eligibility are much lower than for WIC. Postpartum WIC clients may have been recruited into WIC because of poor pregnancy outcome and may have been less motivated to seek care initially (such as the second control group in Kennedy et al[68]). Other methodologic concerns discussed in the NWE review include confounding the length of WIC program duration with length of gestation, and regression to the mean in studies that simply compared non-WIC pregnancy outcomes with subsequent WIC pregnancy outcomes. Despite these methodologic concerns, the NWE reviewers concluded that a 1% to 2% difference in LBW was attributable to WIC, as was a 30- to 60-gram birthweight increase, findings that are highly congruent with the conclusions of the GAO review.

The NWE used two approaches. The historical study[69] used WIC, vital records, and census data from 1392 counties in 19 states for the period 1972 to 1980, a time during which WIC gradually increased its coverage of the eligible population. Time series analyses indicated that greater WIC coverage was associated with a significant 23-gram birthweight difference, although the 0.5% reduction in LBW rate was not significant.

The NWE's second approach, the longitudinal study,[70] compared WIC pregnant women with non-WIC community controls drawn from a nationally representative multistage sample. The 30-gram birthweight difference was not statistically significant; neither were the rates of births at less than 2500 grams. However, control group women were initially at lower risk, having higher income, education, and employment status. Also, difficulties in building a sufficient control sample size limited study power. However, significant WIC effects on infant head circumference were found, and when measures of local WIC program quality were considered, improved birthweight effects were significant for the higher quality programs.

Caan et al,[71] an evaluation not included in the GAO or NWE reviews, focused on women receiving WIC support both before and during pregnancy. A 131-gram birthweight difference and a 35% reduction in the LBW rate (3.2% vs 5.1%) were reported, with both analyses controlling for length of gestation. The large differences are likely attributable to the extended length of WIC participation across the prepregnancy and pregnancy periods.

Perinatal mortality. A meaningful summary of studies of perinatal mortality was not possible according to the GAO and NWE reviews because of low study sample sizes and great variability in the outcomes examined. The Kotelchuk et al[65] study found fewer neonatal deaths in the WIC group, but Massachusetts WIC rules terminated the participation of women who missed two consecutive visits. Systematic attrition from the WIC group of women delivering premature infants was therefore a potential alternative explanation.[72] Stockbauer[66,67] found a significantly lower perinatal mortality rate for non-White WIC participants versus non-White nonparticipants, but for Whites the non-WIC cases had lower mortality. The NWE reviewers suggest that this difference may be due to a greater degree of initial nonequivalence between the White WIC and non-WIC groups than between the non-White WIC and non-WIC groups.

The NWE, perhaps the only investigation with sufficient power, reported mortality effects. The historical study found a significant reduction in fetal mortality (-2.3 per 1000), and a marginally significant reduction in infant mortality (-1.5 per 1000), both of meaningful magnitude. The longitudinal study, with less power, found a nonsignificant but meaningful fetal mortality reduction (-5.9 per 1000).

Client and program characteristics. There is some evidence that WIC factors interact with maternal and program characteristics. Several studies reported that WIC effects were greater for Blacks, teens, the less educated, and those who possess several WIC risk factors.[65,67,69,73,74] Metcoff et al[73] reported that WIC birthweight differences disappeared with more complete statistical control, except in the case of heavy smokers, where a 168-gram difference was maintained.

Several studies reported that greater levels of WIC participation are associated with better pregnancy outcomes, whether measured by more time in the program[65,67,75] or by greater use of food vouchers.[66,68] Stockbauer[67] indicated that at least 7 months' participation are necessary before birthweight effects emerge. GAO's review also reported "some evidence" for a dose-response relationship.

Cost benefit. Schramm[76,77] analyzed linked Missouri data to provide estimates of financial savings to Medicaid that were attributable to WIC participation. Besides a $100 cost increment for non-WIC Medicaid newborns being identified, $0.83 and $0.49 in Medicaid costs were recouped for every WIC dollar expended in 1980 and 1982, respectively. Mathematica Policy Research,[78] in a five-state study that controlled for prenatal care adequacy as well as other demographic confounds, reported that $277 to $598 (varying by state) in Medicaid costs were saved for every $1 invested in WIC. The Missouri cost-benefit estimates were lower because postnatal costs were tracked for a much shorter period. However, both results are probably conservative; neither considered the long-term childhood morbidity costs associated with LBW.

Community-Based Nutrition Programs

Most, but not all,[79,80] non-WIC supplementation studies have reported birthweight improvements.[81-84] The occasional negative findings seem to be related to incomplete nutrition behavior change and supplement consumption, delivery of supplements late in pregnancy, or insufficient malnutrition among participants at the beginning of the study.[62] Some studies have reported an interaction between supplementation and other risks, as was reported with WIC. For example, Rush et al[80] reported no birthweight effects except among heavy smokers, findings similar to those of the WIC study of Metcoff et al.[73] Villar and Rivera[84] reported birthweight effects of high magnitude when supplementation included the interpregnancy interval as well as pregnancy, as did the WIC study of Caan et al.[71]

Studies of nutrition education without supplementation offer a mix of results. Several have documented improved maternal nutrient intake, others showed attitude and knowledge improvements, and still others reported increases in maternal weight gain and infant outcomes. For example, Orstead et al,[85] using historical controls at a Chicago hospital clinic, reported mean birthweight (100 grams) and LBW rate (4% vs 13%) differences, as well as a 5:1 cost-benefit ratio.

Implications and Future Needs

With the NWE study finally released, and the recent five-state study demonstrating impressive cost benefits for WIC, the debate over this program's effectiveness seems to be largely resolved. Given the general consensus on WIC's effectiveness, it is unfortunate that only about 45% of all eligible women, infants, and children are served at current funding levels.[86] Future efforts need to focus on (1) expanding the program to more eligible women and infants, (2) attracting women into the program earlier in pregnancy, and (3) further using WIC as a mechanism for identifying other health needs (eg, smoking cessation, substance abuse, Medicaid).

HOME VISITING   Home visitors provide direct services to families by linking them to care, providing information and social support, and encouraging risk reduction. In this capacity they can address multiple health and social problems facing high-risk, low-income pregnant women.

Home visiting began in the 19th century in both Europe and the United States as a way to reduce infant mortality and improve child health and development.[87,88] In Western Europe, home visiting is still a routine aspect of maternity care. Home visits are usually provided as a postnatal service by specially trained nurses or midwives.[89] In the United States, home visiting is much less common and is generally provided for targeted families rather than universally available.

Unlike European programs, most United States programs focus on education- rather than health-related goals. In a survey study, more than 4000 United States home visit projects were identified. Of the 1900 projects that responded to the survey, only 9% were focused on health. Education-focused home visiting for preschool-aged children, particularly through Head Start, was the most common program type.[90] It is encouraging that some states are beginning to incorporate health-focused home visiting as part of the recent Medicaid expansions. The National Governors Association has identified 24 states that now provide Medicaid-reimbursed home visiting.[91]

Recent Evidence of Home Visiting's Effectiveness

Recent rigorous investigations have demonstrated a broad range of positive benefits from home visiting, including reductions in LBW and prematurity rates, better use of prenatal care, improved health-related behaviors during pregnancy, improved weight gain by LBW babies, and decreased accidents and child abuse.[92-100] In addition, home visiting has been associated with improved cognitive development for premature, LBW, and malnourished infants.[98,101-105] However, although some projects improved health-seeking or maternal care behaviors, they did not improve other objectives that are more difficult to affect, such as LBW and reported child abuse.[97,104,106-109]

A major strength of home visiting lies in its potential to affect a range of outcomes with a single intervention method. For example, results from the randomized trial of the Prenatal Early Intervention Program (PEIP) included decreases in smoking, home accidents, emergency room visits, and incidents of abuse, and an improvement in birthweight.[92,93] Home-visited PEIP women were also more likely to complete schooling, gain employment, and plan future pregnancies.[94] Stronger effects resulted from combined prenatal and postnatal home visiting.

Similarly, Hardy and Street[100] reported that infants from families randomly assigned to home visiting completed preventive care more frequently, had lower rates of ear infection, made fewer outpatient visits, had less frequent hospital admissions, and had fewer incidences of suspected and documented abuse. Larson[99] reported that home-visited infants experienced fewer accidents, were more likely to be up to date on their immunizations (93% vs 70%), and scored higher on tests of cognitive development and school achievement.

Two projects using quasi-experimental designs reported birth outcome effects. Rural teenagers participating in the South Carolina Resource Mothers Program experienced a 10.6% LBW rate versus 16.3% among matched control patients. The rate of inadequate prenatal care was also significantly lower among Resource Mothers clients.[95] A Michigan project found that the pregnancies of women who were visited at home by nurses resulted in fewer LBW and premature infants and in significantly higher Apgar scores and mean birthweights.[96]

Home visiting can improve the growth and development of preterm and LBW infants. For example, Field et al[98] reported that preterm infants of home-visited teenage, Black, low-income mothers had significantly improved weight gain and scored significantly higher on tests of infant development. Ross[102] reported similar results from a quasi-experimental study, as did Rauh et al[103] and Resnick et al[104] with random design experiments. The Infant Health and Development Project[105]—a randomized, multisite project employing home visiting, a child development center, and bimonthly parent groups—reported significantly higher mean IQ scores at 36 months for home-visited children.

Implications and Future Needs

Although many home visiting projects have been successful, others have not. The following features of home visiting programs appear to be associated with greater effectiveness.

First, effectiveness and client acceptance seem to depend on when services are initiated. Larson[99] found a significantly stronger program effect when home visiting began prenatally and was highly intensive during the immediate postpartum period. Siegel and associates[110] indicated that home visitors reported stronger, more trusting, and more effective relationships with clients if the intervention began in the prenatal period.

Second, visit content must be carefully structured. Effective programs have been more intensive and have combined risk reduction with social support objectives.[92-94,98,102,103,111-114] For example, projects that reported birthweight improvements specifically tailored services to encourage risk-behavior reduction among clients.[92-94] Projects that reported decreased accident and child abuse reported teaching families specific child safety and alternate discipline techniques.[99,100,109] Successful programs to improve child development also carefully structured their services by working with both caregivers and infants, modeling exercises that they wanted the parents to use with the infants and providing information firmly grounded in developmental theory.[98,102,103,105,113,114] Projects spanning the prenatal and postpartum periods were more successful.

Third, training and supervision are central if home visitors are to deliver services effectively.[111] Poor training and supervision are mentioned in many evaluations of less successful programs.[97,115-118] Solid training and supervision are particularly needed for paraprofessionals.[119,120] In contrast to the United States, where training for home visiting varies widely and where no agreed-upon curriculum is used, Great Britain and Denmark have a uniform training system for home visitors above and beyond normal nurse training.[88]

Fourth, home visiting approaches seem particularly germane for groups that are difficult to reach and retain through center-based or other service delivery modes.[121] Several projects have shown success with low-income teenagers and with abusive parents, two groups that are traditionally difficult to access.

Finally, linking women to other needed services is a critical aspect of home visiting. Low-income, high-risk women face many impediments to accessing needed medical and social services, including financial, structural, and personal barriers.[122] Home visitors can reduce personal barriers through education and, equally important, can help reduce structural barriers by serving as case managers.[88] Programs that cannot perform this linking function lack a key element for success.

HEALTH PROMOTION AND UNIVERSAL ACCESS

Our review suggests that health promotion interventions have significant effects on behavioral-dependent variables, but more research is needed to ascertain impacts on health outcomes and costs. Existing research, although indicating modest effects, does not contain sufficient data to allow for definitive health outcome conclusions. Cost-benefit studies, although few in number, are suggestive of meaningful short-term cost savings, but studies of long-term and systems-level impacts are needed. This challenge for future work also exists for health promotion research with other populations and requires using more longitudinal designs and larger sample sizes.

Despite the clear need for additional research addressing the gaps discussed in this review, continued expansion of health promotion is vitally important. To maximize the likelihood of improved perinatal outcomes, we believe universal access to maternity services must incorporate a model of comprehensive care in which health promotion activities figure prominently. This belief is echoed by the 1989 report of the Public Health Service's Expert Panel on the Content of Prenatal Care, which called for the routine delivery of psychosocial and health promotion interventions for high-risk women.[1]

Unfortunately, health promotion within the existing maternity care system can be characterized as uneven at best. Efforts are generally poorly defined and are often excluded from public and private insurance coverage. Programs also suffer from a lack of trained, available personnel to offer services that are known to be useful. Therefore, expanding service capacity is critical for the full benefits of health promotion to be realized. The expert panel noted that health promotion services are sometimes provided in public health and clinic settings but are less frequently available in private settings. Private insurers especially need to recognize the benefits of health promotion coverage, particularly during pregnancy. Although new Medicaid policies have allowed payment for some health promotion services, reimbursement is low and benefits vary widely among states.[91] Recruiting and training personnel to provide health promotion has been an impediment in many instances, suggesting that training programs for nutritionists, health educators, community health workers, and other providers should be broadened.

Besides enlarging the financial and personnel base of health promotion, we must address microlevel issues of integrating these services into existing delivery systems. Because clinic and practice routines will become more complex as additional health promotion components are added, systematic efforts to enhance acceptance and adoption of health promotion need to be fielded. Research should address the organizational challenges posed by adding these new services to traditional medical care. Study of the characteristics of interventions, organizations, and proactive change approaches associated with successful adoption of health promotion in maternity care organizations should become a priority for future research.

Other industrialized nations spend a smaller share of their gross national product on health care than the United States. Yet in these nations, some maternal and infant health promotion services considered costly by many US analysts are routinely available. Given the critical role of health promotion in reducing LBW, the cost and success of services seem to be less the issue than the political and professional will to make them universally available. Health promotion must be an integral part of any universal access program, so that behavioral risk reduction efforts will be financed, staffed, and incorporated into mainstream maternity and infant care.

REFERENCES

1. Expert Panel on the Content of Prenatal Care. *Caring for Our Future: The Content of Prenatal Care*. Washington, DC: US Public Health Services; 1989.
2. Institute of Medicine. *Preventing Low Birth Weight*. Washington, DC: National Academy Press; 1985.
3. Thompson JE. Health education interventions during pregnancy. In: Merkatz IR, Thompson JE, Mullen PD, Goldenberg RL, eds. *New Perspectives on Prenatal Care*. New York, NY: Elsevier; 1990:319–336.
4. Fox SH, Brown C, Koontz AM. Perceptions of risks of smoking and heavy drinking during pregnancy. *Public Health Rep*. 1987;102:73–79.
5. Kleinman JC, Kopstein AK. Smoking during pregnancy: 1967 to 1980. *Am J Public Health*. 1987;77:823–825.
6. Land GH, Stockbauer JW. Who smokes while pregnant? Jefferson City, Mo: Center for Health Statistics, Missouri Department of Public Health; 1986.
7. Streissguth AP, Darby BL, Barr HM, Smith JR, Martin DC. Comparison of drinking and smoking patterns during pregnancy over a six-year interval. *Am J Obstet Gynecol*. 1983;145:716–724.
8. Mullen PD. Smoking cessation counseling in prenatal care. In: Merkatz IR, Thompson JE, Mullen PD, Goldenberg RL, eds. *New Perspectives on Prenatal Care*. New York, NY: Elsevier; 1990:161–176.
9. Williamson DF, Serdula MK, Kendrick JS, Binkin NJ. Comparing the prevalence of smoking in pregnant and non-pregnant women, 1985 to 1986. *JAMA*. 1989;261:70–74.
10. Ershoff D, Mullen P, Quinn V. Women who quit smoking at the beginning of pregnancy: clinical implications in identification and relapse prevention. Presented at the 114th Annual Meeting of the American Public Health Association; Oct. 1, 1986; Las Vegas, Nev.
11. Fingerhut LA, Kleinman JC, Kendrick JS. Smoking before, during, and after pregnancy. *Am J Public Health*. 1990;80:541–544.
12. Prager K, Malin H, Spiegler D, VanNatta P, Placek P. Smoking and drinking behavior before and during pregnancy of married mothers of live-born infants and still-born births. *Public Health Rep*. 1984;99:117–127.
13. Baric L, MacArthur C, Sherwood M. A study of health educational aspects of smoking in pregnancy. *Int J Health Educ*. 1976;19(2):1–17.
14. Bauman KE, Bryan ES, Dent CW, Koch GG. The influence of observing carbon monoxide level on cigarette smoking by public prenatal patients. *Am J Public Health*. 1983;73:1089–1091.
15. Burling T, Bigelow G, Robinson C, Mead A. Changes in smoking during pregnancy. Presented at the Society for Behavioral Medicine; 1984; Philadelphia, Pa.
16. Donovan JW. Randomized controlled trial of anti-smoking advice in pregnancy. *Br J Prev Soc Med*. 1977;31:6–12.
17. Ershoff DH, Aaronson NK, Danaher BG, Wasserman FW. Behavioral, health, and cost outcomes of an HMO-based prenatal health education program. *Public Health Rep*. 1983;98:536–547.
18. Ershoff DH, Mullen PD, Quinn VP. A randomized trial of a serialized

self-help smoking cessation program for pregnant women in an HMO. *Am J Public Health.* 1989;79:182–187.

19. Loeb B, Bailey J, Waage G, Feldman V. A randomized trial of smoking intervention during pregnancy. Presented at American Public Health Association Annual Meeting; Nov. 15, 1983; Dallas, Tex.

20. MacArthur C, Newton JR, Knox EG. Effect of anti-smoking health education on fetal size at birth: a randomized clinical trial. *Br J Obstet Gynecol.* 1987;94:295–300.

21. Mayer JP, Hawkins B, Todd R. A randomized evaluation of smoking cessation interventions for pregnant women at a WIC clinic. *Am J Public Health.* 1990;80:76–78.

22. Secker-Walker RH, Flynn BS, Solomon LJ, Collins-Burris L, LePage S, Mead PB. Attitudes, beliefs, and other smokers: factors affecting smoking cessation in pregnancy. Presented at the American Public Health Association; 1986; Las Vegas, Nev.

23. Sexton M, Hebel JR. A clinical trial of change in maternal smoking and its effect on birth weight. *JAMA.* 1984;251:911–915.

24. Windsor RA, Cutter G, Morris J, et al. The effectiveness of smoking cessation methods for smokers in public health maternity clinics: a randomized trial. *Am J Public Health.* 1985;75:1389–1392.

25. Langford ER, Thompson EG, Tripp S. Smoking and education during pregnancy: evaluation of a program for women in prenatal classes. *Can J Public Health.* 1983;74:285–289.

26. Windsor RA, Orleans CT. Guidelines and methodological standards for smoking cessation and intervention research among pregnant women: improving the science and art. *Health Educ Q.* 1986;13:131–161.

27. Windsor RE, Warner KE, Cutter GR. A cost-effectiveness analysis of self-help smoking cessation methods for pregnant women. *Public Health Rep.* 1988;103:83–88.

28. Ershoff DH, Quinn VP, Mullen PD, Lairson DR. Pregnancy and medical cost outcomes of a self-help prenatal smoking cessation program in a HMO. *Public Health Rep.* 1990;105:340–347.

29. Windsor RA, Dalmat ME, Orleans CT, Gritz ER. *Handbook to Plan, Implement, and Evaluate Smoking Cessation Programs for Pregnant Women.* White Plains, NY: March of Dimes Birth Defects Foundation; 1990.

30. Hebel JR, Nowicki P, Sexton M. The effect of antismoking intervention during pregnancy: an assessment of interactions with maternal characteristics. *Am J Epidemiol.* 1985;122:135–148.

31. Fleisher L, Keintz M, Rimer B, Utt M, Workman S, Engstrom PF. Process evaluation of a minimal contact smoking cessation program in an urban nutritional assistance (WIC) program. Philadelphia, Pa: Fox Chase Cancer Center; 1988.

32. Kretzschmar RM. Smoking and health: the role of the obstetrician and gynecologist. *Obstet Gynecol.* 1980;55:403–406.

33. Lux KM. Good health is good business: prenatal health education in the workplace. *Family Commun Health.* 1989;12(3):77–79.

34. King J, Eiser JR. A strategy for counseling pregnant smokers. *Health Educ J.* 1981;40:66–68.

35. Alexander LL. The pregnant smoker: nursing implications. *J Obstet Gynecol Neonatal Nurs.* 1987;16(3):167–173.

36. Householder J. Infants born to narcotic-addicted mothers. *Psychol Bull.* 1982;92:453–468.

37. Jones CL, Lopez RE. Direct and indirect effects on the infant of maternal drug abuse: component report on drug abuse. In: Merkatz IR, Thompson JE, Mullen PD, Goldenberg RL, eds. *New Perspectives on Prenatal Care.* New York, NY: Elsevier; 1988:273–318.

38. Chasnoff IJ, ed. *Drug Use in Pregnancy: Mother and Child.* Norwell, Mass: MTP Press; 1986.

39. Rosett HL, Weiner L, Edelin KC. Treatment experience with pregnant problem drinkers. *JAMA*. 1983;249:2029–2033.
40. Weiner L, Rosett HL, Edelin KC. Alcohol consumption by pregnant women. *Obstet Gynecol*. 1983;61:6–12.
41. Abel EL, Sokol RJ. Maternal and fetal characteristics affecting alcohol's teratogenicity. *Neurobehav Toxicol Teratol*. 1986;8:329–334.
42. National Institute on Drug Abuse. *National Household Survey on Drug Abuse*. Rockville, Md: US Dept of Health and Human Services; 1989.
43. National Association for Perinatal Addiction Research and Education. A first national hospital incidence survey. Press release, 1988.
44. Besharov D. *Testimony Before the US House of Representatives*. Select Committee on Children, Youth, and Families. April 19, 1990.
45. US General Accounting Office. *Drug Exposed Infants: A Generation at Risk*. Washington, DC: GAO; 1990.
46. Illinois Department of Alcoholism and Substance Abuse. *Illinois Women's Needs Assessment for Alcoholism and Substance Abuse Treatment*. Springfield, Ill: IDASA; 1990.
47. Bean X. Overview of neonatal effects in infants exposed to PCP, cocaine, and other drugs. Presented at Conference on Chemical Dependency and Pregnancy; Oct. 25, 1986; San Francisco, Calif.
48. Clement D. Babies in trouble. *Minn Monthly*. 1989;47–51.
49. Reed BG. *Testimony Before the US House of Representatives*. Select Committee on Children, Youth, and Families. April 23, 1990.
50. Smith BV. *Testimony Before the US House of Representatives*. Select Committee on Children, Youth, and Families. May 17, 1990.
51. Walker J. *Testimony Before the US House of Representatives*. Select Committee on Children, Youth, and Families. April 23, 1990.
52. Halfon N. *Testimony Before the US House of Representatives*. Select Committee on Children, Youth, and Families. May 17, 1990.
53. Chavkin W. Drug addiction and pregnancy: policy crossroads. *Am J Public Health*. 1990;80:483–487.
54. Wilson P. *Testimony Before the US House of Representatives*. Select Committee on Children, Youth, and Families. May 17, 1990.
55. US Department of Health and Human Services. *Crack Babies*. Washington, DC: Office of the Inspector General; 1990. Publication OEI-03-89-01540.
56. Smith IE, Lancaster JS, Moss-Wells S, Coles CD, Falek A. Identifying high-risk pregnant drinkers: biological and behavioral correlates of continuous heavy drinking during pregnancy. *J Stud Alcohol*. 1986;48:304–309.
57. Coles CD, Smith IE, Lancaster JS, Falek A. Persistence over the first month of neurobehavioral differences in infants exposed to alcohol prenatally. *Infant Behav Dev*. 1987;10:23–28.
58. Larsson G. Prevention of fetal alcohol effects: an antenatal program for early detection of pregnancies at risk. *Acta Obstet Gynecol Scand*. 1983;62:171–178.
59. Chasnoff IJ, MacGregor SN. Cocaine in pregnancy: trimester abuse pattern and perinatal outcome. *Pediatr Res*. 1988;4:403. Abstract.
60. Little RE, Streissguth AP, Guzinski GM, Grathwohl HL, Blumhagen JM, McIntyre CE. Changes in obstetrician advice following a two-year community educational program on alcohol use and pregnancy. *Am J Obstet Gynecol*. 1983;146:23–28.
61. Moss KL, Paltrow LM, Crockett J. *Testimony Before the US House of Representatives*. Select Committee on Children, Youth, and Families. May 17, 1990.
62. Worthington-Roberts BS, Klerman LV. Maternal nutrition. In: Merkatz IR, Thompson JE, Mullen PD, Goldenberg RL, eds. *New Perspectives on Prenatal Care*. New York, NY: Elsevier; 1990:235–271.
63. US General Accounting Office. *WIC Evaluations Provide Some Favorable*

But No Conclusive Evidence on the Effects Expected for the Special Supplemental Program for Women, Infants and Children. Washington, DC; 1984. GAO/PEMD-84-4.

64. Rush D, Leighton J, Sloan NL, Alvir JM, Garbowski GC. Review of past studies of WIC. *Am J Clin Nutr.* 1988;48:394–411.
65. Kotelchuk M, Schwartz JB, Anderka MT, Finison KS. WIC participation and pregnancy outcomes: Massachusetts statewide evaluation project. *Am J Public Health.* 1984;74:1086–1092.
66. Stockbauer JW. Evaluation of the Missouri WIC program: prenatal components. *J Am Diet Assoc.* 1986;86:61–67.
67. Stockbauer JW. WIC prenatal participation and its relation to pregnancy outcomes in Missouri: a second look. *Am J Public Health.* 1987;77:813–818.
68. Kennedy ET, Gershoff S, Reed R, Austin JE. Evaluation of the effect of WIC supplemental feeding on birthweight. *J Am Diet Assoc.* 1982;80:220–227.
69. Rush D, Alvir JM, Kenny DA, Johnson SS, Horvitz DG. Historical study of pregnancy outcomes. *Am J Clin Nutr.* 1988;48:412–428.
70. Rush D, Leighton J, Sloan NL, et al. Longitudinal study of pregnant women. *Am J Clin Nutr.* 1988;48:439–483.
71. Caan B, Horgen DM, Margen S, King JC, Jewell NP. Benefits associated with WIC supplemental feeding during the interpregnancy interval. *Am J Clin Nutr.* 1987;45:29–41.
72. Rush D. Some comments on the Massachusetts WIC evaluation. *Am J Public Health.* 1984;74:1145–1146.
73. Metcoff J, Costiloe P, Crosby WM, et al. Effect of food supplementation (WIC) during pregnancy on birthweight. *Am J Clin Nutr.* 1985;41:933–947.
74. Kennedy ET, Kotelchuk M. The effect of WIC supplemental feeding on birthweight: a case-control analysis. *Am J Clin Nutr.* 1984;40:579–585.
75. Edozien JC, Switzer BR, Bryan RB. Medical evaluation of the special supplemental food program for women, infants, and children. *Am J Clin Nutr.* 1979;32:677–692.
76. Schramm WF. WIC prenatal participation and its relationship to newborn costs in Missouri: a cost/benefit analysis. *Am J Public Health.* 1985;75:851–857.
77. Schramm WF. Prenatal participation in WIC related to Medicaid costs for Missouri newborns: 1982 update. *Public Health Rep.* 1986;101:607–615.
78. Mathematica Policy Research, Inc. *The Savings in Medicaid Costs for Newborns and Their Mothers from Prenatal Participation in the WIC Program.* Washington, DC: MPRI; 1990.
79. Adams SO, Barr GD, Huenmann RL. Effect of nutritional supplementation in pregnancy, I: outcome of pregnancy. *J Am Diet Assoc.* 1978;72:144–147.
80. Rush D, Stein Z, Susser M. A randomized controlled trial of prenatal nutritional supplementation in New York City. *Pediatrics.* 1980;65:683–697.
81. Higgins AC, Moxley JE, Pencharz PB, Mikolanis D, Dubois S. Impact of the Higgins nutrition intervention program on birthweight: a within mother analysis. *J Am Diet Assoc.* 1989;89:1097–1103.
82. Lechtig A, Habicht J, Delgado H, Klein RE, Yarbrough C, Martorell R. Effect of food supplementation during pregnancy on birthweight. *Pediatrics.* 1975;56:508–520.
83. Rush D. Nutritional services during pregnancy and birthweight: a retrospective matched pair analysis. *Can Med Assoc J.* 1981;125:567–576.
84. Villar J, Rivera J. Nutritional supplementation during two consecutive

pregnancies and the interim lactation period: effect on birthweight. *Pediatrics.* 1978;81:50–57.

85. Orstead C, Arrington D, Kamath SK, Olson R, Kohrs MB. Efficacy of prenatal nutrition counseling: weight gain, infant birthweight, and cost effectiveness. *J Am Diet Assoc.* 1985;85:40–45.

86. Office of Analysis and Evaluation. Food and Nutrition Service. *Estimation of Eligibility for the WIC Program.* Washington, DC: US Dept of Agriculture; 1990.

87. National Commission to Prevent Infant Mortality. *Home Visiting: Opening Doors for America's Pregnant Women and Children.* Washington, DC: NCPIM; 1989.

88. US General Accounting Office. *Home Visiting: A Promising Early Intervention Strategy for At-Risk Families.* Washington, DC: GAO; 1990. GAO-HRD-90-83.

89. Miller C. *Maternal Health and Infant Survival.* Washington, DC: National Center for Clinical Infant Programs; 1987.

90. Wasik B, Roberts R. Home visiting programs for low-income families. *Family Resource Coalition Report, 1989;*1:8–9.

91. National Governors' Association. *MCH Update: State Coverage of Pregnant Women and Children.* Washington, DC: NGA; 1990.

92. Olds D, Henderson C, Tatelbaum R, Chamberlin R. Improving the delivery of prenatal care and outcomes of pregnancy: a randomized trial of nurse home visitation. *Pediatrics.* 1986;77:16–28.

93. Olds D, Henderson C, Tatelbaum R, Chamberlin R. Preventing child abuse and neglect: a randomized trial of nurse home visitation. *Pediatrics.* 1986;78:65–78.

94. Olds D, Henderson C, Tatelbaum R, Chamberlin R. Improving the life-course development of socially disadvantaged mothers: a randomized trial of nurse home visitation. *Am J Public Health.* 1988;78:1436–1445.

95. Heins H Jr, Nance N, Ferguson J. Social support in improving perinatal outcome: the resource mothers program. *Obstet Gynecol.* 1987;70:263–266.

96. Mayer J. Evaluation of maternal and child health community nursing services: application of two quasi-experimental designs. *Health Action Papers.* 1988;2:38–48.

97. Nagy M, Leeper J. The impact of a home visitation program on infant health and development: the rural Alabama pregnancy and infant health program. Presented at the 1988 Annual Meeting of the American Public Health Association; Nov. 16, 1988; Boston, Mass.

98. Field T, Widmayer S, Stringer S, Ignatoff E. Teenage, lower-class, black mothers and their preterm infants: an intervention and developmental follow-up. *Child Dev.* 1980;51:426–436.

99. Larson C. Efficacy of prenatal and postpartum home visits on child health and development. *Pediatrics.* 1980;66:191–197.

100. Hardy J, Street R. Family support and parenting education in the home: an effective extension of clinic-based preventive health care services for poor children. *J Pediatr.* 1989;115:927–931.

101. Grantham-McGregor S, Schofield W, Powell C. Development of severely malnourished children who received psychosocial stimulation: six-year followup. *Pediatrics.* 1987;79:247–254.

102. Ross G. Home intervention for premature infants of low-income families. *Am J Orthopsychiatry.* 1984;54:263–269.

103. Rauh V, Achenbach T, Nurcombe B, Howell C, Teti D. Minimizing adverse effects of low birthweight: four-year results of an early intervention program. *Child Dev.* 1988;59:544–553.

104. Resnick M, Eyler F, Newson R, Eitzman D, Bucciarelli R. Developmental intervention for low birth weight infants: improved early developmental outcomes. *Pediatrics.* 1987;80:68–74.

105. Infant Health and Development Project. Enhancing the outcomes of

low birthweight, premature infants: a multi-site randomized trial. *JAMA*. 1990;263:3035–3070.

106. Dawson P, Van Doorninck W, Robinson J. Effects of home-based, informal social support on child health. Dev Behav Pediatr. 1989;10:63–67.

107. Spencer B, Thomas H, Morris J. A randomized controlled trial of the provision of a social support service during pregnancy: the South Manchester family worker project. *Br J Obstet Gynecol*. 1989;6:281–285.

108. Barth R, Hacking S, Ash J. Preventing child abuse: an experimental evaluation of the child parent enrichment project. *J Primary Prev*. 1988;8:201–207.

109. Olds D, Kitzman H. Can home visitation improve the health of women and children at environmental risk? *Pediatrics*. 1990;86:108–116.

110. Siegel E, Bauman K, Schaefer E, Saunders M, Ingram D. Hospital and home support during infancy: impact on maternal attachment, child abuse and neglect, and health care utilization. *Pediatrics*. 1980;66:183–190.

111. Chamberlin R. Home visiting: a necessary but not in itself sufficient program component for promoting the health and development of families and children. *Pediatrics*. 1989;84:178–180.

112. Powell C, Grantham-McGregor S. Home visiting of varying frequency and child development. *Pediatrics*. 1989;84:157–164.

113. Shonkoff J, Hauser-Cram P. Early intervention for disabled infants and their families: a quantitative analysis. *Pediatrics*. 1987;80:650–658.

114. Halpern R. Lack of effects for home-based early intervention? some possible explanations. *Am J Orthopsychiatry*. 1984;54:33–42.

115. Halpern R. Parent support and education for low-income families: historical and current perspectives. *Child Youth Serv Rev*. 1988;10:283–303.

116. Chapman J, Siegal E, Cross A. Home visitors and child health: analysis of selected programs. *Pediatrics*. 1990;85:1059–1068.

117. Larner M. Lessons from the child survival/fair start home visiting programs. Presented at the 1988 Annual Meeting of the American Public Health Association; Nov. 14, 1988; Boston, Mass.

118. US Dept of Health and Human Services. Office of the Inspector General. *Evaluation of the Boston Healthy Baby Program*. Washington, DC: DHHS; 1989.

119. Larner M, Halpern R. Lay home visiting programs: strengths, tensions, and challenges. *Zero to Three*. 1987;8:1–7.

120. Halpern R. Home-based early intervention: dimensions of current practice. *Child Welfare*. 1986;65:387–398.

121. Hornick J, Clarke M. A cost-effectiveness evaluation of lay therapy treatment for child abusing and high risk parents. *Child Abuse Neglect*. 1986;10:309–318.

122. US General Accounting Office. *Prenatal Care: Medicaid Recipients and Uninsured Women Obtain Insufficient Care*. Washington, DC: GAO; 1987. GAO/HRD-87-137.

Section 3

Maternity and Infant Care 1990: A Decade of Decline

A basic theme of this book is that pregnant women and infants do not receive adequate amounts of health care and that the care they receive is not tailored to individual risk and need. This section develops this theme more fully by first quantifying the extent of the problem—a necessary first step in taking corrective action.

Charles Johnson presents data on the number of pregnant women not receiving sufficient prenatal care and describes some of the analytic hurdles that must be overcome in arriving at useful estimates of unmet need. A parallel piece by Donald Schiff describes the consequences of inadequate health care for infants.

Sarah Brown and George Ryan discuss the reasons why both pregnant women and infants receive insufficient care. These "barriers" are numerous and vary from place to place, but the authors stress that the financial barrier—or the absence of Medicaid, in the case of very low-income people—is the most pervasive and potent.

One increasingly significant barrier to care for pregnant women is the inadequate number and poor distribution of obstetricians and other obstetric care providers serving poor women. Lorraine Klerman and Sarah Hudson Scholle discuss this growing problem and include an important section on poor provider participation in Medicaid and on the obstetrical malpractice conundrum.

Finally, Samuel Flint and Rachel Gold analyze the shortcomings of private insurance for financing needed obstetric and pediatric services. This chapter is particularly important given the numerous health care reform proposals currently on the table that rely heavily on employer-based private insurance.

CHAPTER 6

Projecting Unmet Need for Prenatal Care

Charles D. Johnson, PhD

Infant mortality and morbidity is widely recognized as a significant problem in the United States. Each year approximately 40 000 infants born here die before their first birthday. This rate of 10.1 deaths per 1000 live births places the United States in a tie for last place among the top 20 industrialized nations,[1] a startling drop from the sixth-place position it held from 1950 to 1955. White infant death rates are higher in the United States than among the populations of other countries such as Singapore, Belgium, Sweden, and Hong Kong, and Black infants die at nearly twice the rate of White infants. The Black infant mortality rate of 17.9 deaths per 1000 live births in 1987 is almost double the surgeon general's goal of 9 by 1990.[2] These statistics reflect the increasing criticality of the problem, although the United States spends more of its gross national product on health care than any other nation in the world.[3]

Infant mortality can be viewed as a fundamental metric of the health of a nation;[4] as such, it is a grim barometer of a population's access to basic preventive care of all types. Yankauer[5] contends that the disparity between Black and White infant mortality rates in the past four decades provides, as clearly as any social history book, essential insight into the social order of our society. Infant mortality is an inescapable bottom line that cannot be altered by persuasive arguments or chic social theories. It responds only to actual changes in the well-being of infants and pregnant women.

The reduction in infant deaths from 32.2 per 1000 live births in 1947[6] to 10.1 in 1987 is obviously cause for some optimism. However, because this decline was primarily due to technological advances such as the advent of antibiotics in the 1940s, which reduced postneonatal mortality, and to reductions in neonatal deaths through neonatal intensive care[5] rather than to any fundamental improvement in primary prevention, our self-congratulations should be tempered with caution.

The United States' continued reliance on technological breakthroughs, although low-cost, well-understood health care alternatives are being practiced around the world, bespeaks something less admirable than devotion to scientific achievement. Like all effective, bottom-line benchmarks, infant mortality stirs the public health field to action by challenging professional folklore and forcing researchers to ground assumptions about health care delivery in empirical fact. Clearly, infant mortality as an indication of adequacy of maternity care has been the driving force behind the increased attention on maternal and infant health in the past decade.

... the disparity between Black and White infant mortality rates ... provides ... essential insight into the social order of our society.

A 1987 study by the General Accounting Office (GAO) reported that low birthweight (LBW) infants are 40 times more likely to die during the first 4 weeks of life than normal-birthweight infants. Further, two thirds of infant deaths during the first 4 weeks of life and half of deaths in the first year are attributable to LBW.

Recent evidence of a slight increase in very low birthweight infants (ie, less than 1500 grams) has been cause for particular alarm. This increase is due in part to the onslaught of drug abuse in American society. Although the rise in LBW attributable to drug abuse is most marked among urban Black populations,[7] White women are evidencing similar problems. In New York City, birth certificate data reveal a threefold increase in the number of drug-using mothers from 1981 to 1987.[8] The prevalence of cocaine use is especially troublesome because some evidence indicates that cocaine may precipitate premature delivery and LBW.[9] A recent GAO study[10] reported twice the incidence of LBW (2500 grams) among drug-exposed infants. At four large city hospitals the rate of LBW infants ranged from 25% to 31% among drug-using women and from 4% to 11% for low-income women not identified as using drugs.

The efficacy of prenatal care for preventing LBW is covered in detail in other chapters and is not extensively discussed here except for a comment that the role of prenatal care in preventing LBW has been well documented.[11] For example, the Office of Technology Assessment reviewed evidence of the effectiveness of prenatal care in reducing LBW and neonatal mortality.[12] In the multivariate studies in which maternal demographics and medical risk were controlled, 18 of 21 studies reported positive effects for infant birthweight attributable to prenatal care. Similarly, of 15 controlled studies of neonatal mortality, 11 found a significant reduction in neonatal mortality among women receiving appropriate prenatal care.

Despite the obvious link between LBW and inadequate prenatal care, one third of pregnant women in the United States do not receive sufficient care.[13] Recently, considerable attention has focused on pinpointing the reasons why (see chapter 8). Although in certain instances an array of variables can be influential, available evidence indicates that income serves as the most powerful determinant of difficulties in accessing prenatal care.[14,15] Although it is feasible to focus needs assessments on nonfinancial barriers to access, and many nonfinancial variables may indeed affect individual access to prenatal care, the widespread predominance of financial barriers makes income the central variable in most such efforts. Given this predominance and the centrality of income as an eligibility determinant for publicly funded services, this discussion primarily reviews needs assessment efforts that focus on income as a barrier.

One of the first questions to arise in discussions of expanding access to maternity care concerns information on the size, salient characteristics, and geographic distribution of the population of women in need. Clearly, the number of women eligible for contemplated services has primary implications for costs and the range of maternity services that might be included in a new programming effort. In *The Forward Plan: Maternal and Child Health 1984–1989*,[16] federal Maternal and Child Health (MCH) leaders emphasized "needs assessment and identification of populations, areas and localities requiring assistance." The direct influence of state and local government in making resource allocation decisions has grown as a result of the MCH Block Grant legislation (Pub L No. 97-35, Title V), which requires states to submit a report describing the population and geographic localities identified as in need of such services. State public health policymakers are now compelled to document in some fashion the problems of women requiring maternity services, thus prompting widespread interest in needs assessment.[17]

IMPORTANCE OF NEEDS ASSESSMENT

Unfortunately, the scientific work of identifying women who are in need of maternity services does not occur dispassionately. Maternal and infant health advocates, in their efforts to sway the undecided, sometimes incorrectly present infant mortality and morbidity as a kind of societal flat tire (ie, a critical impediment to progress, but one that is easily understood and quickly repaired with known remedies). Predictably, their estimates of numbers in need of services are large enough to demand action but small enough to avoid attracting the attention of the guardians of cost containment.

On the other hand, opponents of an expanded government role in ensuring the availability of maternity services frequently advance two counterassertions: (1) There is no unmet need, and hence no need for additional services. (2) Broadened coverage will most certainly unleash an insurmountable demand resulting from a bottomless pit of need. Such incongruities suggest that needs projections are merely a forum for expressing political perspectives. In short, what people have to say about the number of women in need of maternity services often derives more from their political views than from scientific data.

There are two types of data-based strategies for determining needs: secondary data analysis and direct survey techniques. The relative strengths and weaknesses of both are examined in this section.

NEEDS ASSESSMENT METHODS

Secondary Analysis of Social Indicator Data in Needs Assessment

Social indicators such as vital statistics and census data have traditionally been the primary data bases for assessing population health needs.

In the area of maternal and child health services, these data bases necessitate almost universal reliance on secondary analysis. Researchers in maternal and child health planning do not typically collect data to estimate numbers of people in need, but rather use existing data sets that have been assembled for other purposes. As a result, the methodologic emphasis is generally on statistical manipulation rather than on data collection procedures.

The strengths of this approach include widespread availability, populationwide coverage, and low-cost access to information. A major disadvantage of relying on social indicators is that data may not be sufficiently timely to provide a surveillance function. In addition, because social indicator data of the type gathered in the census are not focused directly on maternal and infant health issues, much of the creative energy evident in the literature is directed toward coaxing data sets to answer questions they were not designed to answer.

Klerman and Rosenbach[18] discussed combining different social indicators in MCH planning. Drawing on a content analysis of state block grant applications, they discussed and illustrated techniques for ranking localities by combining different data sources with standardized scores, weighted scores, and factor analytic techniques.

Researchers can project need for specific services by combining datasets that were created for disparate reasons (eg, insurance data and vital statistics). Such projections must be interpreted with caution, however, because they often rest on strong assumptions about pieces of information that are inevitably missing. That different, or at least unconnected, individual records are represented in the combined data sets precludes most cross-tabulations. Further, lack of information on some critical variable (such as income information) may limit the value of the data base for assessing unmet need or estimating the numbers of people who are eligible for a proposed program.

Proxy variables. Payne and Strobino[19] suggested that education could serve as a proxy for the income information that was not recorded on the birth certificate. Because many states record mother's education, this proxy variable has substantial appeal. Payne and Strobino found a correlation of approximately $r = .60$ between education and income for samples of women drawn from Mississippi and Maryland. This approach is limited by the fact that it provides only an estimate of the total population of women who require maternity services; what proportion of that population is having difficulty accessing care is unknown. Payne and Strobino cautioned that applying population relationships to estimating the need for prenatal care requires a critical assumption: that proportions characteristic of the total population are also accurate for the subgroup that is in need of health care services. A further difficulty is that the correlation between education and income for maternity cases may not be as high as noted in the Payne and Strobino study. A 10-state survey[20] of more than 13 000 postpartum women noted that correlations between education and income across participating states were often in the .30's (overall $r = .42$), which decreases the value of education as a proxy for income.

Some states, most notably Massachusetts, are remedying this problem by recording income-related information on the birth certificate. The "payor for delivery" will be included in future Massachusetts vital statistics records. Because not all eligible people are enrolled in Medicaid, this information would not provide a direct measure of income, but it would be useful in projecting numbers of mothers and infants at various poverty levels. The information might be even more useful in monitoring adequacy of care received by Medicaid recipients, because the birth record also has information on prenatal visits and trimester of initiating care.

... 100 000 births per year involved late or no prenatal care.

Social area analysis. Guyer and colleagues[21] used social area analysis to determine need for MCH services in Massachusetts by combining information on birth outcome with poverty data. Based on social indicator data, Guyer created two need indices for each county in Massachusetts. The first index, called the health indicator score, combined (1) LBW, (2) the adolescent pregnancy rate, and (3) the neonatal mortality rate. The second index, called the poverty indicator score, included (1) the percentage of population below poverty level and (2) the unemployment rate. Values for these variables were derived from several archival data sources, including census, vital health statistics, and Department of Labor data bases. These analyses were reported to be helpful in allocating funds more adequately to high-need areas in the state. Social area analysis is subject to what has been termed the ecological fallacy,[22] which draws attention to the fact that relationships among variables at higher levels of aggregation may not hold at lower levels. The key to the ecological fallacy is that it is impossible to reconstruct any individual from multiple data sets. Thus, although it may be true that the average family has 2.4 children and 1.5 automobiles, it is unlikely that any particular family would match this description.

Absence of care. One clear indication of unmet need is the number of women who receive undeniably inadequate prenatal care. One routinely collected vital statistics variable is whether the mother received no prenatal care. Focusing on official records such as those of women who received little or no care establishes a lower boundary on the number of women in need, because it represents those women who experience the worst access problems. This approach is comparable to estimating the number of illiterates, or those with less than an elementary school education, as a measure of the effectiveness of public education. That is, only total failures are enumerated.

Singh et al[23] addressed unmet need for prenatal care at the national level through an analysis of the 1980 National Natality Survey, a survey based on a probability sample of all births. The survey method involves selecting a sample of birth certificates, interviewing mothers, and examining medical records. Estimates from the survey data base indicated that 100 000 births per year involved late or no prenatal care. Women who received no prenatal care are generally viewed as the most extreme cases among women who need maternity services, but one answer to the question how many women receive inadequate care is 100 000 per year.

As a measure of access to care, late entry into care is generally regarded as more adequate than no prenatal care. Prenatal care initiated beyond the first trimester of pregnancy is considered late. Table 6-1 summarizes data on the timing of prenatal care.[24] The numbers and rates are for all women, regardless of race, and thus they summarize overall need for earlier care. Black women are approximately twice as likely as White women to enter care after the first trimester of pregnancy.

TABLE 6-1
Month of Pregnancy in Which Prenatal Care Was Begun, 1985[23]

Age	Month Care Begun (no.)				Unknown (no.)	Total (no.)
	1–3	4–6	7–9	None		
Under 19	248 270	159 356	40 527	15 987	13 565	477 705
	(51.97%)	(33.36%)	(8.48%)	(3.35%)	(2.84%)	(100%)
20–29	1 777 546	392 658	85 982	35 399	51 085	2 342 670
	(75.88%)	(16.76%)	(3.67%)	(1.51%)	(2.18%)	(100%)
30–39	755 232	105 767	20 739	9 363	19 589	910 690
	(82.93%)	(11.61%)	(2.28%)	(1.03%)	(2.15%)	(100%)
40+	20 849	5669	1367	718	893	29 496
	(70.68%)	(19.22%)	(4.63%)	(2.43%)	(3.03%)	(100%)
Total	2 801 897	663 450	148 615	61 467	85 132	3 760 561
	(74.51%)	(17.64%)	(3.95%)	(1.63%)	(2.26%)	(100%)

Financing maternity care. Gold et al[25] in a 1987 report published by the Alan Guttmacher Institute (AGI) address the general issue of financing maternity services in the United States. Drawing on insurance and Medicaid data bases, the report documents several important trends:

- The proportion of families without health insurance is increasing.
- Nearly 15 million women of reproductive age are not covered by private or public insurance.
- One third of mothers get insufficient pregnancy care.
- Maternity and newborn care represent 27% ($2 billion) of unpaid hospital bills.
- The average bill for having a baby constitutes one fifth of a typical young couple's annual income.

The rate of inadequate care was highest among the unmarried (58%), teenagers (56%), Blacks (51%), least educated (53%), and poor married women (47%).

Estimating Newly Eligible Women Under Medicaid

It is not surprising that several recent research efforts have focused on the consequences of expanding Medicaid to serve more women. The number of women who would be newly eligible can be combined with Medicaid reimbursement rates to estimate program costs. In an early effort to arrive at cost estimates of possible Medicaid expansions, the Congressional Budget Office (CBO) developed estimates of newly eligible women up to 150% of poverty.[26] The CBO study drew on the Current Population Survey (CPS) and projections were based on calculations of national fertility rates by income strata. The technique was to estimate the number of women between ages 15 and 44 who were below various poverty cutoffs but not eligible for Aid for Families With Dependent Children (AFDC), which at that time would have precluded Medicaid eligibility. AFDC eligibility criteria varied by state, and these state-level figures were factored into the calculations. Other fine-tuning involved eliminating women who might already qualify for state-level assistance under programs for the medically needy.

More recently,[27] successive reports were prepared by the National Governors' Association (NGA), which, like the CBO study, used the CPS data to arrive at the number of women aged 15 to 44 who were below 100% of poverty. The NGA reports added the refinement of state-specific fertility rates and a subsequent report extended estimates of newly eligibles to 185% of poverty. Numbers of uninsured women who would be eligible for expanded Medicaid coverage at 100% and 185% of poverty totaled 327 827 and 857 203, respectively. These figures represent estimates of women below the specified poverty levels who are not currently on Medicaid. The number among them who may have private insurance is unknown.

Torres and Kenney's study. The study conducted by Torres and Kenney,[13] the most ambitious effort to estimate national need figures, draws on the NGA[27] methodology and extends the needs assessment methodology developed by the AGI for estimating need for family planning services. Although others[28,29] have used multiple and linked data bases for establishing estimates of need, this study provides the best overall national estimate of the number of women in need of maternity services.

Torres and Kenney, augmenting the methodology of the NGA study with fertility by poverty status and more recent CPS data, estimated that if all states extended Medicaid coverage to pregnant women at 100% of poverty, 361 000 newly eligibles would result (see Table 6-2). An expansion to a 185% guideline as allowed by the Omnibus Budget Reconciliation Act of 1987 (OBRA 1987) would add 552 000 more for a total of 913 000 women who would be newly eligible for Medicaid-financed prenatal care. These women would be of two types: those who are under the new poverty ceiling and are uninsured and those who are insured but have no maternity coverage. Uninsured women repre-

TABLE 6-2
Torres and Kenney[13] Need Estimates, in Thousands

State	100% of Poverty		185% of Poverty	
	Total Eligible	Total Uninsured	Total Eligible	Total Uninsured
United States	361	230	913	391
Alabama	10	6	23	9
Alaska	1	1	2	1
Arizona	9	5	18	8
Arkansas	6	5	14	7
California	41	28	96	48
Colorado	5	3	12	5
Connecticut	1	1	6	2
Delaware	1	1	2	1
District of Columbia	1	1	2	1
Florida	19	13	48	23
Georgia	10	6	23	9
Hawaii	2	1	4	1
Idaho	3	2	7	3
Illinois	14	8	37	14
Indiana	9	5	22	9
Iowa	5	3	12	4
Kansas	5	3	11	4
Kentucky	7	5	18	8
Louisiana	13	9	28	14
Maine	1	1	4	1
Maryland	4	2	11	5
Massachusetts	4	2	11	4
Michigan	10	6	26	10
Minnesota	5	2	15	4
Mississippi	8	6	18	8
Missouri	7	5	19	8
Montana	2	1	5	2
Nebraska	3	1	8	2
Nevada	1	1	4	2
New Hampshire	1	1	2	1
New Jersey	5	3	14	5
New Mexico	5	3	10	5
New York	17	11	51	21
North Carolina	10	6	25	10
North Dakota	2	1	4	1

TABLE 6-2 (cont.)
Torres and Kenney[13] Need Estimates, in Thousands

State	100% of Poverty		185% of Poverty	
	Total Eligible	Total Uninsured	Total Eligible	Total Uninsured
Ohio	12	7	35	13
Oklahoma	7	5	15	8
Oregon	5	3	12	5
Pennsylvania	10	6	32	11
Rhode Island	1	1	2	1
South Carolina	5	3	14	6
South Dakota	2	1	4	2
Tennessee	8	5	21	9
Texas	41	29	92	46
Utah	5	3	13	4
Vermont	1	1	2	1
Virginia	6	4	17	7
Washington	6	4	14	6
West Virginia	3	2	9	4
Wisconsin	5	3	16	5
Wyoming	1	1	3	1

sent the additional Medicaid cases under an expansion. National estimates of the number of women who are uninsured, and therefore in need, were 230 000 at 100% of poverty and 391 000 at 185%. On a state level, case loads would grow by fewer than 4000 annually in 18 states and up to 41 000 in California and Texas. The total number of births covered by Medicaid would be 1 to 1.5 million births nationwide. The critical parameter on which this estimate is based is that approximately 24% of the 3.8 million women who give birth each year were assumed to be below 185% of poverty and uninsured. According to Torres and Kenney, approximately 26% of all women of reproductive age had no medical insurance, 64% had insurance coverage, and about 10% were under Medicaid in January 1989.

Although Torres and Kenney relied on the same CPS data base, they arrived at 10% higher estimates of potentially eligible women than the NGA study. The reasons for this difference may be the somewhat different array of fertility multipliers, assumptions, and updated data they used. Because it is the most comprehensive study available for estimating national need, it may be useful to review the complex steps in the methodology:

1. Based on the recent interest in OBRA expansions to 100% and 185% of poverty, the first step was to calculate the number of women below

100% and 185% of poverty. The authors used CPS data from the period 1985 to 1987 to arrive at average state proportions for these groups, which were applied to state-level 1985 figures "obtained from the commercial firm Market Statistics; the results were adjusted to agree with national population projections by the Bureau of the Census."[13] (p21)

2. This total number of potentially eligible women was reduced by selecting only that proportion of women in the CPS with no insurance and with private insurance who would be candidates for the new Medicaid program.

3. To estimate the number of pregnant women in each poverty group by state, the number of children younger than 1 year was used to compute fertility rates by national poverty status.

4. Because the state-level data for the CPS involved too few infants to yield reliable estimates, state-specific rates were adjusted by the national fertility rate (identified in step 3) for women at each level of poverty.

5. The state estimates were further adjusted to exclude an estimated number of women who, although they are uninsured publicly or privately, become covered by Medicaid as a result of pregnancy.

6. Cost figures derived from Kenney et al[30] survey of state Medicaid agencies to determine state hospital reimbursement schedules were used to project program costs under 100% and 185% of poverty.

The overall federal and state expenditures to provide maternity and newborn care to newly eligible women below 100% of poverty were estimated at $654 million annually; another $658 million was required at 185%, for a total of $1.312 billion at current levels of Medicaid reimbursement. Table 6-2 presents overall and state-level projections of the numbers in need at 100% and 185% percent of poverty.

Caution must be exercised in adopting these projections, however, particularly at the state level. As the earlier NGA[27] study pointed out, CPS data are intended to be representative of national, not state, population figures. For example, only 7 states in the CPS are represented by as many as 500 respondents, and 16 states are represented by fewer than 200. Their limited state-level representation in the CPS makes the specific projections for many states—including Connecticut, Delaware, Hawaii, Kansas, Minnesota, and Washington—rather questionable.

Direct Surveys

As an alternative to secondary analysis of social indicator data, some researchers have implemented direct surveys of need for maternity services. Direct survey techniques for assessing need, although quite common in other social problem areas, are relatively less frequent in the maternal and child health area. Important social problems (education, unemployment, workers' compensation, drug use, etc) generally have reporting systems and resultant data bases directly related to policy and corrective action. Survey-based needs assessments allow investigators to select variables that directly reflect identified goals. Unlike social indicator strategies, assessment is immediate rather than historical and can include all variables of concern that may affect eligibility and geographic distribution of need. In addition to numbers, surveys can identify special characteristics of newly eligible women that can effectively guide outreach and enrollment efforts. The relative strengths of social indicators and direct survey approaches to need assessments are summarized in Table 6-3.

Direct surveys of need are nevertheless rare, perhaps because of the cost and effort required and because they rely on samples rather than on the entire population.[31] Data bases such as the national census and vital statistics offer a stability not found in samples. The possibility always exists that the sample may be unrepresentative of the larger population. Survey researchers must contend with estimates of sampling error and confidence intervals, whereas population-level researchers need have no such concerns.

Successful Implementations of Direct Survey Methodology for Need Assessments of Maternity Care

There are many state-level examples of successful implementations of survey methodology for assessing need for maternity care, although only a few illustrative examples can be cited here. Sullivan and

---

TABLE 6-3
Relative Strengths of Social Indicator and Direct Survey Methods

	Survey Approach	**Social Indicator Approach**
Unit of analysis	Individual; ability to aggregate	Typically at higher level aggregation: census tract, minor civil division, county, SMSA, state
Measurement error	Self-report	Self-report
Validity/representativeness	Sample representativeness needs to be documented	Population is represented
Timeliness	Typically short turnaround	Typically lengthy turnaround
Data element selection	Great deal of flexibility	Limited flexibility; use of proxies
Cost	Moderate	Low
Data collection responsibility	MCH personnel	Other professionals
Effort	High	Low

Beeman[32] conducted a mail survey of women who had been identified through Arizona vital statistics records to determine their satisfaction with the prenatal care they received. The Illinois Department of Health,[33] also working with vital statistics records, similarly surveyed women who had received inadequate prenatal care. Approximately 29% of 16 224 women responded to the Illinois survey and indicated that their chief reasons for not receiving care were lack of funds, difficulty finding a provider, belief that care was unimportant, and lack of transportation. Oregon was one of the first states to survey maternity patients[34] for the purpose of identifying women in need. This study, like the Arizona and Illinois projects, relied on a sample drawn from vital statistics records.

The primary focus of the PRAMS is on maternal risk behaviors.

Pregnancy Risk Assessment Monitoring System (PRAMS). In a recent application of survey methodology, the PRAMS[35] began collecting data in August 1988 under the direction of the Centers for Disease Control (CDC). The PRAMS is a continuing study of women in six states—Alaska, Indiana, Maine, Michigan, Oklahoma, and West Virginia—and the District of Columbia. Samples ranging from 1200 to 3000 per year are selected from birth certificate records in each state. The primary method is mail surveys augmented by telephone follow-up for nonresponders. Large high-risk populations that might be less likely to respond to mail surveys are monitored through hospital records and in-hospital interviews. Core questions are augmented by state-specific questions on issues of local interest.

The primary focus of the PRAMS is on maternal risk behaviors. The system description points out that infant mortality is related to "maternal behaviors including smoking, drug and alcohol abuse, and failure to fully use prenatal and pediatric care." Thus, the primary emphasis of this CDC surveillance system is on maternal behaviors that negatively affect pregnancy outcome. This approach is much in the CDC tradition of monitoring behavioral risk factors in the population.

Although several studies indicate that individual factors (eg, drug use, disbelief in the value of care) account for fewer of the causal factors in inadequate care than system obstacles (eg, financial barriers, transportation), the PRAMS system is nonetheless a good example of a state-level surveillance system. Although the states have the option of including questions on barriers to access, income, and other issues beyond patient choice, there is no assurance that they will collect this information consistently. In addition, the manner in which income information is collected prohibits the calculation of poverty levels, thus limiting its value as a means for calculating eligibility for new programs.

The PRAMS does, however, have the important virtue of permitting centralized aggregation of information and a sufficient number of common data elements across states to permit broader level analyses.

Although only six states are currently involved, the PRAMS model has the potential for providing state, regional, and national surveillance information. Changes needed in the model to achieve this potential are broader state participation, sufficient funding to enhance state-level capacity for participation, greater focus on barriers to access, and improved information on respondent income.

Hospital-Based Obstetric Surveys. Blakely and Johnson[36] conducted an early effort to use direct survey data to identify those who needed maternity services in Michigan. Their selection of the direct survey approach resulted from a need to provide the state legislature with information on women who would qualify for a state-sponsored program aimed at women below 185% of poverty who had no third-party source of payment. Best estimates based on previous vital statistics and Medicaid data ranged from 2000 to 35 000 women. A sample based on vital statistics records would have been 2 years old and would have required a mail survey with an anticipated return rate of 30% or less.

The method that was finally adopted called for a 2% sample of all births in Michigan. Postpartum women were surveyed by hospital personnel while they remained in the obstetrical units. The hospital participation rate was 95% and the patient participation rate was 89% for the 1-week sampling window. The representativeness of the 1879 responding women was verified by examining sample proportions of various descriptors (eg, age, race, number of prenatal visits) against the most recent population values for the past year from vital statistics.

As a result of the Michigan obstetric survey, approximately 7.2% of the Michigan population of pregnant women were identified as being in need of assistance in obtaining prenatal care. The legislature implemented the state-funded Prenatal Postpartum Care (PPC) program, specifically targeting the 10 000 women in need statewide. County need figures were established by defining three regional need figures based on population size, and by using the appropriate regional percentage-in-need figure as a multiplier of the county's projected number of births for the following year.

Two years after the Blakely and Johnson survey, the Michigan obstetric survey was replicated.[37] Because of an improved economy, the number of women in need had narrowed to 7%, but virtually all the points of comparison between the first and second administrations were successfully replicated. As part of the PPC program, the Michigan legislature required the state health department to report on the status of Michigan's pregnant women every 2 years.

Ongoing surveys can be responsive to dynamic state-level situations that are often undetectable in archival data bases. For example, during 2 years beginning in 1979 a single Michigan insurance carrier, Michi-

gan Blue Cross and Blue Shield, lost 550 000 subscribers. It was not until 1983, however, after a 1981 increase in infant mortality, that Michigan's MCH data system of linked birth-death records sounded an
alarm. Although the Michigan vital statistics data system was as technologically current and as responsive as any other state's system, it
simply could not detect service deficits until they were reflected in post
hoc body counts.

In response to the unavailability of timely information on access to
care, and because of its earlier successes with direct surveys, Michigan
implemented a statewide prenatal health care survey[38] of access to care.
In vivid contrast to the delayed detection of problems in the 1981 to
1983 era, Michigan's 1989 survey[39] identified 15 Michigan obstetric
units that had closed since 1986 as well as the reasons (some had more
than one) for closing (ie, lack of obstetric providers, n = 6; decline in
patient demand, n = 5; hospital mergers, n = 4; nursing shortage,
n = 2). These closures were unrecognized by existing recording systems
in that time period.

By surveying at 2-year intervals, Michigan has established a low-cost
($17 per respondent), statewide surveillance system focused on the
health of women and infants that can identify developing access problems early enough to permit corrective action. Because the nationwide
focus for service delivery has shifted away from state health departments and toward Medicaid,[39] it will be interesting to note whether
the Michigan Health Department will maintain its watchdog function
for maternity services.

Multi-state Study of Need for Prenatal Care. In a report employing much the same methods as the Michigan surveys, Mayer et al[40] reported the results of 10 state-level surveys of obstetric patients. As in
the Michigan surveys, women responded while they were postpartum
patients but still in the hospital. The 10 states involved in this MCH
Special Project of Regional and National Significance (SPRANS) accounted
for 38% of all births nationally. The SPRANS project primarily involved
providing technical assistance to state MCH personnel in devising and
conducting state-level obstetric surveys. Participating states were Arizona, California, Michigan, New Mexico, New York, Oklahoma, Oregon, Rhode Island, South Carolina, and Texas. Individual sampling
frames aimed at ± 3% measurement error were devised for each state.
Comparisons of sample and population parameters (drawn from the
most recent annual vital statistics report) were conducted on variables
such as maternal characteristics (eg, age, race, education); service variables (eg, number of visits, trimester in which care began); and birth
outcomes (eg, birthweight) to determine sample representativeness for
each state. On the basis of available evidence, the samples appeared to
be representative of women giving birth in these states.

Across the 10 states approximately 13 000 women from 883 hospitals
reported on the prenatal care they received and how they paid for it.

Although the states were free to include questions about local concerns in their surveys, each state included the same 17 core items related to prenatal care, source of payment for prenatal care, and income level of the women. The result was a state-level focus on issues of immediate concern, as well as a multistate data base specifically designed to answer the question How do women pay for prenatal care and delivery?

Need figures were calculated on the basis of each state's percentage of women who were living below various poverty cutoffs and were uninsured for maternity services. These percentages were multiplied by the predicted number of births for the coming year to arrive at the projected number of low-income women in need of maternity care. Each state's need figure was based on several parameters, including the state birthrate, relative fertility of low-income women, extent of insurance coverage for maternity cases, current Medicaid ceiling for maternity cases, and other programs offering perinatal services to low-income women. In brief, states with an abundance of pregnant low-income women, stringent Medicaid eligibility, relatively low rates of private insurance coverage, and few state-funded programs have the highest need figures.

... states may be well served politically by beginning to establish their own need figures ...

Mayer et al found the following two points most noteworthy:
- State MCH personnel were completely capable, with technical assistance, of implementing a valid needs assessment of their obstetric populations.
- Those in need and their specific access problems varied across states, suggesting that sweeping assertions regarding national needs may mask state-level problems and solutions. For example, the conventional wisdom that those most in need are minorities, at the lowest end of the income spectrum, and younger than 16 is not universally true. In Oregon, women who were just below the Medicaid eligibility cutoff were more likely to receive inadequate care than those at the lowest income levels. Women who had no insurance in Texas were more likely to have LBW infants than Medicaid mothers. In Oklahoma neither age nor race was predictive of inadequate care.

Comparative Need Estimates from Social Indicators and Direct Surveys

In congressional testimony based on the Mayer et al data, Johnson et al[41] reported that approximately 152 000 women across the 10 states were living in poverty (ie, below 100% level) and had neither Medicaid nor private insurance to pay for prenatal care. The comparable figure at 185% of poverty totaled 230 000 for the 10 states in 1987. Table 6-4 presents the comparable state-by-state figures from the Mayer et al study and the Torres and Kenney[13] national study. The figures are similar for Michigan, New Mexico, New York, Oklahoma, Oregon, and Rhode Island. Differences in need are mainly in the direction of higher need figures from the state surveys.

TABLE 6-4
Comparative Need Figures for Two Large-Scale Studies

State	Torres[13] (100%)	Mayer[40] (100%)	Torres[13] (185%)	Mayer[40] (185%)	CPS Sample Size*	Mayer Sample Size
Arizona	5000	8724	8000	13 650	228	892
California	28 000	53 245	48 000	87 289	1745	2085
Michigan	6000	5770	10 000	9608	736	1892
New Mexico	3000	5047	5000	8228	391	331
New York	11 000	9342	21 000	17 643	1471	2031
Oklahoma	5000	3980	8000	6352	242	797
Oregon	3000	2130	5000	4790	208	1042
Rhode Island	500	203	1000	585	142	537
South Carolina	3000	5189	6000	10 238	206	1076
Texas	29 000	58 331	46 000	71 792	1135	2032
Totals	93 250	151 961	158 000	230 175	6504	12 715

* Sample sizes are drawn from NGA 1987.[42]

For California and Texas, Mayer's estimates are dramatically larger than the Torres and Kenney estimates. That California and Texas evidence the greatest discrepancy is noteworthy, because these two states have the greatest number of low-income people in the nation and underestimates of need therefore reflect the greatest negative consequences for pregnant women. In both states, Medicaid expansion has proceeded on the basis of the state-developed number, which is the safer course. Overall, the Mayer et al direct survey data produced need estimates for Texas and California that are approximately 50% higher than those of Torres and Kenney.

In the near future an empirical answer will resolve the issue, because the state surveys suggest that more than 50% more women are eligible than the Torres and Kenney projections indicate. Rapid new enrollments approaching the total number that Torres and Kenney predicted in need would provide evidence that their estimates are too low, at least for California and Texas, because Medicaid is extremely unlikely to reach 100% of eligibles. Prottas,[43] in examining 23 studies of the client "cost" of so-called free services, found that organizational impediments generally operate to keep participation rates below 50% of eligible participants. With this point in mind, the observation of new Medicaid enrollments of about 45% to 60% of the Torres and Kenney estimates would increase our confidence in those need figures. In any case, states may be well served politically by beginning to establish their own need figures so that they have a frame of reference for evaluating numbers in need assigned to them from outside.

Although the Torres and Kenney and the Mayer et al studies are not to- tally consistent in their findings, they make the same point in regard to MCH policy. The number of women in need of expanded maternity services is significantly large to warrant alarm but small enough to be effectively served. The estimated numbers of women with neither Med- icaid nor private insurance range from 230 000 to 340 000 at 100% of poverty and 391 000 to 580 000 at 185%. Even if the Torres and Kenney data underestimate the number in need by as much as 50%, evidence arrived at by different methods indicates that serving unmet need for maternity services is a feasible undertaking.

It may be most productive for researchers and needs assessment inves- tigators to focus now on assisting states in developing MCH data sys- tems that are more powerful protectors of the health needs of mothers and infants than existing schemes. In the face of competing issues, po- litical support may erode, states may weary of increased Medicaid ex- penditures (even with the federal match) and, in the absence of effec- tive surveillance systems that specifically target mothers and infants, maternity services will be convenient targets for cuts. Infant mortality is a long-term issue, not a momentary crisis. It reflects basic anomalies in US society.

The slow emergence of the identification of the infant mortality prob- lem stands in mute testimony as an indictment of MCH data systems. The epidemiologic tradition of post hoc sifting through historical records is the basic MCH model, and vital statistics data including matched birth-death records have been extensively referenced in the identification of infant mortality as a national policy issue. Contrary to popular belief, matched birth-death tape analyses revealing excess in- fant deaths do not alert us to the fact that women are having difficulty with access. In truth, all that can be surmised on the basis of such in- formation is that women may have had some problems of unknown origin about 2 years ago. Although body counts figure prominently in recent MCH history, it should be obvious that these data elements have not functioned as particularly strong guarantors of maternal and infant health.

In the absence of other options, research based on vital statistics data has been enormously valuable in highlighting the infant mortality problem. But fixation on this type of archival data may foreclose im- portant alternatives before they have been examined. Moving away from the final calamitous proof of system failure (ie, death) to monitor service accessibility routinely would provide mothers and infants much better protection. The relationship between historical MCH data sys- tems and corrective action is analogous to a highway traffic system in which traffic fatalities (perhaps linked with drivers' license data) are tallied to determine the need for traffic signals. Few unnecessary traffic signals would likely be installed, but the populace might question whether they are best served by such empiricism. Establishing markers for determining traffic volume and flow characteristics makes more

CONCLUSIONS AND RECOMMEN- DATIONS

sense; in fact, it is done with more precision than is evident in the monitoring of MCH needs.

No widespread system provides the surveillance function that is implied in the federal guidelines for the MCH Title V Block Grant program. Because the states are charged with the responsibility under both Medicaid and the MCH Block Grant, they must be in charge of data collection and producing statistical reports on their own populations. Centralized processing of data for national concerns is useful, but for state personnel to wait for reports from Washington or New York on the status of their women seriously debilitates their efforts to serve. The states must be able to cultivate the staff and resource capabilities that will permit the development of surveillance systems aimed at monitoring and protecting the health of mothers and infants. The OBRA 1989 guidelines are a step in the right direction in that they clarify what needs assessment data must be aggregated as part of the state application for Title V funding. Whether sufficient fiscal resources will be provided to allow states to effectively perform this work remains to be seen. Leadership in identifying infant mortality as a social issue emerged at the state level; that initiative should not be dissipated by removing the surveillance function from the states.

Infant mortality is a long-term issue, not a momentary crisis.

Simplistic need formulas based on parameters such as race, income level, or age are not an adequate substitute for state-specific examinations of obstacles to access.[40] The 1987 GAO report on prenatal care[14] noted that identified barriers varied substantially in importance across communities. "A comprehensive effort is needed," stated the report, "to identify the primary barriers in a community, develop programs to overcome those barriers, and evaluate their effectiveness in improving access to prenatal care."[14(p3)] An adequate surveillance system should provide at least the following variables:

- Demographic variables, including geographic information about the location of need.
- Barriers to maternity care.
- Content and adequacy of maternity care.
- Information related to program eligibility, such as income, risk status, and source of payment care.
- Information about special interests related to subgroups of the targeted population, such as ethnicity, age, and employment status.
- Information about pregnancy outcomes.

The proposed solution is the establishment of state-based surveillance systems in which the state MCH office would have responsibility for collecting needs assessment data regularly. In actuality, the MCH Block Grant legislation already requires that states justify need on the basis of specific health problems of their women and children. In *The Forward Plan: Maternal and Child Health 1984–1989*, federal MCH leaders emphasized the importance of "needs assessment and identification of populations, areas and localities requiring assistance." It is not sufficient to offer guidelines. Federal funding sufficient to empower states to conduct ongoing needs assessments must be available.

Required national funding for the proposed surveillance system would be approximately $1.25 million per year ($2.5 million every 2 years) and would be part of a national universal access package. Many models will likely be developed, but at the moment the Michigan prenatal health care survey[38] is probably the best working example of a state-level surveillance system. This longitudinal project is a statewide survey of Michigan obstetric patients conducted postpartum but while the women remain in the obstetric units. The survey is repeated approximately every 2 years and monitors continuing access concerns as well as new challenges that have arisen since the last survey. The result is a cumulative data base that is focused specifically on mothers and infants and that identifies emerging problems before they become crises. Projected national costs for installing a state-level surveillance based on the Michigan survey model, conducted every 2 years, would be approximately $50 000 per state for each survey.

The following recommendations are offered:
- Maternal health concerns need to be defined as sufficiently important to merit their own custom data bases.
- Needs assessments based on historical, archival data should be augmented with current, custom-designed MCH data bases.
- Service availability and access must become an outcome variable just as infant mortality and morbidity are now.
- Funds must be available to allow states to develop their own data collection, analysis, and reporting capabilities.

REFERENCES

1. Committee on Government Operations. *Barriers to Prenatal Care: Can the United States Do More with Less?* Human Resources and Intergovernmental Relations Subcommittee, 100th Congress, 2nd Session. Washington, DC; 1988.
2. American Public Health Association. Report on 1990 objectives highlights victories, defeats. In: *The Nation's Health.* Washington, DC; 1990.
3. *Caring for Our Future: The Content of Prenatal Care. A Report of the Public Health Service Expert Care Panel on the Content of Prenatal Care.* Washington, DC: Public Health Service; 1989.
4. Taylor J. Infant mortality in Michigan. Paper presented at American Public Health Association, Dallas, Tex; 1984.
5. Yankauer A. What infant mortality tells us. *Am J Public Health.* 1990; 80:653–654.
6. Hunt EP, Moore RR. Perinatal, infant, childhood, and maternal mortality for 1955. Washington, DC: US Children's Bureau; 1958. Statistical Series no. 50.
7. Joyce T. The dramatic increase in the birthrate in New York City: an aggregate time-series analysis. *Am J Public Health.* 1990;80:682–684.

8. Habel L, Lee J, Kaye K. Trends in maternal drug abuse during pregnancy in New York City 1978–87. Presented in the 116th annual meeting of the American Public Health Association; 1988; Boston Mass; 13–17.

9. Chasnoff IJ, Burns WJ, Schnoll SH, Burns KA. Cocaine use in pregnancy. *N Engl J Med.* 1985;313:665–669.

10. US General Accounting Office. *Drug Exposed Infants: A Generation at Risk. Report to the Chairman, Committee on Finance, US Senate;* 1990.

11. National Commission to Prevent Infant Mortality. *Death Before Life: The Tragedy of Infant Mortality.* Washington, DC; 1988.

12. US Congress. Office of Technology Assessment. *Healthy Children: Investing in the Future.* 1987.

13. Torres A, Kenney AM. Expanding Medicaid coverage for pregnant women: estimates of the impact and cost. *Fam Plann Perspect.* 1989; 21:19–24.

14. US General Accounting Office. *Prenatal care: Medicaid Recipients and Uninsured Women Obtain Insufficient Care. Report to the Subcommittee on Human Resources and Intergovernmental Relations.* Washington, DC; 1987.

15. Council on Maternal and Child Health. Background paper on universal maternity care. *J Public Health Policy.* 1986;7:105–123.

16. US Bureau of Health Care Delivery And Assistance, Division of Maternal And Child Health. *The Forward Plan: Maternal and Child Health 1984–1989.* Rockville, Md: US Department of Health & Human Services, Public Health Service, Health Resources and Services Administration; 1984.

17. McGee EM, Pratt MW. *Fifty Years of US Federal Support to Promote the Health of Mothers, Children, and Handicapped Children in America.* Vienna, Va: Information Sciences Research Institute; 1985.

18. Klerman LV, Rosenbach M. *Need Indicators in Maternal and Child Health Planning.* Washington, DC: Division of Maternal and Child Health, US Dept of Health and Human Services; 1984.

19. Payne SM, Strobino DM. Two methods of estimating the target population for public maternity services programs. *Am J Public Health.* 1984; 74:164–166.

20. Mayer JP, Johnson CD, Condon JW, Bergquist CB. *Multi-state Prenatal Needs Determination Project. Final Report to the Bureau of Health Care Delivery and Assistance, US Public Health Service;* 1987.

21. Guyer B, Schor L, Messenger K, Prenney B, Evans F. Needs assessment under the Maternal and Child Health Services Block Grant. *Am J Public Health.* 1984;74:1014–1019.

22. Milcarek BI, Link BG. Handling problems of ecological fallacy in planning and evaluation. *Eval Program Plann.* 1981;4:23–28.

23. Singh S, Torres A, Forrest D. The need for prenatal care in the United States: evidence from the 1980 National Natality Survey. *Fam Plann Perspect.* 1985;17:118–124.

24. National Center for Health Statistics. Advance report of final natality statistics, 1985. *Monthly Vital Statistics Report.* vol. 36, no 4 suppl. Hyattsville, Md; 1987. DHHS Publication (PHS)87-1120.

25. Gold RB, Kenney AM, Singh S. Blessed events and the bottom line. New York, NY: Alan Guttmacher Institute; 1987.

26. Rodgers J. *A Methodology for Estimating the Impact of Extending Medicated Coverage to All Pregnant Women and Children with Incomes Below the Poverty Level. A Report Prepared for the Congressional Budget Office.* Washington, DC; 1986.

27. Newacheck PW. Estimating Medicaid-eligible pregnant women and children living below 185 percent of poverty. Washington, DC: National Governors Association; 1988.

28. Buescher PA. Linking administrative data files: research and policy

applications in a state government setting. Presented at 1988 meeting of the American Statistical Society; Aug 24 1988; New Orleans, La.

29. Senner J. Report on the impact of Medicaid expansion on Arkansas. Presented at the 1989 National Governors Association Meeting; March 29 1989; San Antonio, Tex.

30. Kenney AM, Torres A, Dittes N, Macias J. Medicaid expenditures for maternity and newborn care in America. *Fam Plann Perspect.* 1986; 18:103–110.

31. Bloom BL. The use of social indicators in the estimation of health needs. In: Bell RA, ed. *Assessing Health and Human Service Needs.* New York, NY: Human Sciences Press; 1983.

32. Sullivan DA, Beeman R. Satisfaction with maternity care: a matter of communication and choice. *Med Care.* 1982;20:321–330.

33. Illinois Department of Health. *Birth Certificate Survey on Access to Prenatal and Well Child Care.* Springfield, Ill; 1985.

34. Curry MA, Howe CL. *A Survey of the Access to Perinatal Care and the Incidence of Perinatal Morbidity in the State of Oregon.* Portland, Ore: Oregon Health Sciences University; 1983.

35. *The Pregnancy Risk Assessment Monitoring System.* Atlanta, Ga: Centers for Disease Control; 1987.

36. Blakely CH, Johnson CD. *Estimating the Need for Prenatal Care. Report to the Michigan Department of Public Health.* Lansing, Mich: University Associates; 1984.

37. Mayer JP, Johnson CD. *Statewide Need for Prenatal Care.* Lansing, Mich: Michigan Department of Public Health; 1986.

38. Bergquist CL. *Prenatal Health Care Survey.* Michigan Department of Public Health; 1989.

39. Seitz K, holmes D. State program coordination and collaboration. Presented at the National Governors Association meeting; March 29, 1989; San Antonio, Tex.

40. Mayer JP, Johnson CD, Blakely CH, Taylor JR. Pregnant women eligible under medicaid expansion of maternity services. *Evaluation and the Health Professions.* 1989;12:424–436.

41. Johnson CD, Mayer JP, Blakely CH, *Texas OB Survey: Determining the Need for Maternity Services in Texas.* Austin, Tex: Bureau of Maternal and Child Health, Texas Department of Health; 1987.

42. Newacheck PW, McManus MA. Estimating the numbers and Costs of Newly Medicaid-Eligible Pregnant Women and Infants: A Technical Report on Implementing the 1986 Omnibus Budget Reconciliation Act. Washington, DC: National Governors Association; 1987.

43. Prottas JM. The cost of free services: organizational impediments to access to public services. *Public Admin Rev.* 1981;41(3):526–534.

CHAPTER **7**

Health Consequences of Inadequate Access to Maternity and Infant Health Care

Donald W. Schiff, MD

Inadequate access to health care deleteriously affects all people, but no group is more vulnerable to this type of neglect than our nation's children. Lack of adequate access to a range of essential services means that too many of America's children go unimmunized for preventable diseases, suffer unnecessarily from complications of conditions such as asthma and appendicitis, or are injured or abused as a result of lack of parental education. Although these devastating effects are often linked to low socioeconomic status, the crisis in access to child health care is not limited to the poor, but now extends to the middle and upper classes as well.

In this chapter the critical link between income and child health is discussed first, then the consequences of inadequate access to a range of effective preventive and primary health services. The discussion also addresses inadequate use of certain pediatric health services considered essential in meeting contemporary standards of pediatric care, although the evidence of their efficacy is incomplete. Finally, inadequacies in public and private responses to these gaps in access to care are presented.

Although this chapter focuses on primary and preventive care, lack of access to such care creates an environment in which many families use health care less readily for major life-threatening problems as well. Starfield[1] reviewed a select group of serious disorders, including asthma and appendicitis, and found evidence that delay in care resulted in increased mortality, increased morbidity, or an increase in the duration of residual effects. Family stability, educational level, income status, and cultural values also vitally affect the health of children, but discussing these factors would exceed the limits of this chapter, which focuses on comprehensive maternity and infant care and the health consequences (primarily for the infant) of failure to access that care.

Although middle-class children are increasingly facing serious health care barriers, children who live in poverty continue to be more likely to suffer morbidity and mortality than those who come from more financially secure homes. These differences are readily apparent from fetal life throughout childhood (Table 7-1).

INCOME AND ACCESS TO CARE

Surveys of child mortality in Maine from 1976 to 1980[2] and North Carolina from 1985 to 1988[3] reveal that poor children (participants in Aid for Families With Dependent Children [AFDC]) have comparative mortality rates that range from 2.7 times that of the nonpoor (non-AFDC participants) but that rise for specific age-related susceptibility groups to 6.9 times as great (eg, burns). The deaths of poor children from disease (eg, cancer, heart, and pneumonia) and injury, which occur at two to five times the rate for nonpoor children, suggest that parents or other caregivers either postpone seeking medical care until the disorder has become advanced or have no access to health care.

Further evidence of the critical role income plays in access to care is revealed by analyzing patient visits to physicians in relation to family income. On average, children from lower income families make fewer visits to physicians than children from higher income families (Table 7-2). This relationship is exaggerated for children with illness or other impairment. In 1986 Newacheck reported a strong gradient of health status that follows family income levels.[4] Low-income children were reported to spend 64% more illness days in bed than their counterparts from high-income families (Table 7-3). They are also reported to be in fair or poor health 18% more often and are 63% more likely to be limited in their activities over the long term by chronic illness or impairment. Important differences in health care use between higher and lower income families are also apparent when disadvantaged children with health problems are compared with those in good health. A study

---

TABLE 7-1
Morbidity Associated With Low-Income Status*

Low birthweight

Cytomegalic inclusion disease, iron deficiency anemia, lead poisoning, hearing disorders, poor functional vision, psychological problems, otitis media

Chronic conditions interfering with school work and regular school attendance

More disability days per child per year

More hospital days per child per year, higher average length of hospital stay

Lower survival when ill with leukemia

Data from Starfield.[1]

TABLE 7-2
Use of Health Care for Children Aged 17 Years and Younger With Health Problems, United States, 1981

Family Income	Visits*
Low	8.4
With Medicaid Use	9.3
Without Medicaid Use	7.7
Middle	10.0
High	10.5

Source: Microdata tapes from the 1981 National Health Interview Survey, Child Health Supplement.

* Average number of visits per year to a physician for children reported as limited in usual activities or in fair or poor health.

TABLE 7-3
Health Status of Children Aged 17 and Younger, United States, 1981

Family Income	Average Annual Bed Disability (Days)	% Reported in Fair or Poor Health	% Limited in Usual Activities
Low	6.9	7.4	5.2
Middle	5.1	3.4	3.7
High	4.2	2.6	3.2

Source: Microdata tapes from the 1981 National Health Interview Survey, Child Health Supplement.

by Kleinman,[5] using national survey data, suggested that underuse of physician services may be more prevalent for children who are within the least healthy segment of the low-income population (see Table 7-2). Children from low-income families without access to Medicaid had 2.8 fewer medical visits per year than children from high-income families. Furthermore, low-income children with activity-limiting chronic conditions made 18% fewer visits to physicians than similarly limited children from high-income families (Table 7-4). A large proportion of low-income children in poor health or with chronic limitations (more than 40%), not covered by Medicaid, are unable to receive appropriate care.

Financial barriers to access remain a critical obstacle to be overcome. Lack of health insurance for more than 8 million American children effectively denies them crucial health services. Although Medicaid can improve access to health care for economically disadvantaged children in poor health, fewer than half of these children are covered by Medicaid. A few states have made outstanding efforts to reverse the trend by

TABLE 7-4
Visits to a Physician by Children Aged 17 and Younger, United States, 1981

	Family Income		
	Low	**Middle**	**High**
Unadjusted average annual visits	4.5	4.2	4.2
By children with no bed days	3.2	3.1	3.2
Per 100 bed days by children with one or more bed days	22.6	26.3	29.1
By children in good or excellent health	4.1	3.9	4.0
By children in fair or poor health	9.6	12.3	12.4
By children without limitations in usual activities	4.3	4.0	4.0
By children with limitations in usual activities	8.1	8.5	9.9

Source: Microdata tapes from the 1981 National Health Interview Survey, Child Health Supplement.

innovative approaches to both process (ie, complex application forms, unnecessarily restrictive eligibility tests) and reimbursement problems (see Chapters 11 and 12). These improvements have often been rewarded with a renewal of interest in the program by physicians. However, federal mandates such as the Omnibus Budget Reconciliation Act of 1989 (OBRA 1989) have been viewed by most states as yet another costly intrusion to be repealed if at all possible.

The effects of poor access to care are painfully obvious in a number of areas, five of which—asthma, acute appendicitis, infant mortality, immunization levels, and access to screening—are discussed in this section.

CONSEQUENCES OF POOR ACCESS TO CARE

Asthma

Asthma is a condition that has been increasing in frequency and seriousness in the past decade. At present, 2.5 million children are affected, and the annual mortality rate increase is averaging 6.5%. Prevalence rates of 7% to 10% have been found in school-aged children. Asthma is responsible for one third of all chronic illness in children and is the leading cause of missed school due to chronic conditions. Although hospitalization is not usually required, there may be no alternative if ongoing control of the disease is poor and severe attacks are frequent. Hospitalization for treatment of the condition is up 225% since 1969.

Strong evidence indicates that medical care can influence the prevalence and severity of asthma symptoms. Counseling on the avoidance of actions and contacts that produce symptoms or the use of established and recently available medications can produce a major improvement in a child's quality of life. However, to be effective, this type of program requires access to continuing care so that the treatment can be monitored and modified over time.

In Baltimore, children who used the emergency room as their primary source of asthma care had higher hospitalization rates (23% vs 11% hospitalized within the previous 12 months) than those who obtained care from a private pediatrician or clinic.[1] In an urban low-income population, fewer than half of the children reported by parents to have asthma were said to receive regular care for their condition. Forty-five percent of asthmatic children whose regular source of care was a health maintenance organization were reported to receive ongoing nonacute care for their asthma versus 26% for a sample where care was predominantly from a hospital outpatient department.[1]

The pattern of asthma deaths among persons of all ages suggests that a portion might be prevented by timely care or appropriate home medication. In one city in Great Britain, 102 of 143 asthma deaths occurred outside the hospital or upon arrival. Only 17 of the 143 persons had been wheezing for less than 30 minutes before death, and some who died at home had been wheezing for as long as 2 weeks. None of the patients who died had been wheezing for less than 2 hours.

Acute Appendicitis

Acute appendicitis is the most common cause of emergency abdominal surgery in children. It occurs in all age groups, but most cases appear in early adolescence. Recent reports show a continued decline in childhood mortality due to appendicitis in all child age groups except infants younger than 1 year. Despite the improvement in mortality rates, the rate of perforation has not changed in the past 45 years. Delay in admission to the hospital has been consistently associated with increasing likelihood of perforation.

Lansden found that simple acute appendicitis without complications showed symptoms for an average of 30 hours before admission.[1] In contrast, those with perforation or abscess had a mean duration of symptoms before hospitalization of 71 hours. Graham, reporting from Texas Children's Hospital, found that delay in diagnosis was directly related to the likelihood of perforation.[1] The range was from 8% for children who had symptoms less than 20 hours to 87% for those who had symptoms longer than 80 hours.

Further evidence of the effects of access to medical care was provided by comparing rates of perforation with family income. Sher and Coil reported in 1980 that the percentage of children with a perforated appendix rose from 0% in families with incomes over $20 000 to 13% at incomes of $15 000 to $20 000, to 35% at family incomes of less than $10 000.[1] The delay in seeking care that occurs with decreased access or financial barriers to care results in more advanced illness at the time of presentation, including perforation, peritonitis, and prolonged morbidity.

Immunization Levels

The cornerstone of primary care is prevention. Nothing that health care professionals do exemplifies this precept better than the use of immunization to prevent disease. The eradication of smallpox represents the degree of success that we hope to achieve over many other modern scourges such as rubeola (red measles) and polio. Yet immunization rates in the United States (Table 7-5) are lower than in 28 of 38 countries in Latin America and the Caribbean. Although we have achieved desired immunization levels for children aged five and older entering school, the more critical need to immunize children within the first few years of life has not been met. In many communities, 50% of poor children have failed to receive the vaccine for rubeola, a disease that can cause encephalitis and death. Significant percentages of children younger than 2 are also behind in protective immunization against diphtheria, pertussis, and polio.

TABLE 7-5

Percentage of Immunized Children Aged 1 to 4, United States, 1970 to 1985

	1970	1976	1983	1984	1985
Rubella	37.2	61.7	64.0	60.9	58.9
Measles	57.2	65.9	64.9	62.8	60.8
Mumps	–	48.3	59.5	58.7	58.9
Diphtheria, pertussis tetanus*	76.1	71.4	65.7	65.7	64.9
Polio*	65.9	61.6	57.0	54.8	55.3

Source: Centers for Disease Control. Based on information from the U.S. Immunization Survey for respondents answering questions after referring to an immunization record.

* Three doses.

Great progress has been made against the communicable diseases that were the most common causes of death among infants and older children at the beginning of this century. But in the 1980s there was a disturbing resurgence of rubeola, pertussis, mumps, and now rubella (German measles), a clear warning of a breakdown in our system of caring for our most vulnerable population: children aged 2 and younger. In 1983 there was hope that the diminished incidence of rubeola to approximately 1500 cases annually foretold the elimination of that disease from the United States. That hope was clearly premature, however. There were 27 672 cases and 89 deaths in 1990; 49 of the children who died were younger than 5.

Currently there are 19 measles outbreaks in progress in the United States. The greatest incidence of rubeola appears to be in major cities with large populations of poor, ill-educated, and immigrant young families. This finding is not surprising, as these populations tend to be uninsured and to have limited or no access to health care. The recent development of an effective vaccine against *Haemophilus influenzae* type b (which can cause septicemia, meningitis, septic arthritis, and epiglottitis) provides the means to prevent severe, potentially lethal disease in 15 000 to 20 000 children in the United States annually. However, this immunization requires multiple injections and is rather expensive.[6] This breakthrough, which can effectively eliminate a major source of childhood morbidity and mortality in children as young as a few months of age, has been limited because of the lack of an adequate payment mechanism.

The anticipated development of vaccines against chicken pox (varicella) and rotavirus (common cause of childhood diarrhea) underscores the need for access to continuing care to achieve effective protection against common serious childhood disease. Strong educational efforts are needed to promote the use of immunizations, and financial barriers to access must be removed.

Prevention of Infant Mortality and Morbidity

The problem of infant mortality in the United States has been discussed in Chapters 1, 3, and 4. Those discussions clearly indicate that increased access to health care services for pregnant women and infants should result in lower infant mortality rates in this country.

Although the United States has made great progress in reducing its infant mortality rate in the past two decades, it continues to rank twenty-second among the industrialized countries of the world (Fig. 7-1).[7] The 1990 provisional U.S. rate of 9.1 infant deaths per 1,000 live births is the lowest yet, but it nevertheless lags far behind Japan, which ranks first with a remarkable 4.8 per 1,000. The rapid decline in the U.S. infant mortality rate during the 1960s and 1970s slowed for both Blacks and Whites in the 1980s. The infant mortality rate for Black infants remains twice that of White infants.[8]

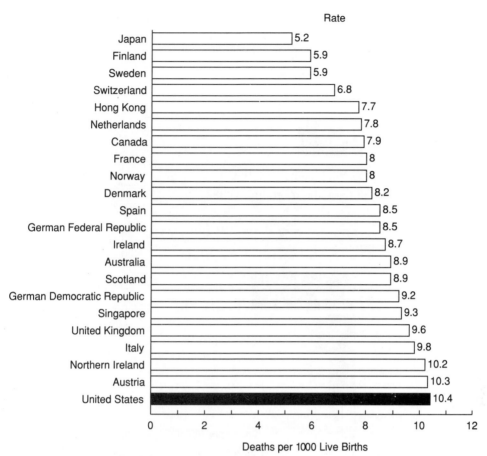

Fig. 7-1.—Cross-national infant mortality ratings: 1986
(Source: Health United States, 1989).

When the causes of infant mortality are divided into neonatal (birth to 28 days) and postneonatal (28 days to first birthday) periods, significant differences appear (Fig. 7-2 and 7-3). Neonatal disorders are invariably associated with the perinatal period and include respiratory distress syndrome, disorders associated with short gestation, low birthweight (LBW), and congenital anomalies. The recent availability of surfactant for clinical use is probably responsible for the improved infant mortality rate because of the 33% decrease in mortality from respiratory distress syndrome. The need for organized, hierarchical perinatal services that guarantee access to sophisticated curative care for at-risk pregnant women and infants are discussed in Chapter 4. The stable LBW rate and Black-to-White infant mortality ratio in the face of declining neonatal mortality provide evidence of the continuing need for preventive health services for all pregnant women.

Postneonatal mortality has come to be dominated by the frequency of sudden infant death syndrome (SIDS). The next four causes of death are congenital anomalies, injuries, pneumonia and influenza, and homicide. After 1 year of age, the leading causes of death drastically

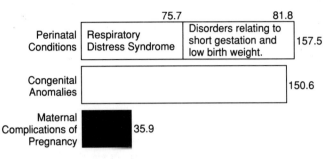

Source: Office of Maternal and Child Health.

Fig. 7-2.—Leading causes of neonatal mortality: 1988

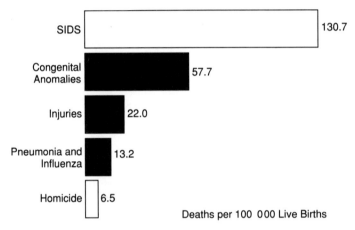

Source: Office of Maternal and Child Health.

Fig. 7-3.—Leading causes of postneonatal mortality: 1988

change; injuries are consistently the leading cause, followed by congenital anomalies and malignancy in the aged 1 to 4 group. These latter two causes are reversed in the age group 5 to 9. Between 10 and 14, homicide, closely followed by suicide, follows neoplasms. Acquired immunodeficiency syndrome (AIDS) is the ninth leading cause of death among children up to age 14 and seventh among young people aged 15 to 24. During the 1990s, AIDS is expected to become one of the top five leading causes of death for children. In most of these areas, comprehensive pediatric services can play a role in improving the health status of infants and young children.

Access to Screening

In 1985 and again in 1988,[9] the Committee on the Psychosocial Aspects of Child and Family Health of the American Academy of Pediatrics (AAP) produced an excellent monograph on health supervision, which is a guide to essential preventive services. The following discussion describes a sample of important selected elements of health supervision, which, if not available to or not used by families, may lead to unhappy consequences later in children's lives. Table 7-6 lists the conditions known to be benefited by health screening in the pediatric care setting.

Newborn screening for metabolic disorders. Newborn screening has become an integral part of public health programs throughout the United States since the first phenylketonuria (PKU) screening test was performed more than 25 years ago. The goal of the newborn screen is prevention of infant mortality, mental retardation, and other potential catastrophes that can occur if the presence of congenital metabolic disorders in infants is not detected early. The exact incidence of inborn errors of metabolism in the neonatal period or in early to late infancy is not known, but cumulatively it may represent more than one in 5000 live births.[10] Early diagnosis and treatment of PKU and hypothyroidism enables those with the defect to live a normal life.

Although treatment for all of the metabolic diseases is not currently available, the possibility of achieving this goal in the future appears promising. Screenings vary widely from state to state, but screenings

---

TABLE 7-6
Conditions That May Be Identified on Screening and Benefited by Early Intervention Services

---

Biologic risk (eg, graduates of neonatal intensive care units, survivors of illness such as meningitis)
Environmental risk
  Impoverished home
  Maladaptive community
  Maladaptive home situation
Chromosomal malformations and other congenital syndromes
Chronic bodily illness
  Endocrine disorders (eg, hypothyroidism)
Major disease of cardiovascular, renal, pulmonary, hepatic, gastrointestinal, or other systems
Severe infections (eg, consequences of human immunodeficiency virus infection)
Defined neurologic disorder
  Central nervous system malformation
  Mental retardation
  Motor disorders (eg, cerebral palsy)
  Neuromuscular disorders
Developmental disorders
  Autism and other pervasive developmental disorders
  Disorders of attention and activity
  Infants and toddlers at risk for learning disabilities
  Language delays
  Motor delays
Metabolic disorders
Orthopedic problems (eg, limb reduction)
Sensory impairment (eg, impaired vision or hearing, pain)

---

for two conditions—PKU and hypothyroidism—are carried out in every state.[11] However, a 1990 review of the screens used by individual states reveals a diverse pattern; 37 states test for galactosemia, 35 for hemoglobinopathies, 20 for maple syrup urine disease, 19 for homocystinuria, and lesser numbers for biotinidase, congenital adrenal hyperplasia, tyrinosemia, cystic fibrosis, and toxoplasmosis.[11] Physicians and public health workers residing in states with developed programs are sometimes lulled into a false sense of security, believing that newborn screening alone is adequate to detect many of these rare abnormalities. In reality, repeated health maintenance visits and continuing care of acute illness are required for complete surveillance of metabolic disease.

Screening for congenital dislocation of the hip. In children born with congenital dislocation of the hip, prompt recognition and appropriate treatment provide the best opportunity for normal hip development. Unfortunately for some children, this diagnosis is not always made during the initial newborn exam. The result is a later diagnosis: abnormal hip due to delayed dislocation.

The incidence of hip dislocation in neonates and infants is 1.3 per 1000 live births. Dislocatable and subluxable hips occur in an additional 1.2 and 9.2 per 1000 births, respectively. Thus, the number of infants with some type of hip instability is approximately 12 per 1000 live births. Females are at higher risk for dislocation of the hip; 70% of dislocated hips occur in girls. Nearly 20% of all dislocations occur in infants born in a breech position. Also at risk and in need of careful examination are infants weighing less than 2500 grams at birth and those placed in intensive care units, because the hip evaluation may be overlooked during the course of treatment for life-threatening problems. Repeat examinations in the 6 months following the newborn period are especially important to detect dislocations that were not detected in the nursery or delayed dislocations. Failure to detect a dislocated femur can lead to permanent significant hip joint dysfunction.[12]

NEED FOR PRIMARY CARE

The emphasis placed on the search for causes of infant and child mortality is well founded, but it must not overshadow the criticality of the need for access to the essential services described as primary care. These programs—carried out by primary care providers including pediatricians, family physicians, and nurse-practitioners—provide preventive care and early detection and treatment of acute diseases in addition to care for children with chronic, often handicapping, conditions. The five problem areas that have been delineated (asthma, acute appendicitis, immunization levels, infant mortality, and access to screening) can be minimized by securing ready access to primary care. Other conditions and issues, a few of which are discussed in the remainder of the chapter, also deserve consideration as aspects of primary care. Among the conditions that can benefit from a continuing relationship with a pediatric care provider are injuries, abuse, and developmental problems.

Injuries

More than half of all children and youth who die do so as a result of injuries. Estimates indicate that for every death that occurs there are more than 100 injuries, many of them severe and possibly disabling. Injury prevention has great potential for reducing child morbidity and mortality. Many injuries previously believed to be accidental and unavoidable are now viewed as preventable. Safety counseling, an important element of primary pediatric care, is a part of each health maintenance visit. Counseling addresses prevention of falls, poisonings, burns and hot water scalds, drownings, and motor vehicle injuries, both passenger and pedestrian.[13]

Susceptibility to injury is determined by the child's developmental stage; consequently, counseling is not effective unless it is targeted at specific types of injuries relevant to the child's developmental level. One example of such a developmentally oriented schedule of injury prevention opportunities is the Injury Prevention Program of the AAP. The role of the pediatric health provider as educator over a span of time is to promote a child-safe environment and to stimulate families to become safety conscious without producing anxiety and overprotectiveness.

Safety advice that requires one-time parental effort for long-term protection (eg, purchasing smoke detectors, childproofing the home, purchasing ipecac, and lowering hot water heater temperatures) is likely to be followed without excessive reinforcement. Pediatricians and other pediatric providers are alert for circumstances that increase the probability of children being exposed to injury.[13] Divorce, death of a family member or friend, remarriage of a parent, or the arrival of a new baby may increase the risk of injury and call for special guidance from the pediatrician.

Child Abuse

Child abuse, known to be a common and potentially damaging experience, remains a hidden morbidity. Most cases are probably still unknown to child protection agencies despite the dramatic increase in cases reported. In 1990 an estimated 2.5 million cases of child abuse and neglect were filed, a 4% increase over the number filed in 1989. Reporting of the incidence of child abuse increased 147% between 1979 and 1989. The number of reported child abuse fatalities has been staggering—1200 cases in 1989, representing a 38% increase since 1985. On average, nearly four victims of fatal child abuse and neglect are reported each day. The risk of death is greatest for children younger than 5; 53% of all children who die from maltreatment are younger than 1 year. Studies of the general population reveal that 15% to 38%

of females and 10% of males were sexually abused as children. Preventing and detecting sexual abuse of children is a critical component of pediatric primary care.

Pediatric providers today are particularly sensitive to children at increased risk of abuse because of the stresses suffered by dysfunctional families. Drug or alcohol abuse, social isolation, or a recent history of behavioral change in caretaker or child alerts the provider to potential problems. Parents and pediatricians may detect symptoms such as onset of sleep or eating disturbances. Physicians must include abuse in the differential diagnosis of many presenting complaints including vaginal discharge, urinary tract infection, rectal bleeding, and new onset of encopresis or enuresis.

Effective intervention by primary care providers to prevent child abuse can include preparing the family to deal with the normal, healthy aspects of childhood sexuality with the dual goal of teaching the parents and children protective behavior and yet avoiding inappropriate fear. Jenny et al used a developmental approach to teaching this material in the child health visit.[14]

Early Detection of Developmental Delay and Handicapping Conditions

Pediatricians and other pediatric care providers are perfectly situated to monitor and counsel families over time on the growth and development of their children from birth through the school years. Knowledgeable about the prenatal history, the health care giver identifies those infants who, because of low birthweight, maternal illness, or other risk factors, require particularly close attention be paid to their developmental status. To detect deviations from established norms usually requires repeated visits to the same health care site, because comparative heights and weights and cumulative developmental and behavioral data are the basis for accurately interpreting the normalcy of the child's development.

The past decade has seen the development of a consensus that early and continuous provision of medical care and intervention services for children who have handicapping conditions confers significant benefits and improved outcomes. The beneficial effects of early identification and intervention were recognized by the Congress in 1986 with the passage of the Education of the Handicapped Amendments (P.L. 99-457) to the original P.L. 94-142. This new legislation relies on cooperative interaction among pediatricians and other professionals to maximize health and other benefits to which eligible children are entitled.[15]

Substance Abuse and Socioeconomic Factors

The frequency of delivery of LBW infants as a result of the lack of prenatal care, further complicated by drug use is clearly related to the incidence of severe life-threatening disorders, including acute and chronic pulmonary disease, in these infants. The necessity of prolonged artificial ventilation and the subsequent development of reactive airway disease and bronchopulmonary dysplasia lead to frequent ambulatory visits, hospitalizations, and an increased incidence of SIDS. Intracranial hemorrhage is also a common event in these very high-risk infants, requiring close monitoring to detect evidence of developmental delays and specific sensory and motor deficits, which affect both child and family.

To this point in the chapter, special emphasis has been placed on the infant at increased risk of having a physical problem, but one must also expect that sociodemographically disadvantaged children born without clinical risk factors are also at risk of health and developmental problems. There can be no doubt that a generalized approach to the detection of abnormalities at the very earliest opportunity is recommended for all children, not solely those at increased risk of health problems.

General Prevention as a Component of Primary Care

The traditional list of hazards to which children are exposed (eg, automobiles, swimming pools, baby walkers, playground equipment, and bicycles) has a relatively new and deadly addition. Firearms have been associated with the deaths of 300 children younger than 14 who die each year of unintentional gunshot wounds. An additional 8000 children and teenagers are injured annually, and 25% of them are left with a permanent disability. The U.S. unintentional firearm fatality rate for children is 5 times that of Europe and more than 2.5 times the rate in Latin America.[13]

Child health advocates can help create an atmosphere in our society in which firearm ownership is not acceptable in families with children. Short of that goal, parents can be helped to avoid firearm injury in their families by pediatric counseling that identifies specific rules for firearm safety: that firearms be unloaded, inaccessible to children, and stored separately from ammunition. The pediatric team must facilitate increased attention to this problem.

Preceding sections have described areas in which lack of access to health care services has compromised child health. Reasons for lack of access are dealt with in detail in Chapter 8, but some reasons bear underscoring.

LIMITATIONS OF PUBLIC AND PRIVATE RESPONSES

Declining availability of private health insurance for the dependents of workers at the lower end of the pay scale is a fundamental and frightening change in our health care system (see Chapter 10). In 1989 the percentage of children under 21 with no health insurance increased to 17%.[16] In addition, private health insurance usually excludes coverage for any services considered preventive. These services for the well child are precisely those health maintenance services and immunizations that have been described in this chapter and recognized as fundamental to child health by most health care authorities.

For that small but ever-increasing percentage of children with established major health problems, private insurance fails to fulfill their needs. By using preexisting conditions as a basis for exclusion; by placing a low, too-easily-reached cap on total expenditures; and by failing to provide catastrophic coverage these programs force the families of such children to seek care in the public sector. Preexisting health conditions become limiting factors for families considering a change of job or location, because the likelihood of remaining with the same insurance carrier is extremely small. The new insurer, invoking the preexisting clause, precludes health insurance coverage for children who are recovering from leukemia or are under treatment for heart disease or cerebral palsy.

This decline in health insurance coverage for our nation's children has outpaced the agonizingly slow increase in the number of families covered by Medicaid. Efforts by Congress and the administration to simultaneously control health care costs (now more than $650 billion per year) and increase access via the Medicaid program have been marked by a confused and variable response at the state and local government levels.

Pediatricians' high level of participation in the Medicaid program (85%) has been the basis for much of that program's success in providing care for poor children since its inception in 1965.[17] Yet, in the past few years, growing problems within Medicaid have turned many pediatricians away from caring for these needy children. The issues of grossly inadequate reimbursement levels and onerous paperwork as well as user-unfriendly administrative procedures have limited the number of pediatricians willing to accept new Medicaid patients or continue serving the ones already in their care.

Expansions of current programs (Medicaid; Early and Periodic Screening, Diagnosis, and Treatment (EPSDT); and Supplemental Security Income and the addition of a potentially significant amendment (P.L. 99-457) that provide for early intervention services for handicapped children have brought new hope to child advocates who have been battling for years to achieve equity in health care for the one third of our population who are our nation's future. However, clearly stated opposition by states to additional federal mandates or expansion of Medicaid has raised yet another barrier to the availability of desperately needed health care. The broad language of OBRA 1989, which requires the EPSDT program to assure that any enrolled child will receive needed medical care regardless of whether or not that care is in a specific state plan, is intended to create new paths through a previously impenetrable health care jungle. Despite the expansiveness of legislative language, promulgating appropriate and clear rules and regulations at both federal and state levels and locating additional funding during a period of recession and state budget deficits continue to be daunting tasks.

CONCLUSIONS

The shameful consequence of our nation's prioritization of care by health insurance coverage status is that too high a price is being exacted from our greatest natural resource—our children. Although some will argue that significant steps have been taken in recent years, it is unclear whether significant progress has been made. Our embarrassing infant mortality and morbidity statistics will not improve until we offer every child and pregnant woman in this country continued access to essential health care services. Current trends and policy developments promise nothing resembling the universal access to care that is needed to ensure the health and vitality of our nation's children. We must take the initiative and achieve equity in health care access for the next generation.

REFERENCES

1. Starfield B. *The Effectiveness of Medical Care: Validating Clinical Wisdom.* Baltimore, Md: The Johns Hopkins University Press; 1985.
2. Nersesian WS, Petit MR, Shaper R, et al. Childhood death and poverty: a study of all childhood deaths in Maine, 1976 to 1980. *Pediatrics.* 1985;75:41–50.
3. Nelson MD Jr. Socioeconomic Status and Childhood Mortality in North Carolina. Raleigh, NC: Center for Health and Environmental Statistics, Department of Environment, Health, and Natural Resources; 1991.
4. Newacheck P, Halfon N. Access to ambulatory care services for economically disadvantaged children. *Pediatrics.* 1986;78:813–818.
5. Kleinman JC, Gold M, Makuc D. Use of ambulatory medical care by the poor: another look at equity. *Medical Care.* 1981;19:1011.
6. Santosham M, Wolff M, Reid R, et al. The efficacy in Navajo infants of a conjugated vaccine of Hemophilus Flu Type B. *N Engl J Med.* 1991;324:1767–1772.
7. Office of Maternal and Child Health. *Child Health USA 90.* Washington, DC: US Dept of Health and Human Services; 1990.
8. Wegman ME. Annual summary of vital statistics 1989. *Pedicatrics.* 1990;86:835–847.
9. *Guideline for Health Supervision II.* Elk Grove Village, Ill: American Academy of Pediatrics; 1988.
10. Ward JC. Inborn errors of metabolism of acute onset in infancy. *Pediatrics in Review.* 1990;11(7):205–215.
11. *Newborn Screening: An overview of Newborn Screening Programs in the United States and Canada.* Springfield, Ill: Illinois Dept. of Health; 1990.
12. MacEwen GD, Millet C. Congenital dislocation of the hip. *Pediatrics in Review.* 1990;11(8):249–252.
13. *Injury Control for Children and Youth.* Elk Grove Village, Ill: American Academy of Pediatrics; 1987.
14. Jenny C, Sutherland MN, Sandahl MN. Developmental approach to preventing the sexual abuse of children. *Pediatrics.* 1986;78:1034–1038.
15. Katcher A, Haber JS. The pediatrician and early intervention for the

developmentally disabled or handicapped child. *Pediatrics in Review.* 1991;12(10):305–311.

16. Foley J. Special Report SR-10. *Uninsured in the United States: The nonelderly population without health insurance—analysis of the March 1990 current population survey.* Washington, DC: Employee Benefit Research Institute. April, 1991.

17. Yudkowsky BK, Cartland J, Flint S. Pediatrician participation in Medicaid. *Pediatrics.* 1990;95:567–577.

CHAPTER 8

Barriers to Access to Prenatal Care

Sarah S. Brown, MSPH
George M. Ryan, MD, MPH

From some vantage points, the 1980s may seem to have been a golden age for maternal and infant health. During that decade the media, the public, and many levels of government became highly attentive to issues of infant mortality, healthy pregnancy, early access to prenatal care, and child health generally. This explosion in public attention was stimulated in part by concern over the nation's slowed pace of decline in the infant mortality rate, reports of actual increases in the infant mortality rates in some cities, and a growing realization that the nation might well not meet many of the maternal and infant health goals set by the surgeon general for the year 1990.[1]

Activism was reported at all levels of American life. Even in the face of an awe-inspiring deficit, the US Congress voted on at least four separate occasions to expand the eligibility of pregnant women and young children for Medicaid, and many states were willing not only to meet required levels of eligibility but also to include optional benefits. The Maternal and Child Health (MCH) Block Grant to states saw several successive years of absolute increases in funding. Other important child health initiatives, such as the Early and Periodic Screening, Diagnosis, and Treatment program of Medicaid, and Head Start, realized striking gains in funding toward the close of the decade. Many states formed statewide blue ribbon coalitions to increase access to prenatal care and reduce infant mortality; the efforts of Michigan in the early 1980s were perhaps the earliest and best-known example. Volunteer groups such as the Junior League became deeply involved in advocacy on behalf of children, particularly those that are low income, high risk, or both. And charismatic leaders in many cities—and even in some rural areas—stimulated the development of a whole new generation of community-based maternal and infant health programs, typically funded by a combination of public and private dollars. Indeed, for a few years the nation seemed awash in programs with such similar names as Baby Love, Be Good to Your Baby, Beautiful Babies, Right From the Start, Better Babies, Healthy Babies, Healthy Start, Birthstart, and so on. Even some corporations focused on the need to promote healthy pregnancies as a means of ensuring a robust work force and reducing the health care resources consumed by employees and their newborn dependents. Perhaps it was, indeed, the decade of the child.

TRENDS IN KEY MATERNAL AND CHILD HEALTH INDICATORS

Unfortunately, not even this outpouring of interest has been enough to make a major improvement in a variety of maternal and infant health indicators. The Public Health Service summarized:

> Although the infant mortality rate is at an all-time low, the pace of progress has slowed. Important measures of increased risk of death, such as incidence of low birth weight and receipt of prenatal care, show no recent improvement.[2] (p364)

Indeed, in some communities key indicators seem again to be going in the wrong direction; rather than being flat or constant, they are deteriorating. In the District of Columbia, for example, the infant mortality rate in 1987 was 19.6 deaths per 1000 live births; final figures for 1988 place it at 23.3, a scenario that is repeated in several other eastern and midwestern industrialized cities (unpublished data, D.C. Office of Vital Statistics, 1989).

Much of the social ferment and activism of the 1980s was squarely directed toward getting more women, especially low-income and high-risk women, to begin prenatal care early in pregnancy. Although many of the community-based programs launched in the 1980s were called infant mortality reduction initiatives, a large number concentrated, in fact, on boosting enrollment in prenatal care.

The focus on prenatal care was based on at least three considerations. First, tackling low birthweight or infant mortality directly has generally proved a complicated goal because the causes and antecedents remain numerous and complicated—participation in prenatal care, by contrast, seems a more attainable goal. Second, the consensus became quite strong in the early and mid-1980s that prenatal care could improve pregnancy outcomes—especially birthweight—and that, therefore, infant mortality could be reduced through the intermediate goal of increasing participation in prenatal care (see chapter 3). This consensus became all the more appealing to policymakers when several reports in the mid-1980s suggested that prenatal care is not only good medicine but also cost-effective.[3, 4] Third, raising rates of early enrollment in prenatal services is a relatively straightforward goal around which a wide variety of groups and interests can rally; it requires little explanation as a concept and appeals to a wide variety of potential players—physicians, nurses, clergy, public health administrators, women's groups, advocates, and others.

Despite such attention, trends in use of prenatal care (see chapter 6) are discouraging. The steady increase during the 1970s in the proportion of women who begin prenatal care in the first trimester of pregnancy has leveled off since 1980, and for some groups has actually reversed. In the late 1980s one quarter of all pregnant women and one half of young Black women still received no prenatal supervision in the first 3 months of pregnancy. Moreover, at present, one third of pregnant women fail to receive the amount of care currently recommended by the American College of Obstetricians and Gynecologists

(ACOG). Even more troubling is that the percentage of women who get no care at all, or only a few visits in the last weeks of pregnancy, has actually increased since 1980. For example, in that year 8.8% of births to Black women were in that category. By 1987 the rate had risen to 10.6%. In fact, 1987 rates of late or no prenatal care for Black women are about the same as in 1976. Improvements in the interim, though slight, have in effect been erased.

Prenatal care is thus a most perplexing preventive service. The consensus is strong that it improves birth outcomes and is cost-effective, and there has been appreciable activity at many levels of society to increase early participation in care; yet the trends are not encouraging. Why, then, are the women not coming in? What are the barriers that keep them away from such an important preventive intervention?

In 1988, the Institute of Medicine (IOM) of the National Academy of Sciences released a report dedicated in part to answering those questions.[5] In studying the nature and magnitude of barriers to care, the IOM defined six types of barriers that stand between pregnant women and prenatal care:

BARRIERS TO PRENATAL CARE

1. Financial obstacles, stemming from coverage gaps in both private insurance and in the Medicaid program, and insufficient funds to pay out of pocket for care when no insurance benefits are available.

2. Inadequate capacity in the prenatal systems relied on by many low-income women, as evidenced by overloaded public health clinics (causing delays of 6, even 8, weeks to get an appointment for prenatal care), decreasing numbers of obstetrician-gynecologists practicing obstetrics, and too few physicians willing to take Medicaid patients, thereby increasing the difficulty such women have in obtaining care.

3. Services that are not consumer or user friendly, exemplified by clinics that require patients to wait many hours to see a provider and then link women to a different provider at each visit; poor coordination among MCH programs, making it difficult to knit together a cohesive set of services; difficult financial aid application forms and other paperwork barriers; difficulty in getting clear information on where to go for care; and frustration in trying to schedule an appointment.

4. The pregnancy's being unintended at the time of conception, or unwanted, or both.

5. A wide variety of personal beliefs and attitudes that make a woman disinclined to seek prenatal care, such as a fear of doctors, hospitals, and anything medical; insufficient understanding of the importance of prenatal care, or even what it is (as is sometimes the case for recent immigrants from countries where pregnancy is managed

127

quite differently); and a belief that if prenatal care was obtained for a previous pregnancy in which the outcome was good (as it usually is), there is no need for prenatal care in the current pregnancy.

6. The persistent, grinding poverty and despair now so prevalent in many inner cities and selected rural areas, resulting in social isolation, apathy, and such self-destructive behavior as profound inability to manage reproduction, pregnancy, and prenatal care in a reasonable way.

... much of the social ferment and activism of the 1980s was directed toward getting more women to begin prenatal care early in pregnancy.

In a given community and for an individual woman, the relative importance of these factors varies, and the mix often changes during the course of a pregnancy. At the community level, enormous variation exists across states and even within states in the nature and importance of individual barriers. In some cities, for example, the network of publicly financed clinics is extensive; in others, services are lodged primarily in the offices of private physicians. In each of these two settings, therefore, the obstacles might vary. In the city, any cutback in the public health funds that support the clinics might limit the availability of care. In the physician's office, obstacles to care depend more on such things as the provider's inclination to care for Medicaid patients and the extent to which some providers might be cutting back on the practice of obstetrics because of recent increases in malpractice insurance premiums.

For individual women also, obstacles vary. One woman may avoid prenatal care in the early weeks of pregnancy, until she reconciles herself to an unintended pregnancy; she may then find that none of her local clinics or providers have personnel who speak her language and give up on prenatal visits in frustration. Another woman in another community may begin care early at the local public clinic, but after two visits that require 3-hour waits to see a provider—with no child care for her 18-month-old—may not return until late in pregnancy, and then only to arrange for a delivery site where her financial status will not be an issue.

Financial Barriers

Given the high cost of having a baby in the United States (currently estimated at about $4500),[6] it is not surprising that financial problems pose major barriers to prenatal care. No matter which category of payment status a pregnant woman falls into—privately insured, insured through the publicly financed Medicaid program, or uninsured and relying on personal funds to pay out of pocket for care—significant problems can arise in financing prenatal services, to say nothing of the hospital charges associated with labor and delivery.

Although privately insured women are more likely to obtain the amount of prenatal care currently recommended than women without such coverage, the mere presence of private insurance is no guarantee that adequate financing is in place. The Alan Guttmacher Institute pointed out recently that among privately insured women of reproductive age, some 14.6 million are not fully insured for maternity care.[6] Policies that cover maternity care may impose waiting periods for benefits to begin, burdensome cost-sharing and copayment requirements, or limitations on services covered that render the policy incomplete at best. Moreover, because many women obtain their private health insurance as dependents of employed spouses, the recent trend for employers to cut back on subsidized dependent coverage as a cost-saving action has directly affected the maternity coverage of pregnant dependents. In addition, because private insurance is an employment-related benefit usually tied to full-time, full-year employment, the disproportionate representation of women among part-time and seasonal workers makes them more likely than other groups to be both employed and uninsured—and also ineligible for Medicaid because their earnings make them too affluent for public insurance. (For more on the role of private insurance in access to maternity care, see chapter 10.)

The steady increase in the proportion of women who begin prenatal care in the first trimester has leveled off...

Medicaid, too, has been found to be a highly imperfect source of health care financing for low-income women. Women covered for pregnancy by Medicaid are known to obtain prenatal care later in pregnancy and to make fewer visits than women with private insurance.[7] Several interrelated factors probably account for these differences. First, because of the bureaucratic difficulties of enrolling in Medicaid, a woman may be well along in weeks of gestation before her eligibility for coverage is established and she is able to begin prenatal care. Second, even with coverage secured, she may have difficulty finding a provider who accepts Medicaid as payment for care, or may face a delay of many weeks between the first call for an appointment and the actual visit. Finally, it is well known that the average Medicaid recipient is characterized by a number of demographic characteristics that are linked to poor participation in prenatal care, such as limited education, being unmarried, and being in poor health. It should not be surprising that the mere presence of Medicaid coverage is unable to produce patterns of health care use similar to those of more affluent women with private coverage.

In the past 6 years, Congress has acted aggressively to expand the scope and reach of Medicaid coverage for pregnant women and young children, and many states have made great efforts to use the new allowances and mandates creatively to draw more women into care early in pregnancy.[8] The results of the congressional actions on prenatal enrollment are not yet known, although several groups are trying to measure the effects on use of health services, including prenatal care.

Some 5 million women of reproductive age with neither private nor public health insurance are among the pool of 37 million Americans judged to be without health care coverage of any kind.[6] For these women, obtaining prenatal care depends on their ability to find free or reduced-cost care from local providers. To the extent that such services are unavailable or overcrowded in a particular community, major gaps in prenatal care may result.

Limited System Capacity

Closely related to the financial barriers just outlined are the problems of limited capacity in the health care systems traditionally used by low-income women (see chapter 9). Although many areas of the country offer networks of community health centers, hospital outpatient clinics, rural and migrant health centers, and various prenatal clinics through local and county health departments, waiting times for appointments at these facilities may be substantial. In the absence of comprehensive state or national data on the capacity and demand for care at these clinics, it is impossible to quantify the extent of system overload. Nevertheless, numerous local and anecdotal reports suggest that in some areas capacity is so limited that the prospect of securing prompt and timely prenatal care is dim.[5] Funding limits and cutbacks in many communities in the past decade have been reflected in, for example, selective cancellation of clinic sessions and the closing of certain services altogether in the District of Columbia (unpublished status report, Mayor's Advisory Board on Maternal and Infant Care, 1989).

Exacerbating this situation is the fact that, in some areas of the country, few or no obstetricians are in private practice or willing to serve in public clinics. In particular, appreciable numbers of obstetricians will not accept patients whose principal source of payment is Medicaid, because of its relatively low reimbursement rates in many states, the paperwork associated with reimbursement claims, and delays in receiving payment. The problem is worsened by the continuing high cost of malpractice insurance. During the second half of the 1980s, partially in response to the malpractice situation, an increasing percentage of obstetric care providers cut back or discontinued obstetrics practice altogether.[9] One particularly unfortunate side effect of the exodus from obstetrics is that publicly financed clinics are having more difficulty recruiting and maintaining an adequate staff of obstetric care providers.[10] In an effort to reverse this trend, some clinics have begun subsidizing a portion of the malpractice fees paid by the obstetricians they employ, and several states are experimenting with ways to subsidize the malpractice premiums of providers who work in public obstetrical clinics.

Service Atmosphere and Procedures

From the perspective of a woman trying to get prenatal services, the tone, procedures, and atmosphere of a health care setting can either facilitate full participation in care or create yet another barrier. Lack of user friendliness may be the obstacle most difficult to measure, but its importance is enormous. Off-putting factors include poor coordination among programs, difficult procedures for securing Medicaid, and a range of classic access barriers such as inadequate transportation, lack of child care, and language barriers.

In theory, a long and comprehensive list of services is available to low-income pregnant women, financed in large part by public funds. Included are services supported by the MCH Block Grant: the Special Supplemental Food Program for Women, Infants, and Children (WIC); Medicaid; and community, rural, and migrant health centers. Yet in many communities, the referral links among these programs are tenuous, and moving among them may involve different application forms, different dates and hours of service, and different eligibility requirements. Regarding the links between WIC and prenatal care, for example, a federal study showed that in several states in which the eligibility for prenatal and WIC services was identical, WIC enrollment among prenatal patients averaged only 58%.[11] Another weak link exists between sites that provide pregnancy tests and those that offer prenatal services, as revealed by studies showing delays of 6 weeks or more between a positive pregnancy test and the first call for a prenatal appointment. Careful follow-up on positive pregnancy tests to arrange appropriate care can increase early enrollment in prenatal services,[12] but anecdotal reports suggest that such procedures are not always followed.

One of the least consumer-friendly aspects of securing prenatal care can be the process of obtaining Medicaid coverage. Numerous studies throughout the 1980s revealed appreciable gaps between the number of individuals eligible for the program and the actual numbers enrolled—the so-called eligibility-enrollment gap.[5] Factors explaining the gap include the failure of most Medicaid programs to advertise eligibility levels and how to apply for benefits and, more important, the difficulty of actually enrolling in the program, particularly for women who are not already enrolled in Medicaid through the welfare program but who are eligible for Medicaid only because they are pregnant. Recent state efforts to institute presumptive eligibility for benefits—an administrative device to shorten the interval between application and coverage—may help to ease this problem.

Additional barriers in this category include a long list of problems that have been repeatedly described in the public health literature.[13] These are the classic access problems posed by lack of transportation to the provider site, lack of child care, inconvenient hours (particularly for women who work or go to school), long hours spent waiting in crowded waiting rooms to see the doctor only briefly, seeing a different doctor at every visit, dreary and uncomfortable surroundings, and poor communication between providers and clients about procedures and about recommended health practices. Even a poor relationship between the doctor-nurse team and the pregnant woman can pose a disincentive to continuing in care. The IOM report referred to the "unfortunate mix of hostility, passivity and evasiveness on the part of the client, matched by arrogance, testiness and indifference on the part of the provider."[6(p76)]

Unintended Pregnancy

It is estimated that just over half of all conceptions in the United States are unintended.[14] Because unintended pregnancy is clearly associated with starting prenatal care late,[15] this factor is of great significance in understanding the nation's poor record for use of prenatal services. A woman who is pregnant unintentionally or who views her pregnancy negatively may start care late for a variety of reasons. She may be inattentive to the early signs of pregnancy; she may be deciding whether to have an abortion; or she may be reconciling herself to the pregnancy before seeking prenatal care.

Cultural and Personal Beliefs

Not all women believe that prenatal care is a useful and valuable service worth the effort to secure it. To many women, pregnancy is seen first and foremost as a normal event, requiring medical supervision only if some problem arises. This attitude may be especially prevalent in women newly-arrived in the United States from countries where medical care is inaccessible and where the prevailing belief is that physicians and nurses have little or no role in pregnancy and childbirth.

Moreover, perceptions about what constitutes a health risk or an emerging problem during pregnancy may vary between medically trained personnel and pregnant women. For example, a study showed that primarily Black, poor women found high-risk behavior in pregnancy to include getting the flu and not taking prescription vitamins; however, they did not consider the previous birth of a low birthweight infant to be a risk factor, nor did they associate risk with already having had more than five children.[16]

Fear deserves special emphasis as a personal barrier to prenatal care. The IOM report defined four types of fear: fear of providers or medical procedures; fear of others' reactions to the pregnancy; fear that one's illegal status in the country will be discovered and deportation arranged if health care is sought; and fear that health-damaging habits such as smoking or drug and alcohol abuse will be detected and sanctions brought to bear. All such worries can be obstacles to prenatal services.

With the recent rise in illegal drug use among pregnant women, principally of cocaine and its derivative crack, the problem of possible sanctions being a deterrent to prenatal care is especially troubling. In the past two years, a number of states and local jurisdictions have tried to impose legal penalties, including criminal sanctions, against women found to be using certain illegal drugs while pregnant. Clearly, if women fear that their illegal drug use will be uncovered during prenatal care visits, they may refuse screening tests, fail to be fully honest in

... over half of all conceptions in the United States are unintended. ... Unintended pregnancy is clearly associated with starting prenatal care late ...

answering questions about their own health habits, or, more important, stay away altogether for fear that they will be detained, perhaps
prosecuted, or have older children removed from their custody. Because of these and other concerns, a recent position statement of the
Board of Trustees of the American Medical Association urged that illegal drug use among pregnant women be handled primarily through
treatment and education.[17]

Persistent Poverty and Social Collapse

All of the many barriers to care described thus far are exacerbated by
the dreadful environments in which the nation's poorest women now
live, where violence and death, poverty, unemployment, and despair
set the tone for daily life. In the poorest inner cities and rural areas, social disintegration can be so profound that admonishing a woman to
seek regular prenatal care is an irrelevant suggestion at best. Throughout the country there are heroic efforts to offer comprehensive health
care and social services in these highest risk communities, including
basic maternal and infant health services, but practitioners report that
much of their time is spent dealing with such basic issues as housing
and food, and that discussing prenatal supervision is often put off repeatedly (J Maxwell; Better Babies Project; Washington, DC; personal
communication, 1988). It is not surprising that women in these circumstances participate sporadically at best in prenatal care, as has been
documented for homeless women in particular.[18]

One factor contributing to the chaos in these communities is the prevalence of drug abuse, particularly the use of cocaine by women of reproductive age. Unfortunately, few data are available to gauge the precise dimensions of illegal drug use among pregnant women; estimates
of the annual number of newborns who are exposed to cocaine prenatally range widely from 30 000 to 375 000.[19] Although the extent of cocaine use by pregnant women and others is not well documented, the
harm and devastation that widespread use of the drug cause to children, parents, and families is indisputable. At a recent workshop convened by the National Forum on the Future of Children and Families,
participants mentioned significant increases in various indexes of social stress and pathology related to high levels of illegal drug use in
communities, including the growing number of child abuse and neglect cases, the increasing load on child protective services, the rising
number and decreasing age of children now in foster care, and (of special relevance here) the rising numbers of women being admitted to
hospitals in labor, with little or no prenatal care.[19]

Relative Importance of Selected Barriers

Although the relative importance of specific barriers to care varies
among communities and individual women (and even during the
course of a single pregnancy for an individual woman), those who
wish to shape public policy to increase early enrollment in prenatal

care frequently ask which of these numerous barriers are the most important. Which ones can policymakers affect, using their available tools of money, programs, education, and bureaucratic manipulation?

To answer these questions, the IOM committee assembled more than 20 studies of barriers to prenatal care from the perspective of women who had recently given birth and had received, in the aggregate, varying amounts of prenatal care. In these surveys the typical procedure was to interview a woman in the immediate postpartum period about whether she had had any trouble obtaining prenatal care and then inquire carefully about reported problems.

These surveys revealed clearly that, from the perspective of care recipients themselves, the most frequently encountered and most important barriers to care were financial, particularly inadequate insurance and insufficient personal funds to pay out of pocket for care. Other especially significant barriers included poorly organized and operated services and problems in arranging transportation to and from service sites. Survey responses also frequently included some variation on "I didn't know I was pregnant," mention of limited provider availability, and dislike or fear of prenatal care. Another finding of these studies was that many women who obtain insufficient care attach a low value to prenatal services.

One of the particularly high-risk groups included in the surveys were women who get no prenatal care at all. Money-related problems were again the most commonly cited barrier to care, along with a low value placed on prenatal care, which suggests that many women who have received no prenatal care are particularly isolated from health services generally and may have only limited appreciation or knowledge of their value. It is also consistent with the view that these women live complicated, highly stressful lives characterized by many daily problems and struggles. It is perhaps not surprising that, for them, prenatal care is of low priority.[6(p97)]

An effort was also made to ask physicians, obstetricians in particular, what obstacles they thought explained the poor use of prenatal care in their communities. A 1987 survey by the ACOG of 2400 of its fellows found that the providers agree with pregnant women that financial barriers to care are the most important. Providers concurred with women that insufficient appreciation of the importance of prenatal care and problems arranging for transportation are also significant barriers to securing adequate prenatal care.[20]

PUBLIC POLICY RESPONSE

Congress has clearly demonstrated that it understands the potency and pervasiveness of financial barriers to care. The steady willingness to expand eligibility to Medicaid for pregnant women is directly responsive to the evidence regarding financial obstacles. Congress has demonstrated that it understands other barriers to care as well by encouraging states to provide presumptive eligibility for Medicaid, by increasing the pressure on states to raise the reimbursement fees for obstetrical care providers, and by encouraging the shortening of application forms. Many states have mirrored the federal commitment by developing a variety of statewide plans to ease problems of uninsuredness in particular (the approaches of Massachusetts, New York, and Hawaii are particularly well-known).

For various reasons, local communities have not demonstrated equal understanding that problems with insurance coverage and other financial issues are critical obstacles to prenatal care. Consequently, community-based programs that squarely address the reduction of financial obstacles are hard to find. Indeed, one of the hallmarks of the 1980s in maternal and infant health was the great proliferation of local-level outreach programs to help women enroll in prenatal care early in pregnancy. These programs, too numerous for even the most dedicated librarian to catalog, typically rely on hotlines linking women with information and care; promotional posters and other graphics announcing programs or clinics; television messages urging pregnant women to get prenatal care; and, above all, community workers to recruit women into care wherever they find them—at home, in the streets, in laundromats, and in unemployment offices. Only rarely are these efforts coordinated with other actions to lower the major financial and administrative barriers to care that have been shown repeatedly to be the principal obstacles to prenatal services.

What [is] required is a fundamental rethinking of the nation's maternity care system, an overhaul that comprehensively addresses the major financial and institutional impediments to care.

Do these outreach programs increase early enrollment in prenatal care? After in-depth reviews of 31 programs that include some form of outreach, the IOM group came to the following conclusion:

> Time and again, the [IOM] learned of communities that have invested in outreach to overcome basic inadequacies in existing networks of prenatal services, rather than changing the system itself. Faced with significant financial barriers, limited service capacity, inhospitable institutional practices, and a basic lack of public understanding about prenatal care, the response is often to hire outreach workers, or organize brief campaigns of posters in buses touting the importance of prenatal services, or arrange for compensatory social support, rather than take on the more challenging task of repairing fundamental flaws. Repeatedly, outreach is organized to help women over and around major obstacles to care, but the obstacles themselves remain. The [IOM] gradually came to the conclusion that organizations whose primary focus is case-finding and social support seem . . . to be "waging guerilla warfare" against institutions that are turning away patients, either deliberately or as an inadvertent consequence of their financial and other policies. Given that outreach programs typically have neither the resources nor the authority to bring about significant improvements in access to care, it is not surprising that their impact, though sometimes positive, is often limited.

Accordingly, [the IOM recommended] that initiatives to increase use of prenatal care not rely on case-finding and social support to correct the major financial and institutional barriers that currently impede access. Rather, outreach should be only one component of a well-designed, well-functioning system and should be targeted toward women who remain unserved despite easily accessible services. Outreach should only be funded when it is linked to a highly accessible system of prenatal services, or, at a minimum, when it is part of a comprehensive plan to strengthen the system.[5(pp150–151)]

CONCLUSION

Despite several consecutive years of sustained attention to improving maternal and infant health, with a special focus on reducing infant mortality and increasing early enrollment in prenatal care, key indicators demonstrate stalled progress. Although infant mortality continues to creep slowly downward, its rate of decline has slowed and, in some communities, increases are again being reported. Use of prenatal care in particular has not increased appreciably in recent years despite the enormous increase in public and media attention to issues of pregnancy, infant mortality, and child survival.

Disheartening though the current situation seems, it holds valuable lessons for policymakers. Recent studies, reports, and experience all suggest that the problem of poor use of prenatal care will not be solved by short-lived, relatively superficial outreach campaigns, nor will it be solved quickly. Even the consistent efforts of Congress to extend Medicaid benefits to more pregnant women and children have yet to produce major changes in rates of prenatal care.

What is required is a fundamental rethinking of the nation's maternity care system, an overhaul that comprehensively addresses the financial and institutional impediments to care. The 1980s saw a notable increase in proposals to reshape the nation's health care system, including maternal and infant health efforts. In the past three years alone, the American Academy of Pediatrics, Congress's own Pepper Commission, the National Leadership Commission on Health Care, and many others have proposed a variety of reforms based on different mixes of public and private financing, responsibilities, and organization.

The likelihood of enacting any single proposal, actual or yet to come, is unclear at best. The current federal budget deficit and a nationwide recession may relegate any notion of reform to fantasy, particularly if any major infusion of public funds is envisioned. On the other hand, as the problems of the uninsured grow, as the public health system shows increasing strain, as health care costs escalate, and as measures of the nation's health show no appreciable improvement, there may yet be action on fundamental health care reform. The clear task of the maternal and infant health community is to articulate the needs of the populations it knows best and to strive to ensure that the interests of these vulnerable groups are well cared for in whatever major reforms are put in place.

REFERENCES

1. Public Health Service. *Healthy People: Surgeon General's Report on Health Promotion and Disease Prevention.* Washington, DC: US Dept of Health and Human Services; 1979.
2. Public Health Service. *Healthy People 2000: National Health Promotion and Disease Prevention Objectives.* Conference edition. Washington, DC: US Dept of Health and Human Services; 1990.
3. Institute of Medicine. *Preventing Low Birthweight.* Washington, DC: National Academy Press; 1985.
4. Office of Technology Assessment. *Healthy Children: Investing in the future.* Washington, DC: US Govt Printing Office; 1988.
5. Institute of Medicine. *Prenatal Care: Reaching Mothers, Reaching Infants.* Washington, DC: National Academy Press; 1988.
6. Alan Guttmacher Institute. *Blessed Events and the Bottom Line: The Financing of Maternity Care in the United States.* New York, NY; 1987.
7. McDonald TP, Coburn AF. *The Impact of Variations in AFDC and Medicaid Eligibility on Prenatal Care Utilization.* Portland, ME: Health Policy Unit, Human Services Development Institute, University of Southern Maine; 1986.
8. Hill IT. *Reaching Women Who Need Prenatal Care.* Washington, DC: National Governors Association; 1989.
9. American College of Obstetricians and Gynecologists. *Survey of Professional Liability and Its Effects. Report of a 1987 Survey of ACOG's Membership.* Washington, DC; 1988.
10. Lewis-Idema D. *Provider Participation in Public Programs for Pregnant Women and Children.* Washington, DC: National Governors Association; 1988.
11. Professional Management Associates. *Improving MCH/WIC Coordination—Final Report and Guide to Good Practices.* Washington, DC; 1986.
12. Jackson CJ, Renner S, Lapolla M. *The Use of Free Pregnancy Testing to Encourage Early Entry into Prenatal Care.* Tulsa, Okla: Oklahoma Medical Research Foundation, Center for Health Policy Research; 1987.
13. Children's Defense Fund. *Dollars and Doctors Are Not Enough.* Washington, DC; 1976.
14. Jones EF, Forrest JD, Henshaw SK, Silverman J, Torres A. Unintended pregnancy, contraceptive practice and family planning services in developed countries. *Family Planning Perspectives.* 1988;20:53–67.
15. Kleinman JC, Machlin SR, Cooke MA, Kessel SA. The relationship between delay in seeking prenatal care and wantedness of the child. Presented at the American Public Health Association annual meeting; Nov. 15, 1984; Anaheim, Calif.
16. Poland ML. Ethical issues in the delivery of quality care to pregnant women. In: Whiteford L, Poland ML, eds. *New Approaches to Human Reproduction, Social and Ethical Dimensions.* Boulder, Colo: Westview Press; 1989.
17. Board of Trustees Report. Legal intervention during pregnancy. *JAMA.* 1990; 264:2663–2670.
18. Chavkin W, Kristal A, Seabron C, Guigli P. The reproductive experience of women living in hotels for the homeless in New York City. *NY State J Med.* 1987 January; 10–13.
19. National Forum on the Future of Children and Families. *Children and Parental Illicit Drug Use: Research, Clinical, and Policy Issues.* Washington, DC: National Academy Press. In press.
20. American College of Obstetricians and Gynecologists. Committee on Health Care for Underserved Women. *Ob/Gyn Services for Indigent Women: An ACOG Survey.* Washington, DC; 1988.

137

Issues in the Provision of Maternity Care

Lorraine V. Klerman, DrPH
Sarah Hudson Scholle, MPH

Maternity care is not an end in itself but a means to achieving a wide range of health objectives. Although professionals and the public usually cite improving the outcomes of pregnancy as the goal of prenatal care, the report of the Public Health Service's Expert Panel on the Content of Prenatal Care expanded the potential of prenatal care to include enhancements in the biologic and social health of pregnant women, their infants, and their families.[1] For maternity care to reach its full potential, however, it must be universally available, include the components of care needed by the population served, and be of high quality.

The first section of this chapter describes the traditional providers of maternity care in this country and the places where such care is offered. It also examines factors that make it difficult for pregnant women to obtain the care they need when and where they need it: shortages and maldistribution of providers and facilities, and medical liability issues. The final sections of the chapter raise two issues often overlooked in analyses of the provision of maternity care: the adequacy of its content and of its quality.

PROVIDERS OF MATERNITY CARE

A universal maternity care system requires enough professionals to provide complete reproductive health services to all women, including family planning, preconception counseling, and prenatal care; to attend women during labor; to deliver and provide immediate newborn care to their infants; and to care for the women in the postpartum period. That an adequate number of trained individuals are in private, public, or quasi-public practice, however, does not in itself ensure that maternity care will be available to all those who need it. The providers must be distributed equitably throughout the country, must care for a reasonable number of obstetric patients, and must be willing to serve poor and high-risk women.

The three groups of professionals that provide most maternity care are obstetrician/gynecologists (ob/gyns), family practitioners (FPs) and general practitioners (GPs), and certified nurse-midwives (CNMs). These three groups vary in number, location of practice, volume of practice, and willingness to serve low-income women, who are currently most likely to receive inadequate care.

Obstetrician/gynecologists

According to the American Medical Association's physician masterfile, 31 364 physicians in the United States identified themselves as ob/gyn specialists in 1986.[2] The American College of Obstetricians and Gynecologists (ACOG), the professional organization for this specialty, counts 29 848 ob/gyns as fellows: 19 111 full fellows; 7273 junior fellows (still in training); 3215 life and founding life fellows (usually inactive practitioners); and 249 affiliate, associate, and honorary fellows (unpublished data, ACOG, 1990). The proportion of medical graduates entering ob/gyn residencies remained stable in the past decade; the number of ob/gyn residents, however, decreased slightly as the total number of medical graduates decreased.[3]

Nearly 400 000 ... women of childbearing age live in areas in 22 states where no ob/gyns are available.

Location. In 1985 the Area Resource File of the US Bureau of Health Professions showed 13 ob/gyn specialists per 100 000 population overall.[4] Like other surgical specialists, however, most ob/gyns work in metropolitan areas. ACOG data for 1988 revealed 35 states with pockets of fewer than 20 ob/gyns per 100 000 women aged 15 to 44. Nearly 4 million women live in these sparsely served areas, which are primarily rural. Nearly 400 000 more women of childbearing age live in areas in 22 states where no ob/gyns are available. Seventeen states, primarily larger states in the southern and western parts of the country, have fewer than 10 ob/gyn specialists per 100 000 population. In general, states with lower ratios of ob/gyns to population have relatively higher ratios of FPs and GPs.[5]

Volume of practice. Ob/gyns work about the same number of weeks per year as other physicians, but they spend more time in professional and patient care activities.[6] In a 1990 ACOG survey, active obstetricians reported an average of 13.4 deliveries per month, or about 160.8 per year. Specific figures varied widely: 24% delivered fewer than 10 babies per month; 34%, 10 to 14; 22%, 15 to 19; and 19%, 20 or more.[7]

It is generally believed that ob/gyns shift from obstetrics to gynecology as they age. A 1985 ACOG study revealed that 54.2% of respondents said they stopped practicing obstetrics before age 55; the figure was 66.8% in 1987 and 61.9% in 1990.[7-9] A recent analysis of national physician survey data showed that younger physicians were more likely than older practitioners to concentrate their practice on pregnancy and childbirth. The findings supported the belief that younger physicians build their practices on pregnancy-related care and then shift to other services as their patients pass their childbearing years.[10]

Employment of nonphysician personnel can increase the volume of practice. The number of such personnel per self-employed ob/gyn increased substantially during the period 1982 through 1988. The largest jump occurred between 1987, when ob/gyns employed 48 100 nonphysicians, and 1988, when the nonphysician staff was 64 400.[11] A 1987 liability survey found that only one quarter of the respondents employed CNMs or nurse-practitioners (NPs) as full- or part-time staff. About half of those employing CNMs carried extra liability coverage for them.[9]

Ob/gyns have traditionally participated in Medicaid less than other practitioners, and nonparticipation appears to be increasing.

Willingness to serve low-income women. A 1987 ACOG survey of members' services for indigent women found that most respondents did not believe that low-income women had difficulty obtaining all ob/gyn services in their communities. Approximately 20%, however, had concerns about access to prenatal care, abortion, and gynecologic surgery and about 10% about access to delivery services and family planning. The respondents believed that financial problems posed the greatest barrier to adequate prenatal care, followed by women's belief that prenatal care is not necessary and difficulties with transportation.[12]

Ob/gyns have traditionally participated in Medicaid less than other practitioners, and nonparticipation appears to be increasing. In a 1984 survey, 72.2% of ob-gyns—the lowest percentage of all physicians except psychiatrists—reported participating in Medicaid, versus 82.8% of all physicians. Substantial regional variations existed in ob/gyn Medicaid participation: fewer physicians in the Northeast (62.2%) and in the South (71.0%) participated, and ob/gyns in these areas devoted a smaller practice share to Medicaid patients.[13]

The ACOG member survey showed that salaried ob/gyns and those in multispecialty group, fee-for-service practice were more likely to provide obstetric services to Medicaid patients and to devote a larger portion of their practice to Medicaid patients. A total of 63% of the respondents who were currently providing obstetric services accepted Medicaid patients (87% of salaried ob/gyns and 81% of those in multispecialty groups), but the percentages decreased to only 58% of those in solo practice and 57% of those in single-specialty groups. Twenty-one percent of those who worked in health maintenance organizations (HMOs) or hospitals versus only 10% of solo practitioners reported that more than half of their deliveries were paid for by Medicaid.[12]

Ob/gyns in small communities were more likely to provide services to Medicaid patients: 85% of those in communities of 50 000 population or less, 60% of those in communities of 50 000 to 500 000 and 52% of those in communities of more than 500 000. In addition, ob/gyns in smaller communities devoted a large share of their practice to Medicaid clients. In 1986, 31% of physicians working in communities of 50 000 or less were paid by Medicaid for 21% to 50% of their deliveries, versus 19% of ob/gyns in communities of more than 500 000 population.[12]

The percentage of ob/gyns providing obstetric services to Medicaid patients also varied among the ACOG geographic districts, ranging from 52% in California to 84% in the Middle North district. California respondents, however, reported the highest mean share of practice devoted to Medicaid patients. Respondents provided obstetric services to Medicaid eligibles chiefly in their offices, but also in health department clinics, community health centers, and on an on-call basis at hospitals for all services or for delivery only. In 1987, about 15% of ob/gyns provided services through local health departments.[12]

Low Medicaid reimbursement was cited as a problem by 78% of those who treated Medicaid patients and by 68% of those who did not. Slow payment and denial of eligibility were also noted by large percentages of ob/gyns who did and did not participate in Medicaid. The belief that Medicaid patients would sue more was the fourth most frequently cited problem, noted by 45% of the Medicaid participants and 41% of nonparticipants. Salaried ob/gyns were less likely to rate this concern as important. Thirty-four percent of Medicaid participants and 27% of nonparticipants mentioned the medical high risk of Medicaid patients as a problem.[12]

Liability issues. National and state surveys of physicians throughout the 1980s indicated that increasing numbers of ob/gyns were decreasing or eliminating obstetrics from their practices. In ACOG's 1990 survey of 1988 and 1989 experience, 12.2% of respondents reported that they had stopped obstetrics practice completely, because of malpractice considerations. Twenty-four percent decreased high-risk obstetric care and 10.4% decreased deliveries. In all, a total of 39% of the respondents reported changes in practice because they were concerned about claims of malpractice. The percentage of respondents reporting they no longer practiced obstetrics because of malpractice risk ranged from 5.6% in the Midwest to 17.6% in Florida.[7]

Changes in the cost of liability insurance, which physicians cite as the primary reason for their changes in practice, suggest that the liability crisis is stabilizing. An ACOG survey found that respondents paid an average of $38 138 for professional liability insurance coverage in 1989 versus $30 507 in 1986 and $37 015 in 1987.[7] (In 1988, the mean net income for ob/gyns after professional expenses and before taxes was $180 700.[14]) ACOG reports (unpublished data, 1990) that premium rates have been holding steady since early 1989 and even decreasing for some specialties and some geographic areas. The St. Paul Insurance Company reported declines in obstetrics malpractice premiums for three areas between 1988 and 1989: from $156 580 to $155 510 in Chicago, from $57 130 to $42 330 in Minnesota, and from $20 620 to $16 270 in North Carolina.[15]

Ob/gyns may leave obstetrics to avoid liability suits as well as to avoid the insurance costs. The 1990 ACOG survey specifically asked about changes due to the risk of malpractice litigation. In this regard, the re-

... 12.2% reported that they had stopped obstetrics practice completely, because of malpractice considerations.

sults of the 1990 survey are less encouraging. A total of 77.6% of the respondents had ever been sued—a statistically significant increase over the 70.6% who reported ever having had a claim in the 1987 survey. Claims experience varied by geographic region.[7]

Malpractice fears have apparently also caused obstetricians to reduce the amount of obstetric care they provide to high-risk patients, although this response appears to be lessening. In 1985, 23.1% of respondents reported they had decreased high-risk obstetrics and in 1987, 27.1%, but in 1990, only 24.2%. ACOG believes that tort reform legislation in California may explain the statistically significant increase in the number of providers of large amounts of high-risk care. Between the 1987 and 1990 surveys, the percentage of ob/gyns devoting 21% or more of their practice to high-risk care jumped from 20.5% to 30.2%. Of the 1990 respondents who handled deliveries, almost half devoted 10% or less of their practice to high-risk care. In 1985, only 2% of respondents devoted 10% or less to high-risk care.

Family and General Practitioners

According to AMA data, approximately 68 000 physicians designate their specialties as family practice or general practice.[2] Almost 28 000 are board certified in family practice. In 1985, there were 27 FPs and GPs per 100 000 population.[4]

The American Academy of Family Physicians (AAFP) has an active membership of about 35 000 physicians.[2] About half of AAFP members have completed family practice residencies and about two thirds are board certified in this field. The rest are probably physicians trained before family practice was designated a specialty in 1969, when the association represented GPs (unpublished data, AAFP, 1990).

Younger FPs and GPs, those who are residency trained, and those in group practice are more likely to include obstetrics in their practices. A 1982 study of the content of family practice stated that it was not clear whether the practice of obstetrics by younger physicians "reflects their ages and the ages of their clients or is an ingrained characteristic that will influence family practice in the future ..." (p 719). The study relied on data collected before obstetric liability issues became a major concern to FPs and GPs; thus the future trends in obstetrics practice by FPs and GPs are unknown.[16]

Data from the AAFP's 1986 membership survey on professional liability revealed that 35% of respondents currently included obstetrics in their practice. Most of those who accepted obstetric patients were residency trained (73%) and board certified (83%). Of these, 23% performed both complicated deliveries and cesarean sections; 43% did complicated deliveries only; and 33% did neither. Those doing complicated deliveries and/or cesarean sections were more likely to have completed residencies and to be board certified.[17]

Location. Among FPs and GPs, the most important factors predicting obstetrics practice are region and urban or rural location. A 1982 survey found that FPs and GPs in the Northeast saw very few obstetric patients (only 0.4% of diagnoses were prenatal or postpartum care), whereas those in the north central states saw relatively many (4.3% of diagnoses). FPs and GPs are more likely to work in rural areas than specialists, and those in rural areas are more likely to practice obstetrics than those in urban and suburban areas. FPs and GPs in rural areas— regions not adjacent to standard metropolitan statistical areas (SMSAs)—were twice as likely to see obstetric patients as those in SMSAs (5.2% of diagnoses versus 2.3%).[16] The AAFP estimates that about one third of its members work in rural areas.

Volume of practice. According to the 1980 National Medical Care Utilization and Expenditure Survey, physicians other than ob/gyns provided 26.0% of office visits for normal pregnancies.[18] Although this care was likely to have been delivered by FPs and GPs, it is widely believed that, in the intervening decade, FPs and GPs have decreased the amount of pregnancy care they provide.

A survey of residency-trained family physicians found that the average number of deliveries in the previous year was 39.2 among those who had practiced obstetrics. This number is about one quarter of the average number reported by ob/gyns in 1990. About one third of the family physicians reported fewer than 25 deliveries; about one third, 25 to 50; and another third, more than 50.[19]

Willingness to serve low-income women. Physicians who identify themselves as FPs are somewhat more likely than ob/gyns to participate in Medicaid. A 1984 survey found that 86.8% of FPs and 80.4% of GPs reported accepting Medicaid patients. These figures compare with 82.8% participation by all physicians. FPs and GPs reported the same practice share devoted to Medicaid: 10.6%.[13]

Liability issues. According to a 1986 liability survey, of those FPs and GPs who had ever practiced obstetrics 18.6% had discontinued because of the cost or availability of liability insurance and 36.1% for other reasons. Those who dropped obstetrics because of liability reasons were somewhat younger than those who dropped it for other reasons (mean age 47.8 vs 52.3 years). Another 8.9% of those who had practiced obstetrics had decreased obstetric procedures because of liability concerns.[17] State surveys have shown that FPs and GPs were more likely to stop practicing obstetrics although ob/gyns faced higher liability insurance premiums.[16,20]

A 1987 survey of residency-trained family physicians found that only 45% of these relatively young and well-trained physicians were currently providing obstetric care, whereas 20% had done so in the past and 45% never had. About half of those currently providing obstetric care were considering discontinuing. The respondents most often cited

The providers must be distributed equitably throughout the country, must care for a reasonable number of obstetric patients, and must be willing to serve poor and high-risk women.

rising malpractice insurance premiums and fear of lawsuits as affecting their decision to avoid obstetrics, but (1) interference with life styles and (2) the number of ob/gyns in the area were also important factors. Those who had never practiced obstetrics were more likely to express concern about the adequacy of their training in this area, about their ability to keep up with changes in the field, and about the interference of obstetrics with their office practice.

An Arizona survey included only rural obstetric providers and found that 29% of FPs, 40% of GPs, and 64% of osteopathic physicians versus only 9% of ob/gyns had stopped or were planning to stop deliveries. The authors commented:

> One likely explanation for higher discontinuation rates among generalist physicians lies in the fact that obstetrical care is only one facet of the generalist's practice. Omission of obstetrical care would not threaten the financial viability of their practice since there are other, less litigious services that they can provide. In contrast, most obstetricians surveyed in this study stated that they could not support themselves on a practice which included gynecology but no obstetrics.[21(p10)]

The 1986 Physicians' Practice Follow-up Survey revealed that 19.5% of ob/gyns, 13.2% of FPs, and 12.1% of GPs had ever had problems with availability of insurance. In these three groups, 25.5%, 31.0%, and 30.5%, respectively, had discontinued certain high-risk cases in the past year because of the cost of insurance. Fifteen percent of ob/gyns reported having discontinued some form of obstetric care in 1986.[22]

Certified Nurse-Midwives

CNMs are registered nurses with additional training in midwifery. They are certified by the American College of Nurse-Midwives (ACNM), which states that

> nurse-midwifery practice is the independent management of essentially normal newborns and women antepartally, intrapartally and postpartally and/or gynecologically. This occurs within a health care system which provides for medical consultation, collaborative management and referral.[23(p2)]

Approximately 4500 CNMs have been certified, but the ACNM believes that only about 3000 practice and only 2900 are members of ACNM. Two hundred to 250 nurse-midwives are certified each year, although in 1989 this number decreased to 179 because of problems with the education programs. The ACNM expected the number of graduates to increase to previous levels in 1990 (unpublished data, ACNM, 1990).

Location. A 1988 survey of ACNM members found that 71% of respondents were engaged in clinical practice. Sixty percent included the management of births in their practice. Fifty-eight percent of respondents deliver babies in hospitals. The type of practice varied significantly across regions: those in New Jersey, New York, and the South were more likely to be involved in full-scope midwifery (including management of births), whereas those in the Midwest were least likely to perform deliveries. Nearly one quarter of the respondents were employed by a hospital. Comparisons with previous surveys show that fewer CNMs are involved in independent CNM practice (either in office-based or freestanding birth center practice) and fewer are practicing in hospital and public health departments. CNM employment is increasing in HMOs and in private physician practices.[24]

Volume of practice. CNMs care for an estimated 2% to 4% of US births and provide prenatal care to even more.[25] The number of births attended by midwives has risen substantially: midwives attended 3% of births in hospital in 1988 versus 1.4% in 1980.[26] The proportion of births attended by midwives varies greatly from state to state. In 1986, midwives attended 4% or more of hospital deliveries in 12 states and the District of Columbia, and in 9 states they attended 0.1% or less of deliveries.[27] The exact number of deliveries conducted by CNMs is unknown because vital statistics data do not distinguish between CNMs and other midwives. All of the hospital births and most of the out-of-hospital births probably were conducted by CNMs. Yet, even this may be an underestimate, because a number of midwives do not sign birth certificates for the infants they deliver.

Liability issues. Problems relating to the cost and availability of liability insurance have affected CNMs as well as physicians. In 1985 the ACNM lost its professional liability coverage through its standard insurer. After much effort, the association was able to negotiate a policy through a consortium of commercial carriers and now offers limited coverage for its members. The policy offers CNM coverage at $1 million per claim and $1 million aggregate coverage. Some hospitals require coverage of at least $1 million per claim and $3 million aggregate, thus preventing CNMs from practicing in those facilities. The amount of coverage and premiums are set nationally; there are no variations in premiums by type of practice or by geographic area.

Although the crisis of availability of insurance has been resolved, the cost of insurance has continued to pose an obstacle to CNM independent practice. Malpractice premiums now represent 14% of the average CNM salary versus 2% in 1983.[28] Although the mean annual income of CNMs increased by $10 000 between 1984 and 1988, CNM incomes are still only a fraction of average ob/gyn incomes. Full-time CNMs averaged $33 000 to $38 000 depending on the area of the country.[24]

CNMs report other practice changes due to liability concerns, including loss of hospital privileges and discontinuation of physician collaboration. CNMs also state that they are ordering more diagnostic tests, spending more time documenting their work, and changing patient eligibility criteria.[28]

PLACES WHERE MATERNITY CARE IS OFFERED

Most maternity services are offered on an outpatient basis, except for care in the immediate perinatal period (ie, labor and delivery and postdelivery hospitalization).

Prenatal and Postpartum Care

Women may receive their prenatal and postpartum care in the office of a private physician who also supervises labor, performs the delivery in a hospital, and offers postpartum care. A substantial number of women, however, especially poor women, seek care in public and quasi-public facilities and may not have continuity of care (ie, their babies may not be delivered by the same individual who supervised their prenatal care).

About one in five women receives prenatal care from a public or quasi-public provider such as a hospital outpatient department, a community health center, or a health department. Low-income, Black, Hispanic, teenaged, and unmarried women are more likely to use these facilities. Hospital clinics are the most commonly used type of clinic, reported by 9% of women as the source of care for their first prenatal visit. Family planning clinics serve 5%; health department clinics, 4%; community health centers, 3%; and military clinics, 3%. Low-income women are more likely to rely on these sources of care: 46% of low-income women report doing so versus 17% of higher income women. Public facilities provide services not only to the uninsured and those ineligible for Medicaid, but also to Medicaid recipients who have difficulty finding private physicians who accept Medicaid.[18]

Public and quasi-public providers have also reported liability problems that have decreased or may decrease their availability to poor, high-risk women. Facilities that usually provide liability coverage for their practitioners or rely on private practitioners with their own malpractice coverage to staff obstetric clinics are concerned about increased malpractice costs. Many government-operated services, however, have limited immunity from liability suits.

Hospital clinics. Despite the large contribution of hospital clinics to prenatal care, especially for poor women (15% of whom make their first prenatal visit at a hospital clinic), very little is known about the care provided in this setting. No national data source on hospital clinic use separates outpatient visits for obstetrics or gynecology from other clinic visits. In general, the number of nonemergency outpatient visits is increasing for all types of community hospitals.[29]

In 1988, 749 (14.3%) of community hospitals reported having a women's center. Although the American Hospital Association's (AHA's) definition of a women's center does not require that the center include obstetric services, it is likely that these centers include outpatient obstetric care. The number of women's centers increased between 198 and 1989 in government and private not-for-profit hospitals but de-creased in for-profit hospitals.[29]

In its report on prenatal care in the United States, the Alan Guttmacher Institute (AGI) used AHA data to project the number of nonfederal hospitals that would probably provide prenatal care. Hospitals were considered probable prenatal care providers if they had at least 400 deliveries annually and if they had an outpatient department and ob/gyns on staff. Twenty-nine percent of nonfederal short-term general hospitals, 45% of which had outpatient departments, met these criteria; 810 of these hospitals are private and 156 are public. (The AGI report does not distinguish between for-profit and not-for-profit hospitals.) Hospitals that do not meet these criteria may provide prenatal care through contracts with Title V Maternal and Child Health (MCH) programs.[30]

Public health programs. A 1986 Children's Defense Fund survey of public health officials representing the 51 state agencies (including the District of Columbia) that receive MCH funding under Title V of the Social Security Act found that 48 states offered some prenatal care for indigent women, usually through clinics operated by local health departments. Eligibility requirements and distribution of services varied widely from state to state. Eleven states based eligibility on specific conditions, offering services to high-risk, unmarried, teenaged, or un-employed women. Thirty-six states used uniform financial eligibility criteria, which usually means that services were provided without charge to certain groups, such as those with family incomes below 100% of the federal poverty level. Services were often available on the basis of a sliding fee to other women.[31]

Women in nonmetropolitan areas may have difficulty obtaining maternity care because they are more likely to be poor and uninsured.

A 1989 AGI survey of state MCH program directors identified 2017 service delivery sites operated by health departments. In addition, the state MCH programs funded 289 sites operated by other agencies such as community action groups and family planning clinics. Physicians may be employed to work in clinics or in their offices under contract with local health departments or state MCH programs. CNMs and NPs often deliver prenatal care under the supervision of physicians in health department clinics. Local health departments also may contract with other sources of care to provide prenatal care.[30]

Women who receive prenatal care at clinics subsidized by the state Title V agencies are likely to have incomes below the federal poverty level, to be young, and to be uninsured. An AGI survey of directors of state Title V agencies (25 states reporting) found that 64% of prenatal patients had incomes below the federal poverty level, 34% between 100% and 200% of poverty, and 2% above 200% of poverty. Sixty-four percent were uninsured, 27% received Medicaid, and 9% were privately insured although not necessarily insured for prenatal care. Sixty-two percent were between 20 and 34 years of age, 34% were teenagers, and 4% were 35 and older.[25]

Community and migrant health centers. Community health centers (CHCs) and migrant health centers (MHCs) are federally funded institutions that provide primary health care services, including perinatal services, to medically underserved and disadvantaged populations. Standards for CHCs and MHCs, which have been established by the Department of Health and Human Services (DHHS), require that the centers either provide or arrange for prenatal care and delivery services and that they develop a referral relationship with at least one hospital.

Currently, there are 525 CHC and MHC grantees, all providing prenatal care. The DHHS Office of Primary Care estimates that these grantees provide services at about 1200 sites. In fiscal year 1989 the centers served about 1.5 million women of childbearing age. Of the estimated 200 000 women who received perinatal care at the centers, only about half had their babies delivered by health center providers; the rest were referred to local physicians or hospitals. Many women, especially those at high risk, are referred early in the course of pregnancy (unpublished data, Office of Primary Care, Bureau of Health Care Delivery, 1990).

More than half of the CHCs and MHCs are currently receiving grants to provide comprehensive perinatal services under a program started in 1988. In fiscal year 1991, a total of $36 million was allocated to 285 centers, supplementing their regular funding. The funds must be used to augment existing perinatal systems, particularly to improve care coordination. The Office of Primary Care estimates that approximately 130 000 women received intensive case management services through the program in fiscal year 1989. Some centers also used the special funding to target substance-abusing, human immunodeficiency virus-infected, and homeless women.

CHCs and MHCs serve many poor, young, and uninsured women. AGI reported that in 1986 almost two thirds (64%) of the centers' prenatal patients had incomes below the federal poverty level and another quarter (24%) had incomes between 100% and 200% of poverty. Forty-four percent of the prenatal patients were covered by Medicaid, 42% were uninsured, and 14% were insured privately (although this insurance may not have covered prenatal services). Sixty-five percent were between ages 20 and 24, 27% were teenagers, and 8% were 35 and older. About one third of the CHCs and MHCs did not serve high-risk patients, and only one fifth of these paid for care at a referral agency. Only 16% of responding centers that provided prenatal care paid for delivery. Whether or not centers paid for delivery, their staff (or personnel paid by the agencies) attended almost half of the deliveries (unpublished data, Office of Primary Care, Bureau of Health Care Delivery, 1990).

Some centers are reporting decreases in the amount of obstetric services provided. One reason for the service cutbacks is the cost of liability insurance. The cost to CHCs and MHCs of malpractice insurance has increased rapidly in the past few years, despite the favorable claims experience of center practitioners. Only 16% of ob/gyn specialists in CHCs and MHCs were named in liability claims filed in 1985, but the cost of malpractice insurance increased from $800 to $900 per center that year to $12 000 per center in 1986. The allocation of greater resources to professional liability insurance has meant decreased funds for patient services. The Anchorage (Alaska) Neighborhood Health Center's malpractice premium for six obstetricians rose from $40 000 to more than $200 000 between 1985 and 1986. The center, which expected 500 deliveries in 1986, cut its staff to two obstetricians and its deliveries to 150.[32]

Attention must be paid to the conditions under which providers will care for rural, poor, and high-risk women.

Another reason for decreasing obstetric services in CHCs and MHCs is the declining number of National Health Service Corps (NHSC) personnel. Many CHCs and MHCs, as well as state and local health departments and the Indian Health Service, depend on the NHSC for physicians and other personnel. The NHSC provided scholarships for medical school and required recipients to serve 1 year for every year of training they received under NHSC funding. As of June 1988, of the 1297 NHSC physicians who were CHC and MHC employees, 419 were FPs, 104 were ob/gyns, and 50 were GPs. Another 212 NHSC physicians (including 50 FPs, 69 ob/gyns, and 13 GPs) were federal employees, either civil servants or commissioned Public Health Service officers. More than half of NHSC placements were in rural areas (unpublished data, NHSC, 1988).

The NHSC scholarship program was terminated in the early 1980s. About 115 ob/gyns and 278 FPs who provide obstetric services are due to complete their obligation between 1990 and 1993; only 20 ob/gyns and 69 FPs were available for placement in 1990. The NHSC is using two approaches to improving the supply of health personnel in underserved areas. The first is to attempt to retain personnel in these areas, although not necessarily in the same positions, after their obligation is met. Currently, the retention rate is between 30% and 40%. The second is a new program that offers loan repayments to physicians and others who will serve in underserved areas.

Labor and Delivery Services

Although the total number of hospital obstetric beds increased during the 1980s, the number of beds in hospitals operated by state and local governments decreased. Most hospital beds, as well as obstetric beds, are found in nongovernment, not-for-profit hospitals, and their number increased slightly. The number of obstetric beds in investor-owned (for-profit) hospitals increased more rapidly during this period. More births are occurring in hospitals that have more than 1500 births per year and fewer in hospitals that have fewer than 500 births in part because many of these smaller facilities are closing.[29]

The decrease in public hospital beds is important because public hospitals are more likely to serve poor patients. About 30% of all deliveries in government hospitals are paid for by Medicaid versus 18% in nonprofit, 17% in proprietary, and 16% in church-affiliated hospitals. Government hospitals also have more no-charge deliveries.[25]

A study in Los Angeles County found insufficient delivery capacity in area hospitals. A mathematical model of determining hospital delivery capacity suggested that the capacity of county hospitals was 189 300 in 1989 although births in that year numbered 193 517. This insufficient delivery capacity was present in four county facilities as well as 21 contract facilities. If the number of births continues to grow, the facilities are expected to have been at 110% of capacity in 1990.[33]

In 1988, 1% of all births occurred outside hospitals: 0.2% were attended by a physician, 0.4% by a midwife, and 0.3% by other attendants. Out-of-hospital births include births in freestanding birth centers, physicians' offices, homes, and other sites.[26] The setting may reflect the mother's decision to avoid the hospital because of personal preference or financial pressure, or emergency or unexpected deliveries rather than a shortage of delivery facilities.

PROBLEMS IN PROVIDER AVAILABILITY

The data that have been presented suggest that there are sufficient maternity care providers overall and enough labor and delivery beds in most locations. Yet many rural, low-income, and high-risk women have problems obtaining maternity care.

Coverage of Rural Areas

Women in nonmetropolitan areas may have difficulty obtaining maternity care because they are more likely than their metropolitan counterparts to be poor and uninsured. They are less likely to have Medicaid coverage, because many rural, poor states have restrictive Medicaid eligibility standards. In rural areas, physician availability may be a problem because family physicians have withdrawn from obstetric care rather than because of nonparticipation in Medicaid.

Higher infant mortality rates in nonmetropolitan areas may be related to reduced access to care before and after birth. Although neonatal mortality rates are comparable in rural and metropolitan areas, nonmetropolitan areas have more fetal deaths, possibly because of reduced access to prenatal care. Postneonatal mortality may be elevated because of reduced access to primary and specialized infant care.[34]

This theory appears to be confirmed by a Washington State study that examined the proportion of women in rural areas who received obstetric care in a local hospital. Communities where more than two thirds of deliveries occurred in local hospitals were designated low obstetric outflow areas and those where fewer than one third occurred in local hospitals, high outflow areas. The high and low outflow areas had similar socioeconomic characteristics. In high outflow areas the average distance to a level 2 nursery was 41 miles; in low outflow areas, 79 miles. The largest difference between the groups was the closing of obstetric facilities in the high outflow areas, which was attributed to the decision of local physicians to discontinue obstetrics practice. In these high outflow areas, women were more likely to have complicated and premature deliveries and higher neonatal care costs than in communities where most patients gave birth in the local hospital.[35]

Providers for Low-Income and High-Risk Populations

Even when adequate numbers of providers are present in a community, low-income and high-risk patients may have problems obtaining care. Many ob/gyns restrict the number or percentage of low-income or high-risk patients in their practices, whereas other practitioners may not have the appropriate training to deal with complex obstetric problems.

The National Governors' Association (NGA) conducted a survey of state Medicaid and MCH agencies to assess the extent of problems related to provider participation in maternity care for poor women. Thirty-five states reported problems in provider participation in maternity care. All of these noted that problems existed in rural areas; only three cited problems in finding providers in suburban or urban areas.[36]

In 484 counties in 21 states, officials reported that low-income women had limited access to prenatal and delivery services because there was no provider, because there was a single provider for many counties, or because public programs had difficulty obtaining physician backup or support. Fourteen states reported 246 counties without obstetric providers, and three states reported the closure of 42 hospital obstetric units. These reports came in response to an open-ended question, so they probably underestimate problems that exist.[36]

The NGA findings are supported by the AGI study, which reported that as many as 799 counties (26%) were without a hospital or clinic prenatal provider, although a number of these may be served by private practitioners or by other government programs such as the Indian Health Service.[30]

A Chicago study found that, despite Medicaid coverage, pregnant women in the inner city could not obtain prenatal care because of the lack of physicians. The volume of care reported by the few office-based obstetricians who still practiced in the city's depressed areas made the researchers question the quality of care provided.[37]

For maternity care to be effective, not only must providers be available to all women, but the care they provide must also be appropriate to the needs of the women being served. Although few studies of the suitability of care for middle- and upper-income women have been con-

**ADEQUACY OF
THE CONTENT
OF PRENATAL
CARE**

ducted, several have shown that low-income women benefit from an augmented service package and that such a package is not always available. (For more on preferred content of maternity care see chapter 13.)

California's Ob Access project tried to increase the number of providers in 13 obstetrically underserved counties, but it also required that the contracted providers, largely clinics, provide an enhanced service package. The evaluation found that low birthweight rates among women served in Ob Access facilities were lower than those among matched women who received care elsewhere under Medi-Cal, California's Medicaid program. That Ob Access women were less likely to receive first-trimester care than women in the comparison group suggests that quality of care may have been more important than quantity.[38,39]

> *Studies of the quality of prenatal care or of labor and delivery services are almost nonexistent.*

In a study in one North Carolina county, Medicaid-eligible women were served by obstetricians in office-based practices while poor women without Medicaid or other forms of insurance were served by the health department clinic. With potential confounders controlled, low birthweight rates among the health department group were lower than among the private obstetrician group, although the health department group started care later and had fewer visits. The differences were believed to be due to level of participation in the Special Supplemental Food Program for Women, Infants, and Children (WIC), use of NPs, and case management and coordination of services.[40]

A reanalysis of the General Accounting Office's (GAO's) 1989 and 1990 study of prenatal care found that the infants of women who received prenatal care through state outreach programs weighed more than those who received care through Medicaid. Women who reported that a hospital outpatient department or a community clinic was their regular source of care were delivered of heavier infants than those who used a private physician. The authors attribute these differences to the content of care in the public and quasi-public facilities.[41]

Several other studies also have found that women whose prenatal care is financed through the Medicaid program may have poorer outcomes than other women. A Tennessee study showed that low birthweight and neonatal mortality did not improve when Medicaid eligibility was expanded among married women.[42] A Michigan study found that pregnant women whose care was covered by Medicaid had higher social and behavioral risks and often poorer outcomes than insured and uninsured women.[43] Clearly, Medicaid alone is not the solution to the problems of poor pregnant women; this group also needs a package of care different from the one needed by women with more resources.

THE ADEQUACY OF THE QUALITY OF MATERNITY CARE

Studies of the quality of prenatal care or of labor and delivery services are almost nonexistent. Two of three classic ways of studying the quality of medical care—structure and process—are infrequently applied to maternity care.[44] Pregnancy outcomes are not examined by the qualifications of the staff who provide prenatal care, nor are hospitals examined in terms of the percentage of deliveries conducted by board-certified obstetricians. Differences in prenatal outcomes are usually analyzed by region, state, or county, not by type of facility (clinic vs hospital). These large-scale analyses may hide real discrepancies in the quality of the care provided at different prenatal care or delivery sites within a region.

The Health Care Financing Administration has listed hospitals with excess mortality rates for Medicare patients, even after case mix is controlled, but not for maternity patients. Not since the studies of neighborhood health centers, Maternity and Infant Care projects, and other public and quasi-public providers in the 1970s has there been any major attempt to examine differences in prenatal care by provider,[45] although cesarean section rates have been examined this way.

The third classic measure of quality of care—outcomes—has been adequately studied but is almost always linked to the characteristics of the woman (ie, age, race, education, and similar factors) and to her behavior (ie, when prenatal care was initiated and how many visits were made). Researchers often appear to be blaming the victim for adverse outcomes rather than examining the structure and the process of care first and turning to compliance issues only after the other factors have proved insufficient to explain differences. One exception is a recent study of birthweight in which the major source of prenatal care was used as a measure of the quality of care. The categories were (1) no care; (2) walk-in clinic or emergency care facility where no appointment was necessary and at which women said they were "checked by a doctor"; and (3) hospital clinic, public clinic, or private office requiring an appointment and staffed by obstetricians or family physicians. Even among poor, mostly Black women the source of prenatal care affected outcomes, although the findings clearly reflect the woman's motivation as well as the care source.[46] The reanalysis of the GAO study also suggests that the site of care may be important.[41]

Various recommendations have been proposed for increasing the number of providers and facilities providing adequate maternity care, especially to rural, low-income, and high-risk women.

RECOMMENDATIONS

Medicaid Reimbursements

Increasing provider reimbursements has been suggested as one way to improve access and care. The GAO reanalysis found that a 10% increase in Medicaid reimbursement relative to prevailing private fees was associated with a 1.5% increase in average birthweight.[41]

Most states increased Medicaid payments for deliveries in the second half of the 1980s, and such changes were mandated in the 1989 revisions. Although many expect these increases to improve provider participation in Medicaid, the experience of some states casts doubt on that assumption. The differential between public and private payment levels appears to have greater influence on provider participation than the absolute level of the public payment.[36]

States are also implementing streamlined procedures for filing claims, changing fee structures to allow differential billing for certain services, and eliminating global billing for prenatal care and delivery services. Such changes in Medicaid policies may increase private providers' participation rates.

Medical Liability

In 1989 the Institute of Medicine's (IOM's) Committee to Study Medical Professional Liability and the Delivery of Obstetrical Care recommended a variety of solutions to the liability problem, including a search for an alternative to the tort claims system for malpractice. The IOM committee proposed that the federal tort claims act be extended to obstetric practitioners in CHCs and MHCs to relieve practitioners of malpractice insurance costs while still providing legal recourse to plaintiffs. In addition, the IOM committee recommended that states contribute to professional liability coverage for Medicaid providers by subsidizing professional liability premiums.[47]

Of these recommendations, only the last has been implemented. It is not clear yet what its impact has been or will be on access to maternity care. The stabilization of malpractice premiums for ob/gyns in certain areas may help alleviate some of the access problems. Broad changes in the tort system, however, should not threaten the rights of patients to high-quality care and to appropriate redress in case of malpractice.

Rural Access

The IOM committee recommended that the NHSC be expanded to increase the number of physicians and other providers in underserved areas. This recommendation has been echoed by a number of experts in the field, in addition to proposals to require a period of community service by each newly trained physician. Proposals are needed to address the low retention rates and to increase the number of trained minority and rural individuals who return to rural areas to practice.[48]

Another alternative may be to improve opportunities for education and practice of nurse-midwifery. Currently, the number of CNMs is relatively small compared with ob/gyns and other physicians. But CNMs have shown more willingness to locate in rural areas and to work with low-income patients. The number of training programs for CNMs has recently decreased because of cuts in federal funding. These training programs should be restored and expanded. Proposals for training direct-entry midwives (practitioners with 3 years of postbaccalaureate midwifery training but no nursing) should be evaluated in the context of the diverse needs of maternity populations, especially in rural areas.

High-Risk Women

Finally, a redistribution of maternity care resources is needed to ensure that the women who are at highest risk of pregnancy complications receive more intensive services. This viewpoint is embodied in the report of the Public Health Service's Expert Panel on the Content of Prenatal Care, which recommended that the standard number of prenatal visits be reduced for low-risk women but that additional services be offered on an individual basis to those women who need them.[1] The adoption of these recommendations could theoretically free a large portion of the time of highly trained practitioners to deal with high-risk obstetric cases.

Rosenblatt has noted:

CONCLUSION

> The basic incongruity in American perinatal care lies in our superb ability to care for the individual patient and our dismal failure to address the problems of the larger society. We tend to allocate resources—and, conversely, ration care—based upon the specifics of individual patients, not upon a predetermined attempt to optimize national outcomes. The individual anguish of the patient searching publicly for a liver transplant is more likely to influence public policy than are grim but impersonal statistics about rising rates of infant mortality.[49(p159)]

Making appropriate, high-quality maternity care available to all women is a complex task. Although funding additional women under Medicaid is essential, it will not be enough to improve pregnancy outcomes or meet the other goals of maternity care. Attention must be paid to the conditions under which providers will care for rural, poor, and high-risk women. The content of care must be enhanced for these women, and the quality of care for the poor and for those at high risk must be guaranteed.

REFERENCES

1. US Public Health Service. Expert Panel on the Content of Prenatal Care. *Caring for Our Future: The Content of Prenatal Care.* Washington, DC: US Dept of Health and Human Services; 1989.
2. Roback G, Randolph L, Seidman B, Mead D. *Physician Characteristics and Distribution in the US.* Chicago, Ill: American Medical Association; 1987.
3. American College of Obstetricians and Gynecologists. Residents in Obstetrics-Gynecology. *Obstetrics and Gynecology Manpower Planning Study.* Washington, DC: American College of Obstetricians and Gynecologists; 1987.
4. US Bureau of Health Professions. *Area Resource File System, US and State Summaries of Selected Geographic Resources and Trends in Resources.* Silver Spring, Md: Applied Management Science, Inc.; 1987.
5. American College of Obstetricians and Gynecologists. Map of number

of Ob/Gyns providing patient care per 100,000 women age 15–44 by Zip Code sectional area. In: *Obstetrics and Gynecology Manpower Planning Study.* Washington, DC: American College of Obstetricians and Gynecologists; 1988.

6. Gonzalez ML, Emmons DW, eds. *Socioeconomic Characteristics of Medical Practice, 1989.* Chicago, Ill: American Medical Association; 1990.

7. American College of Obstetricians and Gynecologists. *Professional Liability and Its Effects: Report of a 1990 Survey of ACOG's Membership.* Washington, DC: Opinion Research Corporation; 1990.

8. American College of Obstetricians and Gynecologists. *Professional Liability and Its Effects: Report of a Survey of ACOG's Membership.* Washington, DC: Needham, Porter, Novelli; 1985.

9. American College of Obstetricians and Gynecologists. *Professional Liability and Its Effects: Report of a 1987 Survey of ACOG's Membership.* Washington, DC: Opinion Research Corporation; 1988.

10. Baumgardner JR, Marder WD. Specialization among obstetrician/gynecologists: another dimension of physician supply. *Med Care.* 1991; 29:272–282.

11. Gillis KD, Willke RJ. Employment patterns of physicians, 1983–1989. In: Gonzalez ML, Emmons DW, eds. *Socioeconomic Characteristics of Medical Practice, 1989.* Chicago, Ill: American Medical Association; 1990.

12. American College of Obstetricians and Gynecologists. Committee on Health Care for Underserved Women. *Ob/Gyn Services for Indigent Women: Issues Raised by an ACOG Survey [1987].* Washington, DC: ACOG; undated.

13. Mitchell J. Unpublished data. In: US Congress. Office of Technology Assessment. *Healthy Children: Investing in the Future.* Washington, DC: US Govt Printing Office; 1986. Publication OTA-H-345.

14. Department tracks ob/gyn income data, plans own survey. *ACOG Newsletter.* 1991; 35:10.

15. US General Accounting Office. *Medical Malpractice: A Continuing Problem with Far-reaching Implications.* Testimony Before the Subcommittee on Health, Committee on Ways and Means, House of Representatives, April 26, 1990. Publication GAO/T-HRD-90-24.

16. Rosenblatt RA, Cherkin DC, Schneeweiss R, et al. The structure and content of family practice: current status and future trends. *J Fam Pract.* 1982; 15:681–722.

17. American Academy of Family Physicians. *Family Physicians and Obstetrics: A Professional Liability Study.* Kansas City, Mo: American Academy of Family Physicians; 1987.

18. Alan Guttmacher Institute. *The Financing of Maternity Care in the United States.* New York, NY: Alan Guttmacher Institute; 1987.

19. Kruse J, Phillips D, Wesley RN. Factors influencing changes in obstetric care provided by family physicians: a national study. *J Fam Pract.* 1989; 28:597–602.

20. California Medical Association. Professional liability issues in obstetrical practice (part 2). In: *Socioeconomic Report.* vol 25. San Francisco, Calif: California Medical Association; 1985.

21. Gordon FJ, McMullen G, Weiss BD, Nichols AW. The effect of malpractice liability on the delivery of rural obstetrical care. *J Rural Health.* 1987; 3:7–13.

22. Rosenbach ML, Stone AG. Malpractice insurance costs and physician practice, 1983–1986. *Health Affairs.* 1990; 9:176–185.

23. Adams C. *Nurse-midwifery in the United States, 1982.* Washington, DC: American College of Nurse Midwives; 1984.

24. Lehrman EJ, Paine LL. Trends in nurse-midwifery: results of the American College of Nurse Midwives division of research mini-survey. *J Nurse Midwifery.* 1990; 35:192–203.

25. Knoll K. Certified nurse midwives, nurse practitioners, and family practice physicians in the delivery of prenatal care. In: Merkatz IR, Thompson JE, eds. *New Perspectives on Prenatal Care.* New York, NY: Elsevier Science Publishing Co; 1990.

26. National Center for Health Statistics. Advance report of final natality statistics, 1988. *Monthly Vital Statistics Report.* vol 39, no 4 suppl. Hyattsville, Md: Public Health Service; 1990. PHS 90–1120.

27. National Center for Health Statistics. Advance report of final natality statistics, 1986. *Monthly Vital Statistics Report.* vol 37, no 3 suppl. Hyattsville, Md: Public Health Service; 1988. DHHS publication (PHS)88–1120.

28. Patch FB, Holaday SD. Effects of changes in professional liability insurance on certified nurse-midwives. *J Nurse Midwifery.* 1989; 34:131–136.

29. American Hospital Association. *Hospital Statistics.* Chicago, Ill: American Hospital Association; 1989.

30. Singh S, Forrest JD, Torres A. *Prenatal Care in the United States: A State and County Inventory.* vol I. New York, NY: Alan Guttmacher Institute; 1989.

31. Rosenbaum S, Hughes DC, Johnson K. Maternal and child health services for medically indigent children and pregnant women. *Med Care.* 1988; 26:315–332.

32. Rosenbaum S, Hughes D. The medical malpractice crisis and poor women. In: Brown S, ed. *Prenatal Care: Reaching Mothers, Reaching Infants.* Washington, DC: National Academy Press; 1988.

33. Richwald GA, Morrison K, DeVane DM. *Obstetrical Delivery Service Capacity in Los Angeles County: An Analysis of the Current Crisis.* Los Angeles, Calif: UCLA School of Public Health; 1990.

34. Hughes DC, Rosenbaum S. An overview of maternal and infant health services in rural America. *J Rural Health.* 1989; 5:299–319.

35. Nesbitt TS, Connell FA, Hare LG, Rosenblatt RA. Access to obstetrical care in rural areas: effect on birth outcomes. *Am J Public Health.* 1990; 80:814–818.

36. Lewis-Idema D. *Increasing Provider Participation.* Washington, DC: National Governors Association; 1989.

37. Fossett JW, Perloff JD, Peterson JA, Kletke PR. Medicaid in the inner city: the case of maternity care in Chicago. *Milbank Q.* 1990; 68:111–141.

38. Lennie JA, Klun JR, Hausner T. Low-birth-weight rate reduced by the obstetrical access project. *Health Care Fin Rev.* 1987; 8:83–86.

39. Korenbrot CC. Risk reduction in pregnancies of low-income women: comprehensive care through the OB access project. *Mobius.* 1984; 3:34–43.

40. Buescher PA, Smith C, Holliday JL, Levine RH. Source of prenatal care and infant birth weight: the case of a North Carolina county. *Am J Obstet Gynecol.* 1987; 156:204–210.

41. Schlesinger M, Kronebusch K. The failure of prenatal care policy for the poor. *Health Affairs.* 1990; 9:91–111.

42. Piper JM, Ray WA, Griffin MR. Effects of Medicaid eligibility expansion on prenatal care and pregnancy outcome in Tennessee. *JAMA.* 1990; 264:2219–2223.

43. Schwethelm B, Margolis LH, Miller C, Smith S. Risk status and pregnancy outcome among Medicaid recipients. *Am J Prev Med.* 1989; 5:157–163.

44. Donabedian A. *The Definition of Quality and Approaches to Its Assessment.* Ann Arbor, Mich: Health Administration Press; 1980.

45. Morehead MA, Donaldson RS, Seravalli MR. Comparisons between OEO neighborhood health centers and other health care providers of ratings of the quality of health care. *Am J Public Health.* 1971; 61:1294–1306.

46. Poland ML, Ager JW, Olson KL, Sokol RJ. Quality of prenatal care; selected social, behavioral, and biomedical factors; and birth weight. *Obstet Gynecol.* 1990; 75:607–611.
47. Institute of Medicine. Committee to Study Medical Professional Liability and the Delivery of Obstetrical Care. *Medical Professional Liability and the Delivery of Obstetrical Care.* vol I. Washington, DC: National Academy Press; 1989.
48. Rosenbaum S, Klerman LV. Recommendations to the Council on Graduate Medical Education. 1990.
49. Rosenblatt RA. The perinatal paradox: doing more and accomplishing less. *Health Affairs.* 1989; 8·158 168.

CHAPTER 10

Private Health Insurance Coverage of Maternity and Infant Care

Samuel S. Flint, PhD
Rachel Benson Gold, MPA

Private health insurance plans are the principal source of insurance for Americans younger than age 65 and infants to age 1. In 1985, the most recent year for which data are available, 73% of the 56 million US women of reproductive age—41 million women—had some form of private health insurance coverage.[1] In 1988, 63% of infants were covered by private insurance, including 55% by parents' employer plans and 8% through other sources.[2]

Private health insurance is rooted in the historic tradition of life, property, and casualty insurance. These insurance products offer financial compensation to beneficiaries for expenses incurred as a result of rare and unpredictable events such as fires and hurricanes. High levels of coverage can be purchased for relatively modest premiums because an insurable event is so unlikely to occur. Thus, private health insurance plans, which began only 50 years ago, created financing systems designed to reimburse insured individuals for expenses incurred for inpatient care and surgical procedures, events that are unpredictable and costly. Predictable preventive care and other lower cost ambulatory care are frequently not covered benefits.

PRIVATE HEALTH INSURANCE

Unlike Medicaid, the Maternal and Child Health Block Grant, and other government health care financing systems, private health insurance is not designed to achieve public health goals such as promoting use of preventive care or insuring people who are most in need. Private insurers contribute to society by making medical services more affordable through the organizing of risk-sharing arrangements. However, market incentives are the driving force behind the private health insurance industry.

Private insurance plans are sold by for-profit corporations (ie, commercial insurers, investor-owned preferred provider organizations [PPOs] and health maintenance organizations [HMOs]) and by nonprofit organizations (ie, Blue Cross and Blue Shield plans and some independent PPOs and HMOs). Commercial insurers and other for-profit health care systems, like all other for-profit corporations, are in business to make a return on investment for their owners and stockholders. To do so they attempt to keep their costs as low as possible in order to price their products competitively and maximize profits.

Nonprofit insurers can maintain and expand their market share only if they too price their insurance products competitively. Rather than seek profits to distribute to owners, nonprofit institutions try to create and retain reserves. However, both types of organizations must respond to the same market forces to survive.

Most privately insured children and pregnant women gain coverage as dependents of employees with employer-sponsored plans. In addition to the plans offered by commercial insurers, Blue Cross and Blue Shield plans, HMOs, and PPOs, a large proportion of privately insured employees and their dependents have their medical care financed through employers who "self-insure." Self-insurance means a company directly funds health care expenses for its employees and their covered dependents rather than pay premiums to an insurer. Usually only larger employers have enough employees to take on the risks inherent in this option. Self-insured corporations create their own insurance plans, which are generally quite similar to conventional private insurance plans. Because most employers who self-insure hire an insurance company to administer their programs, employees in self-insured companies are treated like employees in firms that purchase the plans from the administering company.

Self-insurance has been permitted since the enactment of the Employee Retirement Income Security Act of 1974 (ERISA), but its popularity has risen sharply in recent years. Between 1982 and 1988, for example, in firms with employer-sponsored health insurance and at least 100 employees the proportion of workers who were in self-insured firms increased from 22% to 42%.[3]

In general, states—not the federal government—regulate private health insurance. States can specify benefits that must be included, require minimum insurance reserves, and enforce other requirements for commercial insurers, Blue Cross plans, HMOs, and PPOs. However, because of the ERISA exemption, states have no regulatory authority over self-insured corporate plans. Some evidence indicates that avoiding state regulation has been a major motivation of corporations that have opted for self-insurance.[3]

COVERAGE OF MATERNITY CARE

Despite the heavy reliance on insurance to help families afford high-quality medical care when needed, private health insurance has traditionally offered little or no coverage for maternity care. In 1978, however, that situation changed with the passage of the Pregnancy Discrimination Act (PDA), a civil rights measure designed to end the traditional discrimination against women in employee benefit plans. This law requires that most, but not all, employer-sponsored group health insurance policies cover maternity care in the same manner they cover other medical conditions.

This legislation has been extremely effective in assuring that most health insurance policies include coverage of maternity care and that most women with health insurance have such coverage. Before the passage of the PDA, the National Medical Care Utilization and Expenditure Survey concluded that

> Although close to 90 percent of the privately insured in general and women age 15 to 44 in particular were entitled to some benefits for maternity care, only about four out of five were insured for care beyond medical complications of pregnancy.[4(p16)]

By 1986, however, according to the Health Insurance Association of America, 95% of newly written group health insurance policies covered maternity care the same way they covered other services.

Despite these improvements, the protections of the PDA do not ensure that all women covered by private health insurance have coverage for maternity care. The PDA has three major loopholes. First, because the PDA applies only to employer-sponsored insurance policies, its protections are not applicable to so-called nongroup policies that are purchased by individuals independent of the workplace. Three million women—6% of all women of reproductive age—are covered by such policies. These policies are much less likely than group policies to cover maternity care. In 1977, before passage of the PDA, only 51% of women of reproductive age with nongroup coverage had hospital benefits for a normal delivery.[4(p87)]

... private health insurance is not designed to achieve public health goals such as promoting use of preventive care or insuring people who are most in need.

The second limitation of the PDA is that the protections of the law are not extended to people who are insured through firms with 15 or fewer employees. The data indicate that, because of this exception in the law, a considerable proportion of insurance policies written for very small employers do not include maternity care (18% of firms of fewer than 15 employees).

Third, guidelines concerning the PDA issued by the Equal Employment Opportunity Commission make clear that the law requires policies to include maternity benefits for the employee and the spouse of the employee. However, according to the guidelines, "The insurance does not have to cover the pregnancy-related conditions of other dependents as long as it excludes the pregnancy-related conditions of dependents of male and female employees equally" (29 CFR 1604). Thus, even if an employment-related insurance policy includes maternity benefits for the employee and spouse, it may exclude them for nonspouse dependents such as the teenage daughters of the policyholder. Since the passage of the PDA, only eight states have extended dependent children the same protection given their parents. Pregnancy-related care for teenagers in other states often is not covered; 35% of the typical policies written to insure employees and their families exclude nonspouse dependents from eligibility for maternity benefits.[1]

An additional problem for nonspouse dependents is posed by state laws that mandate coverage of newborn infants from the moment of birth. Written in the mid-1970s to prevent delays in the coverage of infants, these laws apply to infants born to the employee and the employee's spouse but not to infants born to nonspouse dependents. As a result, 69% of typical policies do not cover the babies of nonspouse dependents, regardless of whether the teenager herself is covered; only 25% of typical insurance policies cover both the teenager and her infant.[1]

As a result of these loopholes in the PDA, as well as other restrictions in insurance policies such as waiting periods and limitations on coverage of preexisting medical conditions, many women who have some insurance coverage may find themselves with no coverage at all for their pregnancies. Estimates made for 1985 show that about 9% of women of reproductive age—some 5 million women—have private insurance policies that do not cover maternity care, and about 333 000 of the women who give birth each year have private insurance policies that pay nothing for their maternity care.[1]

Even if a woman's insurance does cover her pregnancy, the family may be saddled with significant costs, because insurance often fails to cover all the services mother and infant need. For example, 14% of insurers do not cover Rh immune globulin injections (essential to prevent miscarriage or stillbirth for a pregnant woman whose blood type is Rh negative).[1]

COVERAGE OF INFANTS

Although private plans are the predominant form of insurance coverage for infants, the absolute number and percentage of children under the age of 18 who were insured by private plans declined steadily during the first half of the 1980s.[5] Specific data on infants are not available, but the well-documented decline in coverage for all employee dependents (ie, spouses and children) makes it reasonable to assume that infants were no exception.

Various causes for this trend have been hypothesized, such as the shift in jobs from the manufacturing sector of the economy to the service sector, where health insurance benefits are less frequently offered. However, the data suggest that the principal causes are (1) the increased cost of dependent coverage for employees resulting from escalating health care costs and (2) a growing employee share of family insurance premiums.[6] This issue is discussed in some detail later in the chapter.

Although private insurance is the most common form of coverage for all infants, there is substantial variation in source of insurance by income level. Only one in eight poor infants has private insurance coverage, but the proportion rises significantly as family income increases (Table 10-1). Families with incomes between 125% and 200% of the federal poverty level have roughly the same proportion of privately in-

TABLE 10-1
Source of Health Insurance in 1988 for Infants Under Age 1
by Family Income Level

Percentage of Federal Poverty Level	Population, in millions	Privately Insured, %*	Publicly Insured, %*	Uninsured, %*
All incomes	3.8	63	25	16
Less than 100%	0.9	13	68	23
100%-124%	0.2	49	†	†
125%-199%	0.6	65	19	22
200% or more	2.1	86	6	11

Source: March 1989 Current Population Survey data reported by the Employee Benefit Research Institute (Issue Brief Number 104, "Update: Americans Without Health Insurance," July 1990).

* Percentages do not sum to 100 because some infants are covered by more than one source.

† The number is too small to be statistically significant.

sured infants as the overall infant population. Thus, while Medicaid and other public insurance plans cover most of the insured poor, private plans insure many low-income infants as well as the vast majority of infants in middle- and upper-income families.

Health insurers are continually developing and implementing strategies to contain costs. Many of these practices eliminate unnecessary expenses that provide no medical or social benefits, such as surgical procedures that may not be medically necessary (eg, tonsillectomies). However, other approaches to cost containment, such as excluding benefits or denying coverage, are not in the best interest of infants or pregnant women.

COST CONTAINMENT

Until the late 1970s, for example, insurers were permitted to exclude newborns from private insurance plans for a period of 7 to 30 days, depending on the plan. All states now have passed legislation prohibiting this practice, and self-insured corporations have conformed. However, other practices such as limiting benefits, requiring waiting periods, charging higher premiums, and denying insurance altogether for preexisting conditions are widespread and growing in scope. Among the list of preexisting conditions that may be excluded from coverage are many medical problems that are fairly common among infants, such as chronic otitis media, asthma, and allergies.[7] In addition to denying coverage or requiring waiting periods for specified medical conditions, some 2 million individuals, including many infants, are classified as totally uninsurable.

Twenty-four states have enacted legislation creating high-risk pools for individuals considered uninsurable by private insurers. Because premiums for such insurance are substantially higher than the standard community rates, cost still prevents many people from obtaining coverage. Private insurers have come under increased criticism for systematically avoiding higher risk insureds. To curb exclusions for preexisting conditions, federal legislation (the Federal Health Insurance Equity Act of 1989) was introduced in the 101st Congress. Although the legislation did not pass in the session, recognition of the seriousness of this issue is growing.

CATASTROPHIC COVERAGE

Hospitalizations are much more frequent during the first year of life than at any other time during childhood or young adulthood, although the need for inpatient care is still a relatively unusual occurrence.[8] One lengthy neonatal intensive care stay could bankrupt most families. Thus the need for catastrophic coverage is great for the relatively few families that incur such costs. In addition to the affected families, hospitals (particularly neonatal intensive care units) have a direct stake in this public policy issue. Even well-intentioned families may find that it is beyond their financial capacity to pay for uncovered services, thus forcing these costs to be absorbed by the institution. Most hospitals who serve the highest-risk maternal and infant population are already straining under large, uncompensated care burdens. Without adequate reimbursement from privately insured patients these facilities would have to face very difficult choices, including curtailment of needed care.

Now that the 30-day newborn exclusion has been eliminated, most private insurance plans provide adequate coverage for high-cost, high-technology care. In 1989, approximately half of employer-sponsored private insurance plans had an annual maximum family out-of-pocket expenditure limit of $1000; three fourths had a $2000 limit. Less than 7% had no annual expenditure limit.[9] Most plans, including many of those offered through state high-risk pools, have lifetime benefit limits. In 1989, less than 8% of employer-sponsored private plans had maximum lifetime benefits of $250 000 or less. Most have lifetime limits of $1 million or more, and approximately one in five has unlimited lifetime benefits.[9] Thus, most children and pregnant women who have private insurance are reasonably well covered for catastrophic expenses.

PREVENTIVE CARE

Although private insurance generally covers the high-cost portion of maternal and infant care fairly well, low-cost, low-technology care is often inadequately covered. The single largest gap in coverage is preventive care, also referred to as child health supervision or well-baby care. Given the scope and depth of coverage by benefit category, health insurance would be more appropriately called sickness insurance, because covered medical services are overwhelmingly for disease treatment rather than disease prevention.

In 1988, more than 6% of all infants did not have one preventive care visit. Strong evidence suggests that lack of insurance is a contributing factor.[10] The American Academy of Pediatrics (AAP) and the Canadian Task Force on the Periodic Health Exam recommend six ambulatory preventive visits during the first year of life in addition to two examinations before the neonate leaves the hospital.[11] Some researchers contend that clinical evidence is lacking to support the necessity of more than three visits during the first year (and two in the second year) to provide immunizations against such childhood diseases as polio, measles, and whooping cough, in addition to the newborn exams.[11] All observers agree, however, that some level of ambulatory preventive care is essential. Nevertheless, private insurers resist covering these services although the health insurance premium to cover the AAP preventive care schedule through the age of 2 in the typical private insurance plan is only $2.34 per month per family.[12]

Lack of private insurance coverage for infant preventive care harms young families more than any other group, because these families are more likely to have a lower, less stable income than families with older children. More women are returning to their jobs while they still have infants at home, but many families that normally rely on two incomes have only one breadwinner during the time when one or more infants or toddlers are at home. In addition, parents of infants are generally in the earliest stages of their careers, when earnings are lowest. Job security is also at its nadir because young workers lack seniority and their jobs are vulnerable during economic downturns.

. . . health insurance would be more appropriately called sickness insurance, because covered medical services are overwhelmingly for disease treatment rather than disease prevention.

Although the insurance premium cost is low when spread among all family policyholders, the actual cost of preventive care is substantial during the first 2 years of life, when a large number of vital services need to be provided. In 1991, the national average cost of the AAP's recommended schedule of physician visits, immunizations, and laboratory tests for a baby's first year is $489.[12] The estimated cost for the second year, by which time basic immunizations are completed, is $281. Without insurance coverage for preventive care, young families with little disposable income often must choose between taking an outwardly healthy infant to the doctor or paying for other basic necessities. Some parents consequently defer or forgo preventive care.

Fortunately, this serious underinsurance gap has been steadily declining since the early 1980s as a result of state regulation and market forces in the health insurance industry. Since the early 1980s, private insurers have promoted financing and delivery systems that constrain providers' freedom of choice but offer expanded benefits and lower cost than traditional open-ended health insurance. Prenatal and well-baby care, which have long been standard benefits of HMOs, are now frequently included in PPO and other managed care plans. The coverage of prenatal and well-baby care is a marketing tool for young families who, because of their age, are generally healthier than the overall population and consequently better than average insurance risks.

In 1989 approximately one third of employer-insured workers and dependents were in HMOs (17%) or PPOs (16%). Ninety-eight percent of HMOs covered preventive care for beneficiaries of all ages in 1989.[9] A 1986 PPO survey revealed that 72% covered immunizations for babies to age 2, 75% covered well-baby care other than immunizations, and 85% covered routine prenatal care.[13]

By the mid-1980s, traditional insurance began employing some of the use control techniques that are used in managed care plans (eg, hospital preadmission certification, mandatory second surgical opinions) to keep their premium cost down. They also began offering well-baby benefits to attract lower risk, young families. In 1988, 45% of conventional plans offered at least some well-baby care coverage,[14] and in 1989 this proportion increased to 50%.[9]

Coinciding with health insurance market changes, a number of state laws in the late 1980s were enacted mandating coverage of preventive care for children from birth to ages 3 to 20, depending on the state. In 1986 Florida was the first state to mandate ambulatory preventive care for children in private health insurance plans. Since then, six other states have enacted similar legislation (Table 10-2). In 1989, preventive pediatric care was the second most sought-after private insurance mandate in state legislatures.[15] In addition to mandates for ambulatory infant preventive care, other states require coverage only for "normal newborn" care for infants before they are released from the hospital nursery. Still other states have begun requiring insurance companies to offer preventive care. This regulation has had no discernible effect on employer behavior with respect to insuring preventive care. For example, California has had this requirement since 1980 and there is no evidence that it has led to any increase in preventive care coverage.

INCREASING COSTS

Private health insurance does not always cover the entire charge for the services that are covered. The insured employee is usually required to pay a certain deductible before coverage takes effect; participants also generally have to pay a percentage of most medical bills (coinsurance) or a fixed sum per service (copayments), even after the deductible has been met. Recent data indicate that these costs to the family have been rising sharply. The 1989 Hay/Huggins Benefits Report shows a jump in the percentage of employees with policies that require large deductibles. More than half (57%) of 1989's survey respondents required a deductible of more than $100 versus 33% in 1985. Similarly, fewer employers are paying the entire cost of covered services and are instead requiring employees to pay a percentage of the cost themselves. Only 27% of the companies surveyed by Hay/Huggins paid 100% of hospital and surgical expenses in 1989, versus 35% in 1985.[16] In the decade 1977 to 1987, the percentage of employees with policies that required both deductibles and copayments of 20% or more rose from 60% to 75%.[17]

TABLE 10-2
State Health Insurance Mandates for Infant Preventive Care*

	Hospital Newborn Care	Ambulatory Preventive Care	Must Offer Preventive Care
Arkansas	X		X
California			X
Connecticut		X	
Delaware	X		
Florida		X	
Hawaii	X	X	
Kentucky			X
Massachusetts		X	
Michigan	X		
Minnesota	X	X	
Missouri			X
Montana	X	X	
New York			X
Rhode Island	X	X	
Tennessee	X		
Utah	X		
Virginia			X

* Figures current as of April 1991. The following states and the District of Columbia have no requirements for infant preventive care: Alabama, Alaska, Arizona, Colorado, Georgia, Idaho, Illinois, Indiana, Iowa, Kansas, Louisiana, Maine, Maryland, Mississippi, Nebraska, Nevada, New Hampshire, New Jersey, New Mexico, North Carolina, North Dakota, Ohio, Oklahoma, Oregon, Pennsylvania, South Carolina, South Dakota, Texas, Vermont, Washington, West Virginia, Wisconsin, and Wyoming.

Source: American Academy of Pediatrics.

The cost to the family of insurance coverage itself has also been increasing. Faced with rapidly rising insurance premiums, employers are increasingly passing on at least some of these costs to employees by either requiring them to contribute to the cost of insurance coverage or increasing the size of employee contributions. As a result, the percentage of employers who pay the entire cost of insurance coverage is falling, especially when it comes to family coverage. According to the Bureau of Labor Statistics, fully paid employer coverage for employees declined from 57% to 52% between 1987 and 1988. Fully paid family coverage declined from 36% to 34% during the same year.[18]

Because a large number of women, and all infants, are insured as dependents on their husbands' or parents' policies, the increase in the percentage of employers requiring contributions for dependent coverage is particularly alarming. An equally significant trend is the apparent increase in the number of employers who are making no contribution to dependent coverage. According to a survey by the National Association of Manufacturers, 15% of the large firms surveyed require employees to pay the entire cost of dependent coverage.[19] With the cost of insurance coverage soaring, such requirements might easily place insurance coverage beyond the reach of many families in need of insurance protection, particularly the young families most likely to need maternal and infant care services.

PROPOSED SOLUTIONS

Federal legislation has been proposed that would preempt ERISA and state regulatory authority and require private insurance plans, including the self-insured, to provide adequate coverage for maternity and infant care. These proposals vary widely.

In 1983 and 1984 the Child Health Incentive Reform Plan was introduced in both the House and the Senate. This legislation would have disallowed the cost of employee health insurance premiums or employee medical expenses (for self-insured corporations) as a deduction from federal corporate income taxes unless the plans included full preventive care coverage for employees' children from birth to age 21. The bill did not pass and was eventually abandoned.

Another federal initiative that would preempt the ERISA exemption from state regulatory authority is the Basic Health Benefits for All Americans Act, sponsored by Massachusetts Senator Edward Kennedy and California Representative Henry Waxman. This legislation is designed to expand health insurance to the uninsured through a federally mandated minimum benefit package for all employees and their dependents along with a phased-in expansion of Medicaid. The proposal calls for mandatory coverage of prenatal and well-baby care, but only to age 1. It also would prohibit preexisting condition exclusions and provide a $3000 catastrophic cap for all out-of-pocket expenses.

A third federal proposal was advanced in 1990 by the Bipartisan Commission on Comprehensive Health Care (the so-called Pepper Commission), which recommended a series of major reforms under which all employees in the United States and their dependents would be provided basic health insurance and those without access to employment-related coverage would be eligible for a public program completely separate from Medicaid or welfare. Both the public program and the private insurance policies offered by employers would include coverage for basic physician and hospital care, including maternity and infant care, as well as some other services. As outlined by the commission, private insurance policies would be prevented from excluding people with preexisting medical conditions (including pregnant women and infants) from coverage. Although policies would continue to include annual deductibles for individuals and families, expenditures for prenatal and well-child care would be exempt from deductible requirements.

A fourth proposal under discussion in 1991 is the AAP's plan to ensure universal access for children and pregnant women.[20] This proposal would require employers to provide a comprehensive benefit package to all employees and their dependents who are pregnant or under age 22 or pay 3% payroll tax to a state fund, which would be used to purchase an equivalent private insurance plan. Under the plan, Medicaid funds for pregnant women and children would be redirected to the state fund and all former Medicaid eligibles and the remaining uninsured pregnant women and children would have state-approved comprehensive private insurance plans purchased for them. Full coverage of prenatal and well-child care would be included along with all other medically necessary services.

The path to enactment for any major reform of our health insurance system will undoubtedly be long and tortuous. Millions of Americans, including a disproportionate number of pregnant women and children, have either no health insurance or inadequate coverage. However, in spite of obvious flaws in the financing of maternal and infant health care, a potent constituency seeking fundamental reform has yet to emerge. To the detriment of the next generation, the status quo appears to be acceptable to enough voters to allow health care reform to remain relatively low on the political agenda. Until the American people recognize the risk to the social fabric and the nation's economic viability that the recent pattern of underinvestment and disinvestment in maternal and infant health care represents, government action is unlikely.

Fundamental reform could take the form of mandated employer-based private insurance with residual public sector funding for people who are unattached to the labor force; a single-payer, federally run system; or a plan yet to be devised. However, it is not the absence of agreement about which proposal is most efficient and equitable that is stymieing that reform; it is the absence of a political consensus that incremental reform of private and public insurance is a disservice to the nation. If the battle over the necessity for systemwide reform is won, the debate over how it should be implemented is likely to be a less heated dispute.

CONCLUSION

REFERENCES

1. Gold RB, Kenney AM, Singh S. *Blessed Events and the Bottom Line: Financing Maternity Care in the United States.* New York, NY: Alan Guttmacher Institute; 1987.
2. Employee Benefit Research Institute. *Update: Americans without Health Insurance.* Washington, DC; 1990. Employee Benefit Research Institute Brief no 104.
3. Employee Benefit Research Institute. *Features of Employer-sponsored Health Plans.* Washington, DC; 1990. Employee Benefit Research Institute Brief no 100.
4. US Public Health Service. National Center for Health Services Research and Health Care Technology Assessment. *Private Health Insurance in the United States.* Washington, DC; 1986. Data preview 23.
5. McManus M. Dependent coverage eroding in private plans. *Child Health Financing Report, American Academy of Pediatrics.* 1989;6(2):3-6.
6. US Congress. Congressional Research Service. *Health Insurance and the Uninsured: Background Data and Analysis.* Washington, DC: US Govt Printing Office; 1988.
7. US Congress. Office of Technology Assessment. *Medical Testing and Health Insurance.* Washington, DC: US Govt Printing Office; 1988. OTA-H-384.
8. Kozak LJ, Norton C, McManus M, McCarthy E. Hospital use patterns for children in the United States, 1983 and 1984. *Pediatrics.* 1987;80:481–490.
9. Gabel J, DiCarlo S, Sullivan C, Rice T. Employer-sponsored health insurance, 1989. *Health Affairs.* 1990;9(3):161–175.
10. Bloom B. Health insurance and medical care-health of our nation's children, United States, 1988. *Advance Data from Vital and Health Statistics.* No. 188. Hyattsville, Md: National Center for Health Statistics; 1990.
11. US Congress. Office of Technology Assessment. *Healthy Children: Investing for the Future.* Washington, DC: US Govt Printing Office; 1988. OTA-H-345.
12. Actuarial Research Corporation. *Premiums for Preventive Care Recommended by the American Academy of Pediatrics.* Annandale, Va; 1991.
13. Logsdon DN, Rosen MA, Thadeus S, Lazaro CM. Coverage of preventive services by preferred provider organizations. *J Ambulatory Care Manage.* 1987;10(2):25–35.
14. Gabel J, DiCarlo S, Fink S, deLissovoy G. Employer-sponsored health insurance in America. *Health Affairs.* 1989;8(2):116–128.
15. Demkovich L, Fisher RS. States' interest in mandated benefits remains strong. *State Health Notes.* 1989;92:5–7.
16. Hay Management Consultants. *1989 Hay/Huggins Benefit Report.* Wellsley, Mass.; 1990.
17. DiCarlo S, Gabel J. Conventional health insurance: a decade later. *Health Care Fin Rev.* 1989;10:77.
18. Bureau of Labor Statistics. *Employee Benefits Focus on Family Concerns in 1989.* Press release. 1990.
19. Ham FL. The future of dependent health benefits. *Bus Health.* 1989;7(9):19–26.
20. Harvey B. A proposal to provide health insurance to all children and all pregnant women. *N Engl J Med.* 1990;323:1216–1220.

Section 4

Funding Options for Service Delivery

Section 3 outlined many of the barriers to access to maternal and infant health services. Cost is paramount among those barriers, but others include transportation and both provider and client behavior. In this section we highlight recent federal and state initiatives designed to reduce barriers to care.

Rae Grad and Ian Hill provide an overview of recent federal legislation in the MCH arena. They trace many of the early policies and programs that had significant impact on MCH services but focus most heavily on the MCH Block Grant and the recent Medicaid expansions of the 1980s. These federal policies are examined in light of their influence on maternal and infant services at the state level. The authors describe current federal policy, which has taken some significant steps toward expanding maternal and infant health care access but which remains inadequate to meet current needs.

Chapter 12, prepared by Debra Lipson and Adrienne Puches, presents new information on state initiatives increasing access to care among the poor. Several states have implemented innovative steps to curb the shortage of services. The authors explore the quality of care delivered by these state programs, compare them to services provided under federal Medicaid programs, and address their effect on insurance coverage.

CHAPTER 11

Financing Maternal and Child Health Care in the United States

Rae K. Grad, PhD
Ian T. Hill, MPA, MSW

Most American women give birth at some point in their lives. Each year, nearly 4 million American women—almost 7% of all women of reproductive age—give birth.[1] Most women who have babies are in their twenties, a time when their family incomes are likely to be modest. For many of these women, the average cost of $4300 to have a baby is a sizable percentage of their total family income for an entire year.[2] Most women rely on some form of private or public health insurance or other source of publicly subsidized health care to defray at least some of the costs of childbirth.

In the early 19th century, children were perceived as laborers and, as we can see from the lax child labor laws of the time, a resource to be exploited. Slowly, however, society began to see children as the adults of the future and realized that good health in the early years was crucial to healthy adulthood. Thus, around the turn of the century, attitudes toward children began to change. Individuals and groups began to press for increased federal involvement in developing and administering maternal and child health services.

OVERVIEW AND HISTORY OF FEDERALLY SUPPORTED PROGRAMS

Early efforts met with considerable resistance. Many opponents felt that the federal government was meddling in what should be a private issue and that the well-being of mothers and infants was better left to each individual family. Nonetheless, in the early years of the 20th century many initiatives were launched to promote the health and well-being of mothers and children.

White House Conference on Children (1909)

The children's health themes that were stressed and discussed around the turn of the century are the same ones that are emphasized today: the need for prenatal care, the importance of comprehensive care, and the importance of federal coordination of health services for mothers and infants. These themes were stressed by President Theodore Roosevelt when he convened 200 health care professionals in 1909 at what became known as the White House Conference on Children. Repeated every decade until 1970, these conferences laid crucial background and clarified the financing and service delivery strategies for programs to promote the health of mothers and children.

Children's Bureau (1912)

One of the most lasting results of the 1909 White House Conference on Children was its recommendation to establish the US Children's Bureau. After much heated debate, President William Howard Taft signed legislation creating the Children's Bureau in 1912. The mission of the bureau was to

> investigate and report on all matters pertaining to the welfare of children and child life among all classes of people and . . . especially investigate the questions of infant mortality, birth rate, orphanages, juvenile courts, employment and legislation affecting children in the states and territories.[3]

The Children's Bureau carried out these functions until 1969, when it merged with the Public Health Service and the Office of Child Development of the Department of Health, Education, and Welfare.

Sheppard-Towner Act (1921 to 1929)

Building on the successes of the Children's Bureau, Congress in 1921 passed the Sheppard-Towner Act, which provided grants to states to develop health services for mothers and infants. This program, the first public health grants-in-aid program enacted in the United States, gave matching funds to states for the delivery of a range of services, including prenatal care, well-baby and well-child care, parent education, birth registration, and physician and nurse education.

Although the Sheppard-Towner Act prompted many improvements in the health services available for mothers and infants, its most permanent effect was to establish a precedent for public responsibility for maternal and infant health. Although maternal and infant health services improved considerably during the 1920s, opposition to the Sheppard-Towner Act was strong. It was assailed in Congress as socialistic and denounced as "drawn chiefly from the radical, socialistic, bolshevistic philosophy of Germany and Russia."[4] The American Medical Association opposed the Sheppard-Towner Act, as it opposed any public involvement in medicine. Despite the program's considerable success, opponents succeeded in repealing the Sheppard-Towner Act in 1929.

Title V of the Social Security Act (1935)

Modeled after the Sheppard-Towner Act, Title V of the Social Security Act created programs for maternal and child health and crippled children, with the goal of ensuring the health of all mothers and children, particularly those in rural areas and those suffering from economic distress. Title V moneys generally were allocated to the states, which matched the federal allotment with their own funds and determined how the money would be spent. Federal funds were distributed on a formula basis; the majority of funds were allotted for maternal and child health and crippled children's services.

With the exception of increasing funding levels, few notable changes were made to the Title V program between 1935 and the early 1980s. In 1963 and 1967, Congress authorized (1) Maternity and Infant Care (MIC) projects, (2) Children and Youth projects, (3) intensive infant care, (4) family planning, and (5) dental care for children. Together these projects were called the "program of projects." In 1975 the federal government turned over administration of these programs to the states and allowed them to determine what services were needed, provided they included at least one program in each of the five areas.

In 1981, Title V was amended to establish a block grant; that is, the funds for several maternal and infant health programs were pooled and allocated to the states as one package through a formula grant. Generally, the Maternal and Child Health Block Grant had the same purpose as the previous categorical programs: to enable each state to assure all mothers and children access to high-quality health services, reduce infant mortality, prevent diseases and handicapping conditions among children, and provide special and rehabilitation services for crippled children.

Indian Health Service (1955)

The Indian Health Service was established in 1955 as an agency of the Public Health Service in the Department of Health, Education, and Welfare. The mission of the agency is to provide a comprehensive health care delivery system for Native Americans and Alaska Natives.

Maternity and Infant Care (MIC) Projects (1963)

MIC projects, which resulted from amendments to Title V adopted in 1963, came about primarily because of the findings of President Kennedy's Panel on Mental Retardation. This panel found that a major cause of mental retardation was inadequate prenatal care, resulting in pregnancy complications, premature delivery, and low birthweight babies. The purpose of MIC projects was to identify high-risk pregnant women early in pregnancy so that they and their newborns could be provided with adequate, comprehensive care. Project funds were awarded to local health departments, medical schools, and teaching hospitals. Because many major cities had experienced an increase in infant mortality rates in the 1950s, the program was—unlike Depression-era programs—targeted to urban areas. In addition to reducing infant mortality and morbidity, MIC projects helped communities organize and coordinate services to make them more available to those who needed them. In 1981, MIC projects were merged with other maternal and child health care programs to form the present-day MCH Block Grant.

Children and Youth Projects

In 1965 Congress authorized special project grants for the health of school and preschool children, modeled after the MIC projects. The major objectives of these children and youth projects, called C and Y projects, was to provide comprehensive health services to children and youth living in low-income areas. Health promotion activities were provided, as was medical care, case finding, preventive health services, diagnostic and treatment services, and dental care.

Like MIC projects, C and Y projects were community oriented, employing area residents and involving them on community advisory boards. By 1971, 65 C and Y projects were operating clinics in 30 states, providing care to more than 335 000 children annually. The projects were successful in decreasing the incidence of illness, reducing the need for hospitalization, and increasing school attendance among their young clients. The C and Y projects were consolidated into the MCH Block Grant in 1981.

Although Medicaid was not designed specifically to improve pregnancy outcomes or reduce infant mortality, it is an important safety net program . . .

Medicaid (1965)

The Great Society programs of President Lyndon Johnson increased federal responsibility in areas that had previously been left to the states. Like the Sheppard-Towner Act, Medicaid was opposed by many people, who viewed it as socialized medicine. Although claims of government interference in private affairs were again heard, public sentiment supported a more socially conscious government, and Medicaid was enacted as a landmark change in the financing of health care in America. Passed in 1965 as Title XIX of the Social Security Act, Medicaid was designed as a medical assistance program to improve access to health care services for low-income Americans who were aged, blind, disabled, or members of families with dependent children. Although Medicaid was not designed specifically to improve pregnancy outcomes or reduce infant mortality, it is an important safety net program by which health care is made available to needy women and children.

Unlike other federal programs such as Title V, Medicaid is a financing system, not a service delivery system. States reimburse health care providers for care provided to enrollees and then bill the federal government for a portion of those costs. The federal share of the cost of care, which depends on the state's per capita income, ranges from 50% in more affluent states to 79% in poor states. States are responsible for administering Medicaid funds and can establish income eligibility limits. In general, eligibility for Medicaid is tied to eligibility for Aid for Families With Dependent Children (AFDC).

Comprehensive Neighborhood Health Centers (1965)

Created in 1965 under the Office of Economic Opportunity as part of the Partnership for Health Act, these centers provided family-oriented health care in many communities across the country. The majority of the centers' clients were low-income pregnant women and children. This program was transferred to the Public Health Service in 1971 and is now a part of the community health centers program.

National Health Services Corps (1970)

Established as part of the Public Health Service, this program attempts to attract health service professionals to underserved areas for a specific period of time by defraying some of the costs of a participant's medical or nursing education.

Special Supplemental Food Program for Women, Infants, and Children (WIC) (1972)

WIC was created in 1972 as an amendment to the Child Nutrition Act of 1966. Administered by the US Department of Agriculture's Food and Nutrition Service, WIC distributes funds to the states to provide supplemental food to low-income pregnant women, nursing mothers, and children diagnosed as being at nutritional risk. WIC also provides nutrition education and enhances access to health care services for those who are eligible for the program. Unlike Medicaid, WIC is not an entitlement program and therefore is not required to serve all people who are eligible; WIC reaches only an estimated 40% of the eligible mothers and children. The program's benefits are well documented; WIC participation is associated with increased birthweight and reduction in prematurity among infants born to program participants.

... WIC participation is associated with increased birthweight and reduction in prematurity among infants born to program participants.

Improved Pregnancy Outcome (IPO) Project

Concerned over the slow rate of improvement in infant mortality and the great geographic and socioeconomic discrepancies in infant mortality rates in the mid-1970s, Congress appropriated additional funds under Title V for a new initiative, the IPO project. Its overall goal was to reduce infant mortality through more effective use of existing services and, when necessary, through implementing new services. The projects generally addressed the coordination and promotion of preventive, primary, and referral care for mothers and infants. Grants of up to $400 000 were targeted to states with high rates of infant mortality and teen pregnancy. During the 5-year history of the project, 34 states, the District of Columbia, and Puerto Rico received grants.

The IPO project established a more organized management system for perinatal activities in the states and provided critical seed money to build communication networks and target services. IPO projects were catalysts in the development of a regionalized approach to service delivery, which in turn improved the system of detecting women at risk and arranging for appropriate care. Finally, the IPO project was credited with significantly reducing infant mortality rates in the participating states.

Maternal and Child Health Block Grant (1981)

... health centers reduce the incidence of infant mortality, promote the use of preventive health care, reduce reliance on emergency room care, and respond to public health issues ...

In 1981, seven separate categorical programs were consolidated with existing Title V programs to create the MCH Block Grant. Under the block grant, federal funds are available to the states for providing or purchasing a broad range of maternal and child health services. Within broad parameters, states are free to determine the types and scope of services offered under the block grant. Services often include prenatal care, high-risk pregnancy programs, maternal and infant transport programs, and support for neonatal intensive care units.

Like Medicaid, the MCH Block Grant uses both state and federal money. States provide $3 in matching funds for every $4 in federal funds they receive. Many states supplement their block grant allotment with other state funds for prenatal or delivery services. Eligibility criteria are set by states, which may elect to charge for services that are provided to women whose income is above the poverty level.

Community and Migrant Health Centers

With roots in eight demonstration projects that were begun in 1965, the federally supported community health centers and migrant health centers have expanded over the years into 600 centers operating over 2000 health care sites that provide comprehensive care to nearly 6 million people. Authorized under the Public Health Service Act, the purpose of the health centers is to provide high quality preventive care to the people who are most likely to lack access to health services because of geographic isolation, lack of health care providers, or lack of financial resources. Approximately 1.3 million patients are women of childbearing age, and 2.1 million are children under age 15. Studies have demonstrated that health centers reduce the incidence of infant mortality, promote the use of preventive health care, reduce reliance on emergency room care, and respond to public health issues such as care for the homeless.

In 1987, Congress appropriated funds for comprehensive perinatal care programs to improve the capacity of community and migrant health centers to provide maternal and infant health care. Funding limitations allowed only 206 centers to receive grant awards during the program's first year of operation, but early reports indicate that these centers have been able to significantly expand and enrich their services for mothers and infants.

Childhood Immunization Program

The Childhood Immunization program helps states and localities establish and maintain immunization programs. The vaccine-preventable childhood diseases most commonly immunized against are measles, rubella, polio, diphtheria, pertussis, tetanus, and mumps. The Childhood Immunization program is one of the federal government's most cost-effective programs; every dollar spent on the program saves the government an estimated $10 in medical costs.

During the first half of the 1980s, the research literature demonstrated not only the link between inadequate prenatal care and adverse birth outcomes but also that the single most important barrier to prenatal care facing low-income childbearing women was the lack of insurance.[5] Yet Medicaid—this country's major financing program for health care needs of poor mothers, children, and families—was not meeting the needs of these populations. In fact, Medicaid's capacity had steadily eroded during the preceding decade. The income eligibility threshold for AFDC, to which Medicaid eligibility was linked, stood at approximately 75% of the federal poverty level in 1975. By 1988, however, this average state threshold had shrunk to 48% of poverty level.[6]

RECENT CHANGES IN MEDICAID

Recognizing the slippage in Medicaid and acknowledging the importance of reducing infant mortality in the United States, a strong coalition representing states (the National Governors' Association and the Southern Governors Association), Congress, and consumers (the Children's Defense Fund), explored potential means of separating eligibility rules for Medicaid from those of public welfare programs. These efforts culminated in the passage of the Omnibus Budget Reconciliation Act of 1986 (OBRA-86). This historic act effectively severed the traditional link between Medicaid and AFDC and gave states the power to establish special income eligibility thresholds for pregnant women, infants, and children under the age of 5.

In subsequent years, Congress continued to liberalize coverage of these populations. The Omnibus Budget Reconciliation Act of 1987 (OBRA-87) gave states the option to raise income thresholds for pregnant women and infants to 185% of poverty, and for children up to age 8 to 100% of the poverty level. The Medicare Catastrophic Care Amendments of 1988 (MCCA) transformed what had been optional authority into a mandate; the law required states that had not already expanded coverage to phase in minimum coverage of pregnant women and infants at 100% of poverty over a 2-year period. Finally, the Omnibus Budget Reconciliation Act of 1989 (OBRA-89) superseded MCCA's schedule by requiring states to cover, at minimum, pregnant women and children up to age 6 at 133% of poverty, beginning in 1990.

State Responses to New Flexibility

States responded aggressively to OBRA-86. Within 1 year of the effective date of the law, one half of the states expanded eligibility to 100% of the federal poverty level. By the 2-year anniversary of OBRA-86, 44 states and the District of Columbia had set ceilings of 100% or higher (18 of these states had used OBRA-87 authority to raise thresholds above poverty, usually to the upper limit of 185%). By July 1989, the effective date of the MCCA-mandated coverage, only five states were required to adjust their eligibility levels upward. The impact of OBRA-89 was felt more broadly by states: 32 states did not have thresholds at 133% of poverty and were required to adjust—most from 100% to 133%. Only 15 states were already covering children to age 6 or older at 100% poverty level in April 1990. Thus, OBRA-89 succeeded in establishing uniform, minimum Medicaid coverage of pregnant women and young children across all states at levels never before witnessed by the program.[7]

Legislative provisions in OBRA-86 and each of its progeny opened new doors for the states through which financial access to health care could be extended to thousands of families. However, positive though these developments were, they represented only a first step toward the goal of improving the health status of mothers and children. Although providing families with financial access to care is a critical building block, it simply reinforced the need to address the cultural, behavioral, and systematic barriers that keep women from receiving continuous prenatal care. Moreover, making thousands of new pregnant women eligible for Medicaid exacerbated the current troubling shortage of obstetric care providers who are willing to care for low-income populations. Finally, expanding financial access highlighted the need to reform and redesign not only the services that Medicaid-eligible pregnant women receive but also the existing service delivery system.

Moving Beyond Eligibility Expansions

Acting as a catalyst for comprehensive program reform, OBRA-86 eligibility expansions have stimulated state programs to confront these maternal and child health issues and develop strategies to address them. Unprecedented cooperative, collaborative efforts between Medicaid, MCH, public assistance, and other state agencies promise to have a significant impact on the perinatal needs of families.

Streamlining the Eligibility Process. A growing body of research has demonstrated that the eligibility system for Medicaid can itself be a barrier that inhibits women from enrolling in the program. Although OBRA-86 severed the income linkage between AFDC and Medicaid, it did not separate the process through which persons become eligible for the two programs.

The traditional stigma attached to applying for public aid can discourage many women who might need or want only prenatal care. The fact that Medicaid eligibility workers are typically located in county welfare offices rather than in prenatal care provider sites contributes to this stigma while also posing an access barrier, because applying for the coverage involves separate trips to the welfare office. Medicaid applications, which are often used to determine eligibility for AFDC and many other public programs, are typically complex and require extensive verification and documentation. Finally, states have (and typically use) up to 45 days to make an eligibility determination. This 6-week delay can be a problem for pregnant women, who need access to prenatal care as early as possible in their pregnancy.

Since 1986, a growing number of states have attempted to institute simpler, more accessible eligibility systems and to allow earlier, more timely receipt of care. As a first step, almost all states have taken advantage of two simple yet significant options offered by OBRA-86: states may (1) ignore all personal assets during the eligibility determination process and (2) extend uninterrupted, continuous eligibility to pregnant women throughout their pregnancies regardless of fluctuation of income. By January 1990, 44 and 41 states, respectively, had adopted both of these eligibility options.[7]

Most states have implemented even broader eligibility reforms. Twenty-five states have adopted the complex but promising option of presumptive eligibility. This option, which permits certain prenatal care providers to extend temporary, 45-day eligibility to pregnant women on the basis of a simplified income test, is designed to permit same-day coverage of Medicaid-reimbursable prenatal health care. Because of various administrative complications associated with establishing and overseeing such programs, many states have developed similar but simpler reforms.

By January 1990, 17 states had begun to post official eligibility workers at sites where prenatal care is given to low-income women. This approach precludes the need for women to make a separate trip to a welfare office to apply for aid and eliminates the stigma associated with the welfare eligibility process. Nineteen states have shortened their application forms for children or pregnant women or both. These revised eligibility forms, some of which are as short as one page, are quicker and easier for applicants to fill out and can be processed more quickly by state agencies. In many states, forms have been made so simple that the state welfare agencies have agreed to leave blank forms in provider offices and allow women to complete the entire process by mail. Finally, nine states have given priority status to maternity-related applications and require that eligibility determinations be made within 5 to 10 days of application.[7]

Increasing Provider Participation. The severe shortage of obstetric providers who are available and willing to serve pregnant women on Medicaid threatens to undermine all of the positive advances state and federal governments have achieved. Over the years, low fees, programmatic and bureaucratic complexity, and problems with Medicaid clients' noncompliance have been the principal explanations offered for poor provider participation. Today, new factors—especially the rising cost of malpractice insurance and fear of malpractice suits—are cited as major causes.

Improving the health status of mothers and children requires more than expanding access to care. It requires improving and reforming the content of that care.

States have increasingly attempted to recruit and retain greater numbers of obstetric providers through widely ranging strategies, the most obvious of which is raising provider fees. Between 1987 and 1990, 22 states raised the rates at which they reimburse obstetricians. Nearly one fifth of the states have gone a step further by simplifying and improving billing procedures and claims-processing systems. In addition to addressing low-pay and slow-pay issues, more than half the states have attempted to expand the use of alternative providers such as certified nurse-midwives and nurse-practitioners. Most states have tried to cultivate improved relations with medical societies and obstetric provider associations. Some have hired nursing staff who travel around the state meeting with doctors, explaining new initiatives and trying to persuade them to enroll. Others have designated personnel in the state medical agency to act as provider liaisons who will respond to specific problems and situations.

A few states have attempted to address the malpractice problem directly. Two have set up new no-fault liability funds to cover newborn birth-related injuries. Participation is voluntary for both physicians and hospitals, who pay the fees to support the worker's compensation-type fund. Another state, using its general liability fund for state employees, has adopted a program to cover malpractice claims made against physicians who are under contract with local health departments.[8]

Enhancing the Scope of Prenatal Care. Improving the health status of mothers and children requires more than expanding access to care. It also requires improving and reforming the content of that care. Again, building on the momentum created by expansions of eligibility, states have begun aggressively refining and redesigning the benefit packages that are being extended to Medicaid-eligible pregnant women. As of January 1990, 30 states had implemented broad new programs of enhanced prenatal care services.[7]

Prenatal benefit reforms have been based on the understanding that appropriate prenatal care does not consist solely of medical services. Rather, a package of benefits to meet the diverse needs of high-risk childbearing women combines nutritional, psychological, and educational services with routine and specialized medical care. By working closely with MCH programs, Medicaid agencies typically have added the following core of new services:

- Care coordination (or case management) is considered by many states as the most critical component of enhanced packages. As the glue holding the delivery system together, care coordination services typically consist of determining the needs of a client, developing a plan of care to address those needs, coordinating referral of the client to service providers, and following up to ensure that services are received.

- Risk assessment helps providers identify the various problems being experienced by a recipient and enables providers to plan the various services needed.

- Nutritional counseling includes education on the relationship between proper nutrition and good health, information on special dietary needs during pregnancy, instructions for infant feeding (both breast and bottle), and guidance on weight gain and exercise. Some states specify interventions for women who are at special nutritional risk.

- Psychological counseling attempts to assist women with the numerous stresses that face families and can affect birth outcome. Many families suffer from inadequate income, unsafe housing, insufficient food, and unreliable transportation. Alcohol or drug abuse, depression, and other social and psychiatric problems also need intervention.

- Health education provides women with critical information they need to understand the physiology of pregnancy, healthful behaviors during pregnancy, labor and delivery, basic infant care, and parenting.

- Home visiting is seen as a beneficial perinatal strategy that allows providers to better assess patient needs and to teach healthy behaviors more effectively. States have focused on visiting programs that include both prenatal and postpartum visitation.

- Transportation is critical for effective use of prenatal services. A few states have tried to improve access to care by directly reimbursing families for the costs of transportation.[9,10]

The rapid progress by states to broaden and enhance Medicaid programs for pregnant women and children is very encouraging. In addition to raising income eligibility thresholds up to and above the poverty level, most states have also made their eligibility systems simpler and more responsive, have attempted to recruit greater numbers of obstetric care providers into Medicaid, and have added exciting new benefits to their state plan to make their Medicaid programs' coverage more comprehensive and effective.

CONCLUSION   Clearly, inadequate prenatal care is directly related to poor birth outcomes. The inability to pay for care is one of the most significant barriers women face in obtaining adequate care. Similarly, children's lack of
access to primary health care endangers their health, their learning potential in school, and their capabilities to become productive members
of the work force. Over the years, many public programs have been established to improve access for these populations. Most recently, Medicaid expansions and initiatives undertaken by the states either at the
request of Congress or on their own have shown great promise for significantly enhancing women's and children's ability to obtain timely
and comprehensive care. These groundbreaking changes have begun to
sever the traditional link between welfare and Medicaid, allowing
states and health professionals to coordinate Medicaid with public
health programs already in place.

Progress to date has been impressive, but much work remains. Indicators such as continued high infant mortality rates, inadequate receipt of prenatal care, and poor childhood immunization rates rein-
force the need for further effort. Unfortunately, further progress has
been impeded because of lack of coordination among the myriad
health-related programs that serve women and children, inadequate
funding of key programs such as those discussed in this chapter, and a
lack of awareness on the part of many women about the importance of
preventive health care and how and where to obtain it. Improvements
in maternal and infant health in the United States and the elimination
of barriers to care will come about only as a result of strong leadership
and commitment at all levels of government and in communities
across the country on behalf of pregnant women and children.

REFERENCES

1. Gold RB, Kenney AM, Singh S. *Blessed Events and the Bottom Line: Financing Maternity Care in the United States.* New York, NY: Alan
Guttmacher Institute; 1987.
2. Health Insurance Association of America. *Research Bulletin: The Cost of
Maternity Care and Childbirth in the United States.* Washington, DC;
1989.
3. Bradbury DE. *Five Decades of Action for Children: A History of the Children's Bureau.* Social Security Administration, Dept of Health, Education, and and Welfare. Washington, DC: Government Printing Office;
1962:17. Publication no. 358.
4. Schmidt W. The development of health services for mothers and children in the United States. *Am J Public Health.* 1973; 63:419–427.
5. Institute of Medicine. *Preventing Low Birthweight.* Washington, DC: National Academy Press; 1985.
6. Hill IT. *Reaching Women Who Need Prenatal Care: Strategies for Improving
State Perinatal Programs.* Washington, DC: National Governors Association; 1988.
7. National Governors Association. *MCH Update: State Coverage of Pregnant*

Women and Children, January 1990. Washington, DC: National Governors Association; 1988.

8. Lewis-Idema D. *Increasing Provider Participation: Strategies for Improving State Perinatal Programs.* Washington, DC: National Governors Association; 1988.

9. Hill IT, Breyel J. *Coordinating Prenatal Care: Strategies for Improving State Perinatal Programs.* Washington, DC: National Governors Association; 1989.

10. Hill IT, Bennet T. *Enhancing the Scope of Prenatal Services: Strategies for Improving State Perinatal Programs.* Washington, DC: National Governors Association; 1990.

CHAPTER 12

Maternity and Infant Care Coverage in New State Health Insurance Plans for the Working Uninsured

Debra J. Lipson
Adrienne Puches

Both public and private financing options for maternal and infant health care have undergone substantial improvements in both coverage and scope of benefits in the past several years. Yet significant numbers of low-income women of childbearing age, and children, still lack health insurance coverage. The Alan Guttmacher Institute estimates that approximately 17% of women of reproductive age (about 9.5 million women) have no public or private health insurance and that twice as many poor women (35%) have no health coverage.[1] According to Census Bureau surveys from 1986 and 1988, between 9 million and 12 million children younger than 18 lack health insurance. Nearly 1 in 3 children living below 150% of the federal poverty line lacked health insurance coverage, whereas only 1 in 10 of those who live in families that earn more than twice the poverty level were without health insurance.[2]

Inadequate health coverage persists among low-income women and children despite the existence of the Medicaid program. Designed to ensure access to health care by poor individuals who are eligible for public assistance, the Medicaid program covered only 41% of all the poor in 1987.[3] Because of variations in state-determined eligibility levels for Aid for Families With Dependent Children (AFDC), wide discrepancies in coverage of poor women and children among the states still remain. And despite recent changes in federal law requiring Medicaid coverage of poor and low-income pregnant women and children, many of those who are newly eligible still encounter barriers in gaining access to care.

Even low- to middle-income women and children who have private health insurance coverage are likely to find that many prenatal, maternal and infant, and well-child care services are not covered (see chapter 10). Private policies that do cover these services frequently impose limits on the coverage.

This chapter examines the potential advantages and problems involved in using non-Medicaid strategies, such as those adopted recently in several states, to expand coverage of and improve access to prenatal, maternity, and infant care by low-income women and infants. Although the state programs that were studied in this informal survey are not targeted to women and children specifically, they were designed to help uninsured low-income individuals and families afford private health coverage.

In response to widespread concern that the Medicaid program was not serving those who most needed its coverage, Congress has gradually improved access to health care for uninsured pregnant women and children through a series of expansions in Medicaid's required eligibility categories. As of April 1, 1990, all states are required to cover children up to age 6 and pregnant women in families that were earning less than 133% of the federal poverty level (about $14 000 annually for a family of three). In addition, states may choose to cover pregnant women and infants in families earning up to 185% of poverty. The Omnibus Budget Reconciliation Act of 1990 requires states to provide Medicaid coverage to poor children aged 6 to 18 living in families with incomes under 100% of the federal poverty level on a phased-in, year-by-year basis starting in July 1991.

MEDICAID IMPROVEMENTS AND SHORTCOMINGS

Problems in gaining access to care remain, however. The application process for Medicaid is cumbersome and stigmatizing, requiring applicants to negotiate a complicated, bureaucratic welfare system. In addition, private providers of obstetric care are increasingly unwilling to serve Medicaid patients (see chapters 9 and 10).

Meanwhile, the lack of health coverage for the remaining two thirds to three quarters of the uninsured low-income population—including women who are not pregnant, nonpoor children aged 6 to 18, and working-age adults—continues to place considerable strain on the nation's health care system. As poor pregnant women and children gain access to coverage under Medicaid, states have turned their attention to solving the coverage problem for the rest of the uninsured.

Most people without health insurance are low- or middle-income working people (and their dependents) whose employers do not offer health benefits. More than three quarters (78%) of the 37 million Americans with no private insurance, Medicaid, or other protection against health care costs are workers and their dependents. Workers who make less than $5 per hour are more than three times as likely to be uninsured than workers who earn more.[4]

**COMPARING
MEDICAID WITH
NEW STATE
PLANS**

In recent years, states have pursued various strategies for covering the working uninsured.[5] Most often, states have tried to increase the availability or lower the cost of private health insurance coverage for the low-income population. For example, many programs directly or indirectly subsidize the purchase of private health insurance for people who cannot afford it or are not offered a group plan by their employers. Not only does the state subsidize this arrangement; often the state plans provide a marketing and administrative link between low-income people and private insurance plans.

Most of the state plans for the low-income working uninsured have not specifically targeted pregnant women and infants for coverage because in many cases they are eligible for Medicaid. But women in low-income working families who are enrolled in state-subsidized insurance plans may become Medicaid eligible at pregnancy, and their infants may be eligible at birth. Given a choice between Medicaid and a state-subsidized private plan, pregnant women and their infants face a dilemma. Under a private insurance plan, the payment rates to providers of prenatal and maternity care are usually much higher than Medicaid's reimbursement rates, thus reducing the reluctance of providers to serve low-income women. By helping low-income pregnant women gain access to private coverage that pays higher rates, state-subsidized plans may be able to lessen provider access problems that are common among Medicaid patients.

But private insurance plans are also more likely to place limitations on coverage of maternity care that present major obstacles for low-income women. These limitations include treating pregnancy at the time of enrollment as a preexisting condition ineligible for coverage, imposing high deductibles and copayments, and not covering physician care for newborns.[1] Thus, significant changes in private insurance policies would be necessary for the private sector approach to constitute an improvement in access to comprehensive maternity and infant care for low-income women and infants.

Pregnant women who are eligible for both Medicaid and a state-subsidized private insurance plan should be able to compare coverage; for example, they should know whether special benefits such as genetic testing and counseling, mental health services, and nurse-midwife services, which are increasingly covered under state Medicaid programs, are covered by the state plan. Such differences can prove significant to low-income pregnant women who are at higher risk of experiencing complications or premature delivery.

In comparing Medicaid with a state plan, it is also prudent to determine whether the state plan has an adequate number of obstetricians and pediatricians participating in its provider network and whether those providers also participate in Medicaid; if the family's income drops to the Medicaid level and the providers participate in both Medicaid and the state plan, the chances for continuity of care improve.

To address these issues of comparability, the authors informally surveyed state plans for the working uninsured to answer three questions
about maternity and infant care coverage:

**SCOPE AND
METHODS OF
THE STUDY**

1. Are the new state-subsidized private insurance plans offering pregnant women and infants more reliable access to medical care providers than Medicaid provides?

2. Are the state plans improving on the maternity and infant care coverage typically provided by the private sector?

3. What lessons do these new state plans offer to national policymakers who are interested in designing a universal health insurance system that meets the special needs of low-income pregnant women
   and children?

The six states selected for study (Table 12-1) were simultaneously implementing the Medicaid eligibility expansions for poor pregnant
women and infants and launching new state-subsidized insurance
plans for low-income uninsured working families. For each state, the
following three points were surveyed:

1. How prenatal, maternity, and infant care are covered and delivered
   under the new state plan.

2. How comparable the plan's benefits are with Medicaid's coverage;
   whether there were any referral relationships between them; and, if
   so, how easy it was to transfer back and forth.

3. Whether the new state plan is removing the limitations that are
   commonly imposed on maternity benefits by private insurance policies.

The six states in the study were selected because they met the following three criteria:

1. By June 1989 the state had a health plan for working uninsured
   families whose incomes were below 200% of the federal poverty
   level.

2. By September 1989 the state had adopted a Medicaid eligibility
   standard for pregnant women and infants that was above 75% of
   poverty (all pregnant women whose family incomes were under
   this level had to be covered by state Medicaid programs by July
   1989) and below the maximum 185% of poverty.

3. By June 1990 (the time of this survey) the state had been implementing the health plan for nearly a year, providing some experience on which to base an assessment of program operations and effects.

TABLE 12-1
June 1990 Survey of Selected State Health Insurance Plans for the Working Uninsured
(surveyed by the authors, June 1990)

State	Program Name	Date Enrollment Began
Maine	MaineCare	December 1988
Massachusetts	Center Care	Fall 1988
Michigan	One Third Share Plan	May 1988
New York	Individual Subsidy Plan	November 1989
	Employer Incentive Plan	May 1989
Washington	Basic Health Plan	March 1989
Wisconsin	Small Employer Health Insurance Maximization Plan	February 1989

The presence of all three criteria would increase the chances that women enrolled in the new state plans who became pregnant would also be eligible for Medicaid (by virtue of overlapping income thresholds), raising questions about the relative benefits of the state-subsidized private plan versus Medicaid.

The survey was conducted during the summer of 1990 and information was collected from several sources. Materials published by or about state uninsured initiatives, requests for proposal (RFPs), and pertinent contracts between states and private insurance companies were collected and analyzed. Administrators of the state plans and, in some states, the contracting insurance companies, were interviewed (eg, Health Insurance Plan of Greater New York, Blue Cross Plan in Washington State). In states where the state plan was coordinated with Medicaid agencies, Medicaid officials were also interviewed.

FINDINGS

Overlapping Eligibility

The six state health plans for the working uninsured in this survey target low- to middle-income families. Each of the six plans sets the maximum family income eligibility at 175% or 200% of the federal poverty level. To participate, individuals or families may not have any other form of health coverage. Each state plan, whether targeted to individuals and families or to employers, has qualifying income guidelines that are just above Medicaid income limits for pregnant women and infants (see Table 12-2). The plans' eligibility policies potentially cover the same group of women who would be Medicaid eligible if they became pregnant (and their infants at birth). As of September 1989, the maximum income that would qualify pregnant women and infants for Medicaid was 185% of the federal poverty level in Maine, Massachu-

TABLE 12-2
Maximum Income Eligibility Levels for State Health Insurance Plans and Medicaid*

	% of Poverty	
State	**State Plan**	**Medicaid**
Maine	200	185
Massachusetts	200	185
Michigan	200	185
New York		
Individual plan	200	185
Employer plan	Not applicable	185
Washington	200	185
Wisconsin	175	130

* As of September 1989; only pregnant women and infants under age 1.

setts, Michigan, New York, and Washington and 130% in Wisconsin. Thus, women who were not Medicaid eligible before their pregnancy and whose family incomes are below 185% (130% in Wisconsin) would be eligible for either the state plan or Medicaid once pregnant.

Another feature of the state plans strengthens the overlap in potential eligibility. Like Medicaid, the state plans do not use assets or resource tests to determine eligibility for coverage of infants and pregnant women.

Ease of Enrollment

In view of the overlap in income eligibility criteria between the state plans and Medicaid, program managers were asked about relative ease of enrollment. One Maine official cited the stigma attached to the Medicaid application process as a deterrent to many women who are eligible for Medicaid. The MaineCare program, on the other hand, allows for telephone and mail-in application forms, which have proved more attractive to low-income people.

Nearly every program manager interviewed, including those who work in the state's Medicaid program, called the removal of stigma associated with Medicaid application a major advantage of state health plans for the working uninsured. States offering employer-based initiatives cited the importance of marketing their programs through job sites as another advantage to enrollees and key to the state plans' enrollment success. Meanwhile, in Massachusetts, where outreach and enrollment are performed at individual health centers, program managers also cited ease of enrollment as a major advantage.

None of the states surveyed, however, has compared the effectiveness of such marketing and enrollment techniques to Medicaid agencies' more aggressive outreach and enrollment efforts targeted at pregnant women, such as "out-posting" eligibility workers at prenatal care sites. Therefore, it is not yet known which of these enrollment strategies is more effective in reaching pregnant women.

. . . the removal of stigma associated with Medicaid application [is] a major advantage of state health plans for the working uninsured.

Coverage of Prenatal, Maternity, and Infant Care Benefits

To determine the scope and coverage of prenatal, maternity, and infant care benefits under the state plans versus Medicaid, plan administrators were asked to list and describe the minimum benefits that private insurance plans contracting with the state must cover. Generally, the six states require a core of basic benefits similar to that found in most comprehensive insurance plans: doctor's office visits, X-ray and laboratory testing, emergency care, and basic inpatient hospital services.

In addition, states almost always require coverage of preventive services that are not normally covered by major medical policies, such as routine physical exams, well-baby care, and immunizations, without significant cost sharing or deductibles. An exception is Michigan's One Third Share Plan, as offered by Blue Cross and Blue Shield, which does not cover routine physicals and immunizations. Coverage of preventive services is often designed to reduce the need for costly acute care.[6]

Often excluded from state plans' requirements for contracting insurers are dental care (in Washington, Maine, Michigan, and New York) and prescription drugs (Washington and New York). Coverage for outpatient mental health services are either limited (as in Wisconsin and Maine) or completely excluded (in New York, Michigan, and Washington). New York requires that contracting insurers cover at least 60 outpatient visits for alcohol and substance abuse rehabilitation.

A few contractors reported that some of the benefits they cover exceed the requirements of the state's minimum benefit package. For example, the Health Insurance Plan of Greater New York (one of the contractors operating in the state) permits twice as many well-baby visits as the state requires.

Four of the state plans require contracting insurers to cover prenatal and maternity care (Maine, Michigan, New York, and Washington). In Massachusetts, the state does not specify what benefits must be offered; Center Care enrollees instead receive all of the benefits offered by community health centers (CHCs), most of which offer prenatal, maternity, and infant care. The Wisconsin program also fails to cover prenatal, maternity, or infant care, although some contractors may do so without requisite.

Except for Washington's Basic Health Plan (BHP), more specific information about benefit limitations on prenatal, maternity, or infant care could not be obtained to make comparisons with Medicaid benefits. Washington's required maternity care services appear comprehensive yet do not include prescription drugs. Other states' plan administrators were generally unaware of any visit limits or specific maternity service exclusions; the typical "amount, scope and duration" limits common to Medicaid were not found in the state plans. For example, New York's RFP specifies that no limits can be placed on prenatal and childbirth care or any other conditions related to pregnancy. One disadvantage of many of the state plans, however (except Maine's and Washington's), is that, unlike Medicaid, benefits are subject to copayments. Medicaid law prohibits requiring copayments for prenatal services and for any services provided to children.

Although the private plans cover well-child visits, it is highly unlikely that they would cover the broad scope of benefits available under recently enacted Medicaid requirements for Early and Periodic Screening, Diagnosis, and Treatment. Infant health benefits were not specified in sufficient detail to permit closer reexamination.

Improvements on Private Coverage

Private health insurers often consider pregnancy at the time of enrollment a preexisting and therefore noncovered condition, fail to cover pregnancy of a nonspouse dependent, impose significant copayments and deductibles, and lack coverage for physician care for newborns.

Several of the state plans reviewed are removing some of these limitations. For example, neither Maine nor Washington permits contracting insurers to view pregnancy as a preexisting condition. In Michigan, insurers must provide maternity care and it is therefore assumed that pregnancy will not be considered a preexisting condition. There is no specific policy language stating so, however, which may explain why one of the two private plans in Genesee County considers pregnancy a preexisting condition, although only for employee groups of four or less. New York's RFP does not prohibit insurers from considering pregnancy a preexisting condition, and at least one insurer treats it as such. This practice is permitted in Wisconsin also, because the state has not addressed the issue explicitly.

In Massachusetts, exclusion of pregnancy-related services is unlikely because the plan is run by health promotion-oriented CHCs rather than by insurance companies. If specific prenatal services are not available at one CHC, pregnant women are referred to another that does offer them.

Prenatal and maternity care services are not subject to copayments in Maine or Washington (in Washington, neither are laboratory and X-ray services, emergency ambulance transportation, and preventive care services). In other states, copayments for these services are relatively low, averaging $5 to $10 per outpatient visit.

In the Massachusetts plan, enrollees are not charged a premium but must pay any copayments or deductibles that a CHC would normally charge. The Wisconsin plan does not require coverage of prenatal, maternity, or infant care, but some contracting insurers cover these services subject to the usual deductibles and cost-sharing requirements; total out-of-pocket costs may not exceed $1000 per year for an individual and $2500 per year for families.

Finally, coverage of newborns from the moment of birth is required by Washington and Maine, not addressed in the New York RFP (although some contractors may do so), and not required in Wisconsin or Michigan. Although CHCs in Massachusetts are not required by state law to provide services to infants, they would not likely limit services for newborns, because they are obligated under federal law and funding requirements to provide services to all low-income people.

Access to Obstetric and Pediatric Service Providers

Because access to maternity and infant care has been a difficult problem in the Medicaid program, we sought to determine if the state-subsidized insurance plans were helping to improve the availability of providers for low-income women.

One of the factors that might influence access is the use of managed care plans to provide services to the enrolled population. Managed care is a system for containing excessive or unnecessary use of services, often by requiring prior authorization for hospital admissions and specialized care. The use of managed care by participating private insurance plans may be required by states as a method of controlling the costs of state insurance plans for the working uninsured. States may also pay contracting insurers a predetermined amount per person (called capitation) to hold down costs.

The use of prepaid managed care arrangements to serve low-income pregnant women enrolled in Medicaid has been a problem. A study of Medicaid managed care plans showed them unable to overcome the drawbacks of the traditional Medicaid fee-for-service system (ie, insufficient number of participating obstetric and pediatric providers and low reimbursement rates). These plans also experience a few new problems of their own, such as restricted access to specialized services, leading enrollees to seek out-of-plan services.[7]

This experience suggested that the managed care contracts and prepayment arrangements in state health plans for the uninsured might also be detrimental to non-Medicaid-enrolled low-income pregnant women. If the managed care system limited access to specialized services that women at risk of adverse birth outcomes might require, low-income women would have fewer resources to obtain these services outside the plan. These problems could be obviated by requiring the contracting insurers to include a sufficient number of maternity care providers such as obstetricians, nurse-midwives, or other specialists to accommodate all pregnant women in the plan. If this step were taken, managed care contracts might actually increase access to maternity care.

All the state plans examined in this study employ contracting arrangements with managed care plans. Three states that subsidize the purchase of private insurance policies (Michigan, New York, and Wisconsin) contracted with managed care plans although they were not required to do so. Two states (Maine and Washington) limit contracts only to managed care providers, primarily health maintenance organizations (HMOs). The sixth state (Massachusetts) contracts with an HMO, which then subcontracts with CHCs.

State plans that contract with managed care plans involve both traditional closed-panel HMOs, in which health professionals are directly employed by and accountable to the plan, and other contracting arrangements between insurers and health care providers who agree to serve patients enrolled in the plan for a negotiated fee.

. . . the current policy environment at the federal level indicates that state governments will remain key actors in efforts to increase access to such care.

After approximately a year's experience, administrators of three of the six state insurance plans (Maine, Michigan, and Washington) claimed that the private care plans improved accessibility to obstetric and pediatric care for enrolled pregnant women and infants who, if enrolled in Medicaid, would have greater access problems. Program managers cited a shortage of available Medicaid providers or an unwillingness of providers to take Medicaid patients.

It was not, however, the managed care system that improved providers' willingness to serve low-income women. Rather, by helping low-income women obtain private insurance coverage, which reimburses providers at rates closer to market rates, the state enables women to gain access to care that would be more difficult to obtain through Medicaid. For example, Washington State's contracting managed care plans pay on average about 50% more than Medicaid for a normal delivery.

Unfortunately, state managers' assertions about improved accessibility were not based on any hard evidence nor on any conscious effort by state policymakers to ensure that contracted insurance plans demonstrate adequate obstetrician and pediatrician participation. In addition, the contracts between states and insurers did not contain any assurances that specialized services that are not provided by the contractor and might be needed by low-income pregnant women and infants would be available, although many managed care plans report the use of specialty referral lists.

One additional factor influencing access to care for a low-income population is the participation of providers in both private insurance plans and Medicaid. That the low-income population is subject to frequent changes in income (due to unemployment, part-time and seasonal work, and related reasons) results in periodic on-and-off eligibility for Medicaid. Thus, the survey sought to determine whether provider participation in both Medicaid and the state plan was required or encouraged to ensure continuous service for pregnant women. Only Washington State attempted to ensure that at least one participating insurer or provider group in each area served by the BHP participated in both Medicaid and the state plan. This was based on explicit consideration for the population served by the program—a population whose income varies frequently, altering their eligibility status.

Coordination with Medicaid

Finally, we sought to determine if any of the state plans had worked out an explicit relationship with the Medicaid program for any reason, including accommodating the needs of pregnant women who needed additional benefits, specialized services, or access to a broader network of providers than those contracting with the state program. State programs might also try to coordinate with Medicaid to save the state money. For example, the state's Medicaid matching rate might make enrolling in Medicaid more favorable than enrolling in the state plan for women who need costly services.

Only one of the states surveyed (Washington) had established a coordinated system of referral with Medicaid for those individuals who are dually eligible for the state plan and Medicaid. In Washington's BHP, if a pregnant woman or a woman with a newborn infant appears to be Medicaid eligible, she or her infant or both are referred to the state's First Steps program, the Medicaid expansion program for pregnant women and infants. If a BHP enrollee becomes pregnant, she is encouraged to enroll in Medicaid because it has more extensive benefits, but she is not required to do so. If the woman enrolls in Medicaid for the duration of her pregnancy, she may request that her placement in BHP be reserved.

Michigan and Maine do not have similar arrangements even though the state plan and Medicaid are administered by the same agency in these two states. Although the state administrators in both states were aware of the overlap in eligibility, their primary focus was on enrolling eligible individuals in the state plan.

In Maine, a referral to Medicaid is made only if an individual is found to be ineligible for MaineCare. If a referral is made, the woman must make contact with Medicaid and begin the application process on her own. If a potential enrollee is dually eligible, MaineCare enrolls her in the state plan and does not risk making a referral to Medicaid, under which she may or may not be approved for coverage. If a woman applies for and receives coverage under Medicaid, she can be quickly transferred back to MaineCare later.

The survey revealed no referral relationship between Michigan's One Third Share Plan and the state's Medicaid agency, even though the plan targets former Medicaid recipients. Similarly, neither of New York's two demonstration projects showed evidence of coordination or referral with its local Medicaid agencies.

Wisconsin's Insurance Maximization Plan has an explicit policy that enrollees cannot receive both Medicaid benefits and state plan benefits. However, there is no mechanism for checking the Medicaid eligibility of potential enrollees. The ability to screen for Medicaid-eligible individuals is lost because eligible employees enroll in the state plan on the work site and local private insurance agents market the product.

In Massachusetts' CenterCare plan, the CHCs could refer Medicaid-eligible women and infants to the Health Start program (that state's Medicaid expansion program for pregnant women and infants), but it is unclear whether they do. Apparently, the CHCs get paid regardless of whether they make referrals to Medicaid, so there is little incentive to encourage women to enroll in Medicaid.

Finally, even though states are very concerned with containing the costs of these programs,[8] there appeared to be no attempt to make case-by-case or general policy decisions to screen out high-cost patients from the state plans. This point was true even in states whose contribution toward the premium might exceed their Medicaid contribution for normal maternity and infant care; and it was still true for complicated or premature birth.

SUMMARY OF FINDINGS

On the basis of early assessments by program administrators in six state-subsidized health plans for the working uninsured, it appears that some progress is being made in improving access to maternity and infant care for low-income pregnant women and children. Although participation in the plans is still relatively modest, the state subsidies are to some extent helping women and infants obtain critically needed care.

The study also shows that some of the worst offenses of the private insurance system's handling of pregnancy (such as completely excluding it) have been remedied through requirements in five of the six states that prenatal, maternity, and infant care services be covered by the private plans. However, many services needed by low-income pregnant women, such as prescription drugs, mental health or substance abuse counseling, and other specialty care, are not likely to be covered.

In three state plans (Michigan, New York, and Wisconsin), women may find that they cannot obtain coverage for prenatal and maternity care under the new plan at all, because pregnancy can be treated as a preexisting condition subject to coverage exclusions. Pregnant women find that few provisions, if any, have been made to help them obtain quick Medicaid eligibility determination. The reason is that, among the six state plans, only Washington's BHP informs pregnant women that they can receive prenatal, maternity, and infant care benefits either under the state plan or Medicaid if their incomes are below 185% of the federal poverty level and that Medicaid benefits may well be more generous. Only in the Washington and Maine systems are women who choose to be covered by Medicaid for the duration of pregnancy reinstated easily in the state plan afterward.

How much will state efforts to improve access to health care for the uninsured contribute to reaching the ultimate goal of universal coverage? . . .

Although cost containment considerations often drive Medicaid programs' benefit packages, service delivery modes, and reimbursement features, the state plans do not attempt to steer pregnant women to the less expensive plan to save the state money. Rather, the primary concern has been to improve access to care, which state plan administrators believe is more likely to be ensured through private insurance plans than through Medicaid. More study is needed, however, to determine whether the state-subsidized private plans are indeed more successful in achieving this result than Medicaid eligibility expansions combined with Medicaid provider fee increases would be.

The experiences of these plans are providing important lessons for state and federal policymakers who are developing proposals to subsidize health insurance premiums for the low-income uninsured. In particular, they highlight some important principles to follow in designing a program that builds on the private insurance system and coexists with Medicaid. Policymakers should be mindful that some individuals may be eligible for both programs because of overlapping income eligibility guidelines. In the interest of promoting improved pregnancy outcomes, low-income pregnant women and women of reproductive age who are eligible for both Medicaid and state-subsidized private insurance plans should be able to choose the program that better suits their needs and guarantees access to comprehensive, high-quality obstetric services. The following guidelines for achieving this objective are based on state experiences to date:

1. **Eligibility determination and application process.** Provisions should be made for previously uninsured women who are pregnant when they enroll in a state-subsidized or federally subsidized health plan to obtain expedited eligibility and assignment to an obstetric care provider. Women who do not have a regular provider should be given a list of benefits and participating providers in each plan for which they qualify, allowed to choose, and then assisted in obtaining an appointment. For women who already have a provider, waivers should be granted to continue that source of care on a contractual basis, regardless of whether that provider participates in the chosen health plan, in order to assure continuity of care.

2. Benefits. To enhance access to the specialized services that are more likely to be needed by pregnant women at risk of poor birth outcomes, maternal and infant benefits in private plans subsidized by the government should be at least as generous as those now offered by Medicaid. Because private insurance plans and HMOs tend to limit the scope of care or range of special services, explicit consideration should be given to covering additional services for pregnant women that may not be included in the regular plan—for example, nutritional supplements, psychosocial counseling, diagnostic testing services, substance abuse treatment, and other services needed to improve the chances for the birth of healthy infants.

Copayments and deductibles should be waived to prevent the imposition of any barriers to prenatal, maternity, and infant care, and in no event should pregnancy be treated as a preexisting condition that is ineligible for coverage. Such cost-limiting strategies may not harm women with higher incomes, but they may well deny cost-effective care to low-income women.

3. Provider Participation. The development of new publicly subsidized private insurance coverage and use of managed care are not enough to remedy the shortage of qualified obstetric providers or ensure access to specialized providers. Provisions must be included to ensure that sufficient numbers of participating maternity and pediatric care personnel are available. Regardless of whether enough private obstetricians and pediatricians are available, special consideration should be given to contracting with nurse-midwives, CHCs, and other qualified providers that have demonstrated their commitment to serving the low-income population.

CONCLUSION

In spite of the lessons learned from these six state programs, a question—perhaps the most important one—remains unanswered: How much will state efforts to improve access to health care for the uninsured contribute to reaching the ultimate goal of universal coverage, whether for maternity care or for broader health care benefits? For although some women and infants are benefiting in the short term, serious inequities are created when some states take the initiative to fill health coverage gaps for low-income families while less generous states let the uninsured fend for themselves.

Even those states that are able to afford programs without federal help may be hard pressed to maintain funding support when state finances are tight—a situation likely to be faced by most states during the next few years. Already, many states that enacted authorizing legislation for state subsidy programs to help the uninsured are delaying implementation or scaling back because of economic downturns. Fluctuations in state economies lead to great instability in these programs.

The inconsistency and inequities caused by variations in Medicaid eligibility and benefits among the states fueled federal reforms in the past decade that are slowly eliminating variations in access to maternity care under Medicaid for poor women and children. Replacing this source of inequity with another—namely, state plans that use different, though slightly higher, income thresholds—would represent little progress. Furthermore, as this study shows, programs that compete or coexist with public programs such as Medicaid may create another type of inequity: women enrolled in a private insurance system are preferred by private physicians even though their income is on a par with that of women in the public insurance system.

Although continued state flexibility in the design of approaches to health care access for the uninsured may diminish the sense of urgency for a uniform and fair national health care program, it can be argued that state experimentation with various financing and delivery arrangements for the low-income uninsured is a necessary step in the development of a national health plan. Although state-by-state approaches are often modest demonstrations that affect limited numbers of people, such small-scale strategies may be needed to test various approaches and guide a larger statewide or national program.

One might disagree with the need for this state-level experimentation, but until national policymakers decide on a plan for financing and delivering comprehensive prenatal, maternity, and infant care for every child and pregnant woman in this country, the current policy environment at the federal level indicates that state governments will remain key actors in efforts to increase access to such care.

REFERENCES

1. Gold R, Kenney A, Singh S. *Blessed Events and the Bottom Line: Financing Maternity Care in the United States.* New York, NY: Alan Guttmacher Institute; 1987.
2. US Department of Commerce. Bureau of the Census. *Current Population Survey.* 1987 and 1989.
3. Congressional Research Service. *Medicaid Source Book: Background Data and Analysis.* Washington, DC: US Govt Printing Office; 1988. US House of Representatives Committee on Energy and Commerce, Subcommittee on Health and the Environment Committee Print 100-AA.
4. Short PF, Monheit A, Beauregard K. A profile of uninsured Americans. *National Medical Expenditure Survey Research Findings 1.* 1989. US Dept of Health and Human Services publication (PHS)89-3443.
5. Lipson D, Donohoe E. *Recent State Initiatives for Covering the Uninsured.* Washington, DC: Intergovernmental Health Policy Project, George Washington University; 1989.
6. Alpha Center. *Program Update, Health Care for the Uninsured Program.* No 10. Washington, DC: Alpha Center; 1990.
7. Rosenbaum S, Hughes D, Butler E, Howard D. Incantations in the dark: Medicaid, managed care and maternity care. *Milbank Q.* 1988;66(4):661–693.
8. Alpha Center. *Program Update, Health Care for the Uninsured Program.* No 8. Washington, DC: Alpha Center; 1989.

Section 5

Implications for a National Policy

To this point we have examined the current state of maternal and infant health care in the United States both in terms of access to care and its relative impact on health outcomes and from the social justice perspective. We have outlined the importance of care for pregnant women and infants and have identified a number of interventions that seem to make a difference in health outcomes. Current shortages in availability of care and barriers to access to care—including financial, provider, and ancillary issues—have been identified. This final section presents our own views on what should be done and discusses implications for a national policy.

Craig Blakely, Frankie Wong, Ezra Davidson, and Lynne Hudson start off the section with a description of the services that should be included in a national maternal and infant health program. The authors describe a package of services that augment existing medical practice with a comprehensive array of preventive services supplemented by activities to draw clients into care. Arden Handler, Janet Perloff, and Joan Kennelly then discuss the importance of ensuring that quality care is delivered. The authors base their standards for care on an extensive review of the Medicaid experience and discuss implications for a national maternity care program.

In the final chapter, Jonathan Kotch and Rosemary Barber-Madden identify the limitations of existing practices and current proposals to improve the availability and accessibility of maternal and infant care in the United States. This policy analysis considers four leading policy alternatives from the perspective of 11 analytical criteria. Kotch and Barber-Madden then map out a blueprint for Universal Maternity Care in the United States.

CHAPTER 13

A Comprehensive Model of Maternal and Infant Health Care Services

Craig H. Blakely, PhD, MPH
Frank Y. Wong, PhD
Ezra C. Davidson, MD
Lynne Hudson, MPH

This chapter presents the content of the Universal Maternity Care (UMC) package that is proposed in this volume. The rationale behind the package of services we describe is the conviction that a multidisciplinary set of services is essential for women and their infants to achieve and maintain optimal health. Therefore, although traditional medical services will remain the cornerstone of the hybrid package of services,[1-6] this discussion focuses on the comprehensive psychosocial and ancillary components of care.[7] Such an approach is not intended to reflect the relative importance of the components,[8] but rather to shed light on the ones that have only recently begun to receive adequate attention.

The proposed comprehensive set of services is based on the following objectives of a national maternity care program:

- Reduce the number of unintended pregnancies.

- Reduce maternal mortality and morbidity.

- Reduce risk to maternal mental health.

- Reduce the incidence of preterm and low birthweight infants.

- Reduce infant mortality and morbidity rates.

- Promote a healthy family environment.

- Prevent neglect and abuse.

- Systematically develop a population-based data bank to guide future policy-making.

These objectives can be met by three basic service strategies: (1) early and continuing assessment of risks, (2) education and health promotion, and (3) medical and psychosocial intervention and follow-up.[3] In addition, adequate, accurate, and uniform data collection procedures are essential.

The UMC system detailed here goes well beyond traditional maternity services. The model begins with family planning services and continues through preconception, prenatal, intrapartum, and postpartum care; infant care ends when a child is 18 months old. This upper age cutoff was chosen with the aim of reducing infant mortality rates and was linked to the fact that a number of critical immunizations are scheduled to have been completed by 18 months of age. Recent outbreaks of mumps, measles, and other childhood diseases have focused attention on the need to reemphasize national immunization programs (see chapter 7).[9,10]

Most of the services described in this model maternity care system are neither new nor innovative. Their aggregation in a comprehensive package of services, however, represents an important step toward achieving universal maternal and infant health nationwide.[3]

THE CYCLE OF MATERNITY AND INFANT CARE SERVICES

Figure 13-1 illustrates the proposed cycle of comprehensive maternal and infant services. Care components included in this package of services can be clustered. Boundaries that have traditionally separated these clusters are viewed as somewhat arbitrary (eg, family planning

Fig. 13-1. A model of comprehensive maternal and infant health care services. The following assumptions are made: (1) Family planning care incorporates ongoing gynecologic services, general health promotion, and preventive health care services. (2) The woman could pass through the pregnancy cycle additional times following the interpartum period (ideally at least 2 years) or continue indefinitely with family planning care during her childbearing years.

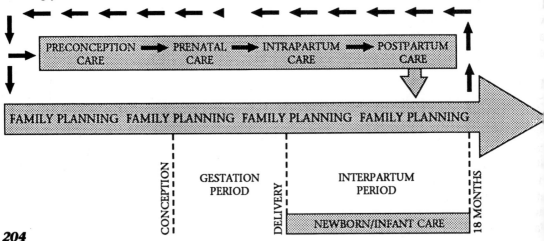

versus preconception care, preconception care versus prenatal care). These boundaries exist more for heuristic value because existing financing mechanisms have dictated their presence than because of any functional reasons for continued separation. A UMC program could and should blur these boundaries.

Continuity of services throughout the cycle of care is critical to the overall success of the model. The cycle begins with family planning services, which coincide with the onset of puberty and the commencement of regular gynecologic services. Women who elect not to have children would continue to receive family planning care.

Women who are actively planning to bear children move on to preconception care. If pregnancy is achieved, they enter the prenatal care phase. When unplanned pregnancies occur, they may well miss preconception care services and may elect abortion. If neither miscarriage nor induced abortion occurs, women then pass through pregnancy, labor, and delivery to the postpartum and infant care period, during which they can decide about future childbearing. Women who elect to retain the ability to conceive return to ongoing family planning care after pregnancy. An important goal of family planning care at this stage would be to foster adequate interpartum intervals and minimal unplanned conceptions. For women who do not wish to have more children, sterilization could be considered.

In keeping with the purpose of this volume—delineation of a health care system for the reproductive continuum—the proposed model implies a focus limited to family planning, preconception, prenatal, intrapartum, postpartum, and infant care. Thus, this model ignores the much broader perspective—the health of women and children generally, environmental health, or general health care access—that affects the whole population. This approach is not intended to imply that other health care concerns are less important or that contextual issues such as income or housing do not constrain the utility of maternity services. Rather, we simply mean to identify the services that we believe are critical for the proposed system of care. Ideally, general preventive health care should be available to all women of childbearing age and all children. With this end in mind, we believe that UMC is an appropriate place to start.

The following sections describe the service delivery components in the cycle of services depicted in Figure 13-1.

FAMILY PLANNING AND PRECONCEPTION CARE

Family planning is a critical component of any multi-faceted maternity care program. Nine of ten women of childbearing age in the United States are sexually active. Two thirds are at risk of an unwanted pregnancy (ie, physically able, sexually active, but not desiring pregnancy at the time).[11] At the heart of family planning programs are services to help women control pregnancy, preserve fertility, and safeguard health. Family planning thus encompasses more than the historical short-term effects of birth control; it also incorporates the long-term perspective of health promotion and protection.[11]

Preconception care functions as a bridge between family planning and prenatal care. The 1989 report of the Public Health Service's Expert Panel on the Content of Prenatal Care[3] identified preconception care as an important planning and preventive health care component of the prenatal care package. We are proposing a slightly different tack—aligning preconception care more closely with family planning than with prenatal care—in part because we have elected to address maternity care within a larger context including both family planning services and infant care. This distinction is important for three reasons.

First, to the extent that UMC substantially increases the numbers of women who receive family planning care either from private physicians or from public clinics, most women will be in the care of or at least known to family planning providers. Most women receive family planning services from private providers or health maintenance organizations (HMOs). Many will undoubtedly provide both preconception care and prenatal care anyway.

Second, when women receive family planning services from a family planning clinic a barrier between family planning and preconception care is reduced; that is, the need for women to seek a new provider when they decide to plan a pregnancy is eliminated. Given our dismal performance at getting women into early prenatal care, one can assume that involvement in preconception care would be worse, particularly in light of the fact that more than half of all pregnancies are unintended.[11,12]

Third, placing preconception care in the prenatal care component only worsens the schism between family planning and maternal and infant health care, a discontinuity that must be alleviated. Family planning care should include the practice of planning for a family and subsequently of preparing for conception, thus providing a natural tie between family planning and preconception services.

Family Planning Services

Family planning services involve a number of components, each designed to help participants make educated decisions about reproduction. A primary goal of family planning is to prevent unwanted and mistimed pregnancies and to make women fully aware of the reproductive process, risk factors related to negative outcomes, and strategies for minimizing those risks. Family planning is also aimed at preventing sexually transmitted diseases (STDs) (eg, acquired immunodeficiency syndrome (AIDS), syphilis, chlamydia); providing health promotion instruction and risk assessments (eg, Pap smears, breast exams, and essential gynecologic health care); preventing unwanted pregnancies; planning for wanted pregnancies; dating pregnancies (ie, fixing the date of the last menstrual period); and initiating women's involvement in maternity services early. Family planning services should include the following:

- Health history.

- Physical examination.

- Pregnancy test (if indicated), laboratory tests (eg, blood, urine, Pap), hypertension screening, and STD screening.

- Health education (including sex education) and counseling.

- Contraceptive counseling and supplies.

- Sterilization services or referrals.

- Abortion counseling and referrals.

- Specialty services (eg, genetic screening, infertility counseling).

- Psychosocial intervention and follow-up as necessary; home visiting.

- Preconception services.

- Enabling services (eg, outreach, care coordination, referral and follow-up, transportation, and child care).

Family planning services for nulliparous women should begin at puberty and be linked to school-based sex education courses as appropriate. For the sexually inactive, the focus is on education and health promotion. The sexually active receive contraceptive services.

For women who have just given birth or otherwise terminated a pregnancy, family planning services should begin in the hospital before discharge to ensure that contact occurs between the woman and the provider. Basic concepts (eg, pregnancy prevention and spacing, fertility preservation, and health promotion) should be presented as part of the hospital discharge process, and both the postpartum visit (if relevant), and a more formal family planning session should be scheduled.

Family planning services can play a major role in curbing the consequences of STDs. Although AIDS deservedly receives most of the media attention, other prevalent diseases such as pelvic inflammatory disease, gonorrhea, chlamydia, syphilis, and herpes continue to have devastating effects on women and infants. Traditionally, health services in the United States have taken the form of secondary prevention interventions (ie, minimizing morbidity once the disease is present).[13] Implementing the proposed family planning procedures would provide ongoing screening and would also offer education on safe sex strategies in a primary prevention format. These infections can best be prevented in children by preventing STDs in their mothers, so priority must be given to providing services to women who are at risk of exposure to STDs.

Preconception Care

Access to care and information on reproduction should be available long before conception occurs. We propose that family planning become preconception care at the point when conception becomes planned. Preconception care focuses on the early detection and management of risk factors before pregnancy, the need to alter behaviors that can affect a fetus (even before conception is confirmed), and the need for regular health care. Preconception services should also address the issue of effective parenting. Preconception care should include the following types of services:

- Extensive medical history (eg, obstetric, genetic, nutritional, and surgical histories).

- Psychosocial history (eg, sociodemographic setting, substance use history, family history including abuse and neglect, and psychosocial stress assessment).

- Occupational history and status assessment.

- Physical exam, including general health assessment, blood pressure, height and weight profile, and breast and pelvic exams.

- Complete series of laboratory tests (eg, hemoglobin and hematocrit, Rh factor, rubella titer, urine dipstick, Pap smear, and tests for STDs, hepatitis B, and drug screens as appropriate).

- Health promotion activities (eg, nutrition counseling and vitamin and iron supplements as indicated; education about the effects of smoking, drinking, and use of illicit drugs; safe sex strategies; the need for continuity in health care throughout the prenatal period; and the risk of X-rays).

- Psychosocial intervention and follow-up as necessary, and home visiting.

- Referral for management of risk factors and, ultimately, for prenatal care.

- Enabling services (eg, outreach programs and services targeting women who are not participating in family planning services, care coordination, and transportation and child care services to facilitate attendance at scheduled appointments).

A number of risk factors can be identified and addressed before conception. Evidence shows that with adequate preconception care a number of medical risk factors can be brought under control, eliminated, or identified and addressed before conception in both nulliparous women and women in the interconception period (between pregnancies). Foremost among these are management of insulin-dependent diabetes,[14] substance abuse (including both illicit and prescription drugs), poor nutritional status, alcohol and tobacco use, chronic illness, short interpregnancy intervals, occupational exposures, and stress.[3] Technologic advances in the past decade have also resulted in the increasingly prominent role of genetic counseling in planning for pregnancy.[15]

Substance abuse. Data have indicated that illicit drug use is relatively common: about 14% of women use illicit substances during pregnancy.[16] The adverse affects of cocaine[17] and its derivatives, heroin and methadone,[18] methamphetamines,[19] and alcohol[20,21] on the fetus, newborn, and growing child have been documented[22] (see chapter 5). This arena has received considerable federal focus during the past few years in the form of the Office of Substance Abuse Prevention's demonstration projects for pregnant substance abusers. Given the evidence regarding the adverse affects of substance abuse during pregnancy, these behaviors should be brought under control before conception through a combination of environmental and counseling interventions.

Smoking. Smoking cessation should also be addressed during the preconception period. Cigarette smoking has been shown to be linked to several negative birth outcomes including premature birth and retarded fetal growth.[23,24] Some women quit smoking on their own once they discover they are pregnant.[25] These women, who typically are better educated and begin prenatal care earlier in pregnancy, generally quit early in pregnancy. Fewer women quit later in pregnancy, and too many women never quit. Although the proportion of women in smoking cessation programs who do quit is not large, the cost-effectiveness of the interventions appears to be impressive[26-28] (see chapter 5).

Psychosocial and behavioral risk services. Although limited research is available on the impact of psychosocial and behavioral risk factors on pregnancy, these factors must be recognized as significant. Although it is impossible to eliminate these risks from a woman's environment, some can be identified and avoided or minimized and others can be planned for in advance.[3] Whenever possible, efforts must be made during the preconception period to identify women who are likely to experience psychosocial stress. Stress can lead to elevated blood pressure or altered uterine blood flow, or it may affect the pregnancy more indirectly by introducing emotional crises that make it difficult for a woman to follow through with scheduled care sequences.[29]

Specialized Services

Mainstream family planning services involve traditional birth control and risk reduction services. However, technologic advances have increased the utility of genetic screening and infertility services. In addition, abortion is an important part of family planning, albeit a politically sensitive one. These topics are addressed in this section.

Genetic screening. Genetic screening should be a major component of family planning and preconception care, available to those who need it. The health status of relatives and the presence of any potentially inheritable disorders should be carefully assessed. Pedigree analyses for such disorders as phenylketonuria (PKU), Tay-Sachs disease, or sickle cell disease have been in practice for years.[15] Extensive data have been gathered in the past 10 years regarding the relative risk of recurrence of many disorders, and mathematical formulas can be used to determine the probability of certain outcomes in view of familial histories.[30] On the basis of the portion of genetic variability we understand, genetic screening can therefore help couples decide on the best course of action. However, genetic screening strategies that are implemented after conception raise the issue of terminating pregnancy when the presence of disorders is confirmed.

Little legislation currently exists mandating genetic screening or testing; for example, PKU and hypothyroidism tests are required for newborns because the conditions are treatable. A UMC program, however, must provide certain basic genetic services such as routine screens for populations at risk and more comprehensive assistance and referrals where individual family histories indicate a more thorough response is warranted. Many chromosomal disorders are detectable in utero; however, it is inappropriate to routinely conduct invasive procedures such as amniocentesis. Where family history indicates the potential for the presence of disorders, these procedures may be warranted. Other factors that may indicate a need for screening include advanced maternal (or paternal) age, race and ethnicity, and drug usage.

Infertility services. A wide variety of infertility services is currently available, ranging from relatively straightforward counseling on the best time to have intercourse based on ovulation cycles to the application of fertility drugs and surgery. Although precise numbers are not readily available, it is estimated that more than 100 000 new cases of infertility occur each year and that as many as 1 million are being treated per year.[31,32]

To date, female infertility is more readily treated than male infertility; available procedures vary considerably in cost.[2] Complex procedures cost thousands of dollars and are therefore inaccessible to a large segment of the population. UMC should provide for initial counseling and screening services. Women with identified complications should be made fully aware of the services available, the likelihood of success

of various procedures, and the steps necessary to locate and obtain infertility services.

Trends in the Practice of Family Planning

The proportion of women of childbearing age participating in family
planning services is dismally low and has not changed significantly
during the past decade.[33] Roughly 20 million women had at least one
family planning visit of some sort at some setting (public clinic or private physician's office) during the year before the 1988 cycle 4 National Survey of Family Growth by the National Center for Health Statistics (NCHS). This number represented about 35% of women aged 15
to 44 years, a drop from 37% in 1982.[34] Figures represent those women
who reported a service contact for "getting a new method of birth control, renewing a prescription for a method already being used, checking for side effects of method use, counseling on birth control methods, and other services."[33(p4)]

However, some methods of birth control do not require frequent or
regular system contact. For example, some women choose not to engage in sexual activities, and others are trying to conceive or practice
forms of birth control (eg, condoms) that do not require regular physician contacts. Although physician contacts have declined, contraceptive use patterns in the United States have increased. In 1982 nearly
56% of all women practiced some form of birth control.[35] By 1988 that
proportion had increased to just over 60%.[35] However, comprehensive
family planning and preconception care, as conceptualized here, is
viewed as a set of services thât goes far beyond simple birth control
and should therefore be universally available.

However, contraceptive use is driven by the age, childbearing plans,
and educational awareness of the participants. Younger women are
most likely to use the pill as a method of birth control.[35] The pill requires regular physician and family planning contact simply to renew
prescriptions. On the other hand, older women, particularly married
women, are more likely to use other methods of birth control that do
not require such frequent system contact. Only 4% of women aged 35
and older reported use of the pill,[35] whereas as many as 60% of older
women who do not intend to have more children have elected sterilization or their partner has had a vasectomy.[11,36] This pattern is reflected in substantially reduced rates of family planning access among
older women (6%).[33]

The Role of Education

The most logical conclusion to be drawn from the dismal pregnancy
prevention and health protection behaviors of a sizable proportion of
sexually active men and women in the United States is that many are
simply unaware of the consequences of their behaviors. Only recently
in the chronology of public health has health promotion become

*... the services
described ... in
[this]
comprehensive
package ...
represent an
important step
toward
achieving
universal
maternal and
infant health
nationwide.*

prominent. Although primary prevention interventions are among the most difficult to evaluate, common sense indicates that information dissemination, educational programs, and screening services should affect maternal and infant health care in both a primary and secondary prevention manner. In this context, schools have become an important source of both reproductive health instruction and sex education. Unfortunately, recent data suggest that roughly 25% of U.S. schools offer no sex education at all.[37,38]

General health promotion—including reproductive health, risks to a healthy pregnancy, and effective means of minimizing risks before conception—must be integrated into school-based curricula, ongoing women's health care programs, and public information campaigns "as major themes, not minor agenda."[6(p123)] High school sex education in particular should be directly linked to family planning services. Students must be informed about the risks both of and to pregnancy before they become sexually active, because many of those risks occur before pregnancy is confirmed. Our goal should be to reach 100% of the women of childbearing age in the same way we seek to inoculate all children. However, it is essential that services go beyond education and include counseling, contraceptive supplies, and follow-up examinations. These strategies are critically important for schools, because recent data confirm that 53% of women are sexually active by age 19.[11]

Unmet Need for Family Planning Services

Women experiencing unwanted pregnancies are by definition less invested in their pregnancy outcomes. A 20-year longitudinal research project in Czechoslovakia suggests that women who do not have the legal option to terminate their unwanted pregnancies are significantly more likely to experience psychological trauma than those who have the option. Also, the former group of women experience more problems with their children than the latter do.[39]

National natality data indicate that indigent and teenage women in the United States are more likely to experience unwanted pregnancies and have infants with low birthweights.[40] As of 1988, more than 10% of all pregnancies were labeled unwanted (mistimed pregnancies were not included).[41] Pregnancies were so classified if the woman reported she had not wanted to have a child "at the time of conception or at any point in the future."[41(p2)] The proportion of women reporting unwanted pregnancies was 26% among those below 100% of the federal poverty line. Some studies indicate that this proportion is as high as 36% at delivery in indigent populations and that nearly two thirds are unplanned at conception.[42] The Alan Guttmacher Institute's (AGI's) most recent figures suggest that 57% of all pregnancies in the United States each year are unintended.[11] All these events are occurring as the contraceptive choices available to American women are shrinking.[43]

These data combine to paint a striking picture of the unmet need for family planning services. To achieve significant impact on negative birth outcomes, a reduction in the proportion of unwanted pregnancies is imperative. Both school-based sex education and more individually targeted family planning services are critical elements of UMC.

Issues Clouding the Future of Family Planning

We have argued that one way to reduce infant mortality rates is to make family planning universally available. Unfortunately, this country's attitudes toward family planning are becoming increasingly volatile because they are intertwined with abortion issues. Obviously, today's sociopolitical milieu is complex. Because fewer contraceptive choices are available to women in the United States than in other industrialized countries,[43] the family planning component of UMC must include access to safe, inexpensive abortions. However, the abortion rights controversy must not be tied synonymously to the more general issue of family planning. Abortion is only one component of a full set of family planning services. Whatever the outcome of the abortion debate, the United States must invest additional resources to encourage women to actively participate in some form of family planning.

Summary

Family planning is a multifaceted set of services with diverse goals. Ultimately, however, family planning is designed to reduce the prevalence of STDs and unplanned and unwanted pregnancies and to prevent adverse outcomes linked to inadequate planning by minimizing the impact of modifiable risk factors. Whenever possible, risks should be identified and addressed before conception.

Family planning services should be universally available to all women throughout their reproductive life span. Finally, family planning services should be linked to preconception and prenatal care, school-based sex education curricula, and various health promotion and media campaigns.

PRENATAL CARE

We use *prenatal care* to define services delivered during the pregnancy period. The maternity care program we have defined for UMC would include family planning, preconception, intrapartum, postpartum, and infant care in addition to prenatal care. Ongoing prenatal care should include the following types of services.

1. Early and continued assessment of risks.
   - Updated interim medical history.
   - Psychosocial history (eg, sociodemographic setting, substance use, family abuse and neglect, etc—updated from the preconception screen if available to prenatal care provider).
   - Physical exam (including blood pressure, height and weight profile, fundal height and weight, fetal presentation, and breast and pelvic exams).

- Series of scheduled lab tests (eg, hemoglobin and hematocrit, urinalysis, rubella titer, tests for STDs, drug screens as appropriate, maternal serum alpha-fetoprotein, hepatitis B, and ultrasound *only as medically necessary*).

2. Education and health promotion.
   - Health promotion activities (eg, nutrition counseling and vitamin and iron supplements as indicated; education about the effects of smoking, drinking, and use of illicit drugs; safe sex strategies; need for continuity in health care throughout the prenatal period; childbirth classes; and education regarding signs and symptoms of preterm labor and what to do about it).
   - Parenting instruction.

3. Psychosocial intervention and follow-up as necessary; home visiting.

4. Care coordination.
   - Early referral to a place of delivery (if not integrated with source of prenatal care).
   - Transportation and child care services to facilitate attendance at scheduled appointments.
   - Coordination with specialty services, other human service agencies, state and federal programs such as the Special Supplemental Food Program for Women, Infants, and Children (WIC), Food Stamps, etc.

Medical Risk Assessment and Services

When a woman enters prenatal care, a full pregnancy history, laboratory tests, a medical risk assessment, and pelvic and physical examinations must take place.[4] The physical and pelvic examinations, including weight and blood pressure, provide a general determination of physical and reproductive health. The complete medical history includes a genetic history, an infection history, obstetric and contraceptive histories, and family and social histories that provide important contextual information. Combined with a series of standard laboratory tests including blood typing, blood count, Coombs test, Pap smear, STD tests, urinalysis, and so on, and critical psychosocial, nutritional, and health promotion information (see the next section), these data equip the health care provider to make decisions about how best to treat the pregnancy.

Regardless of whether significant risks have been identified during either the preconception visit or the initial prenatal care visit, the main focus of the prenatal care package should be ongoing risk assessment, health and nutrition education, and continuing support and encouragement. If risks have been identified, more intensive assessments are justified and significant interventions may be tailored.

Nonmedical Risk Assessment and Services

Nutritional and psychosocial services are vital components of prenatal care. Nutritional assessment provides an indication of current dietary practices and includes identifying nutritional risks through the medical and social history, the laboratory (blood) tests, and the physical examination.[44] The psychosocial assessment provides demographic data such as economic status, educational status, and family composition and addresses the impact of the pregnancy on the family and its social support network.[3,45]

In cases where nutritional services and/or psychosocial counseling are not available on site, women should be referred to other sources. Women who are eligible for programs such as WIC should also be referred to those programs. These referrals and nonmedical interventions should be tailored to meet the needs of the woman.

The Link Between Preconception and Prenatal Care

Participation in preconception care or family planning services should significantly shorten the length of the first prenatal care visit if records are transferred properly. Many assessments would have already been completed at this stage and only the specific pregnancy-related and follow-up services would be necessary. A medical history update since the woman's enrollment in preconception care and a current pregnancy assessment are essential. Other services should include blood typing and determination of hematocrit levels, a pelvic examination for uterine size and dating, urine cultures, weight measurement, etc.

Extensive follow-ups should be conducted on all risks that were identified in preconception care, and records should be transferred to the prenatal care provider. A UMC system would target the completion of adequate assessments during preconception care and would ensure that records are forwarded to the appropriate prenatal care provider. In practice, some duplication of effort will occur. However, the goal should be the establishment of strong working relationships with family planning and preconception care providers to minimize duplication of services.

Trends in Use of Prenatal Care

Since the early goals of prenatal care (to detect and manage preeclampsia and eclampsia) were first put forward, the American College of Obstetricians and Gynecologists (ACOG) prenatal care guidelines have prescribed a series of 13 prenatal care visits beginning during the first trimester and following at increasingly shorter intervals as the pregnancy progresses.[4,46] However, the Public Health Service's report on the content of prenatal care (see the tabular summaries)[3] suggests that seven prenatal care visits should be adequate for the not-at-risk, multiparous woman and nine contacts should be required for the

The interval between birth and ... the first pediatric visit ... is a critical period, particularly for first-time mothers ... the recent trend toward early discharge of mother and newborn increases the need for an early postpartum contact for both mother and infant.

not-at-risk, nulliparous woman (allowing for more visits early in a woman's first pregnancy).

These recommendations, based on the assumption that the pregnancy in question is not viewed as high risk, hold implications for the efficiency of a national system of maternity care. Certainly cost savings could be realized by cutting several prenatal care contacts from the majority of not-at-risk pregnancies. However, this saving would be possible only in a closed system of care in which resources that are shifted from one part of the system are reinvested in another system component—theoretically of greater import and impact. The United States is not operating a system that is adequately supported at this time. By cutting resources (eg, moving some maternal and infant health resources to another categorical area or simply eliminating them), we could directly harm the overall quality of care. By shifting resources (ie, moving maternal and infant health resources within different categories) to more needed service components, we could improve the efficiency of the overall system.

But these recommendations should be considered with caution until more concrete data are available. We must demonstrate that the potential cost savings are worth the tradeoffs in the context of both medical and psychosocial risk factors, particularly when working with populations that are shortchanged on both of these dimensions. Regardless of the frequency and timing of scheduled prenatal care visits, system defaults must be altered immediately when risk factors are discovered that warrant a different approach to maternity care for a particular patient, including referral to obstetric specialists if indicated.

Unmet Need for Prenatal Care

Various estimates of unmet need exist. Torres and Kenney[47] completed one of the more comprehensive studies of the unmet need for prenatal care and concluded that expansion of Medicaid to 185% of the federal poverty level would require serving nearly an additional 1 million women annually. Others have concluded that this number could be significantly higher.[48] (For a more complete discussion of this issue see chapter 6.)

Summary

Universally available prenatal care must provide women with quality services during their pregnancies. The medical services discussed here in the context of UMC do not depart substantially from common practices already in place where high-quality care is provided, but strong nutritional and psychosocial components must be included. In many instances it becomes obvious that home visits are warranted for either medical or psychosocial reasons. Some studies have indicated that home visiting can help achieve many of the objectives of prenatal care with at-risk populations.[3,49] (See chapter 5 for a comprehensive discussion of home visiting.)

Intrapartum care comprises the myriad services that occur during the labor and delivery period. In this section we focus on the links to prenatal care and to care after discharge from the delivery setting. However, we define intrapartum care more broadly to include the entire hospitalization period. Thus, intrapartum care incorporates the following:

INTRAPARTUM CARE AND THE HOSPITALIZATION PERIOD

- Collection of all relevant prenatal care history and risk assessment information.

- An on-site assessment of the maternal and fetal vital signs and risks.

- Ongoing monitoring of maternal and fetal signs throughout the delivery period.

- Delivery.

- An assessment of the mother-infant pair in terms of physical, psychosocial, and nutritional needs.

- Hospital-based predischarge instruction concerning maternal self-care and infant care, and the providing of anticipatory guidance and family planning services.

- Maternal instruction on how to get help in days immediately after discharge on such issues as infant feeding, recovery from delivery, and so on.

- Links to a pediatric provider.

Services must include adequate assessment and monitoring capabilities, including fetal heart rate monitoring, ultrasound, blood and fresh-frozen plasma for transfusions, anesthesia, cesarean delivery capabilities within 30 minutes of a medical decision to intervene, tubal ligation, neonatal resuscitation capabilities, and necessary consultation and referral links. These traditional services are discussed at length in the expert panel's report.[3]

The intrapartum period has traditionally been characterized by the provision of medical services. However, rural hospital closings and reduced or denied access to some hospitals continue to pose problems to patients, particularly indigent patients. Even so, the system of levels of care that has been partially implemented in the United States provides some of the best medical care available in the world (see chapter 4).

Because most women experience no complications during their deliveries, the use of birthing centers or birthing rooms could be integrated into a system of care that could accommodate the changing of risk status, resulting in safe deliveries at lower cost and alleviating the provider shortages that exist in some settings. However, comprehensive medical care must be available for both mother and infant in at-risk pregnancies when complications do occur. A system of linkages among alternative delivery sites—similar to the regional system of levels of care that is being implemented nationally—must be formally established to ensure that adequate care is available for all pregnancies. If a delivery site is not able to provide neonatal intensive care, well-established procedures for transportation to such a site will be necessary. Transporting a high-risk woman in labor to a regional perinatal center is preferable to transporting a fragile preterm infant.[50-52]

Trends in the Provision of Delivery Services

Nearly all births take place in hospitals.[53] These rates of in-hospital delivery have not changed since 1975.[54] Some evidence suggests that women who give birth out of hospital (less than 1% of all births) tend to do so for economic or cultural reasons. For example, nearly 30% of the nation's out-of-hospital births occur in Texas, along the Rio Grande border with Mexico.

Liability concerns, malpractice insurance rates, and other issues have combined to slowly change provider participation trends. See chapter 9 for a detailed discussion of the changing availability of providers of prenatal and delivery services.

Summary

Intrapartum care takes place in a setting where timing is critical and opportunities come and go quickly. One factor affecting infant mortality is availability of access to neonatal intensive care. Intensive care provided by highly skilled health professionals is critical if the fetus or infant is compromised during pregnancy or delivery. Transporting the mother immediately before delivery is preferable to transporting a high-risk infant.[53] Communicating information about care that was delivered before hospitalization and delivery is important to successful delivery. In addition, the hospital setting provides a final opportunity to share useful information with the new mother and infant before discharge.

POSTPARTUM CARE

The postpartum period is a critical transition period for both the new mother and the infant. The goals of this phase of care remain ongoing risk assessment and monitoring of conditions and referrals. Postpartum services have been clustered into three periods: services that should be provided after delivery and before hospital discharge; services that should occur during the lag period between discharge and the traditional 6-week postpartum visit (these may include a 10-day or earlier postpartum visit and additional home visits as warranted); and the 6-week postpartum visit. This entire period provides a window of opportunity during which healthy behaviors for the entire family can be promoted.

The following predischarge and postdischarge components are considered key elements of postpartum care:

- A predischarge, preliminary postpartum visit.

- Initiation of family planning services.

- Scheduling of the postpartum visit.

- Providing postdischarge postpartum care.

Hospital-Based Postpartum Care

The woman's stabilization and recovery are the focus of this phase of care. Before discharge, a number of contacts should occur. Maternal blood pressure and bleeding must be monitored. The contraction of the uterus must also be observed at frequent intervals.

This postdelivery-predischarge period, which is often as short as 24 hours, also provides an opportunity to address a number of important issues with the woman and significant others. First, educational instruction on how to feed and care for the newborn should be provided, particularly for first-time mothers. Breast feeding should be encouraged. Family planning issues should be discussed and a postdischarge family planning visit scheduled if relevant. The follow-up postpartum visit should also be scheduled before discharge. Finally, the pediatrician should visit the infant, discuss the baby's health with the mother, and make arrangements for the first pediatric visit. Because the woman is a captive audience in the hospital after delivery, all efforts should be made before she is discharged to initiate these services and to schedule the more formal contacts to follow.

Another procedure that is increasingly performed during the postdelivery-predischarge period is female sterilization. Surgical sterilization is now more frequently used than the pill as a method of birth control among married couples.[55] Tubal ligation is routinely performed in hospitals the day after delivery. Depending on the time of day delivery occurs and the hospital's discharge policies (eg, 24 hours after delivery), some women may have to remain in the hospital longer if they opt for tubal ligation. Predischarge surgery nevertheless remains a cost-effective and efficient procedure.

Postdischarge Postpartum Care

The usual medical services performed during a postpartum visit include the monitoring of all vital signs and general health stabilization. In an uncomplicated pregnancy and delivery, medical services are a relatively routine continuation of the services outlined as in-hospital services.

However, the postpartum care phase affords health care providers an excellent opportunity to reinitiate family planning with the woman and her family. This planning could range from simple discussions about when to begin contraceptive use to formally scheduled follow-up visits that focus on the merits of sterilization for either the woman or her partner.

The postpartum visit is an opportune time to gather detailed information about how the mother, infant, and family unit are adapting to the new member of the family. Discussions should focus on nutrition and diet, use of vitamins for both the mother and infant, and equally important issues such as sleep deprivation caused by the baby's irregular sleep patterns and general coping skills that can alleviate undue stress, poor parenting behaviors, and other unconstructive activities.

Trends in the Provision of Postpartum Care

Traditionally, the postpartum visit is scheduled approximately 6 weeks after delivery. For certain low-compliance groups, special strategies may be required to ensure that adequate care is delivered. A 10-day postpartum visit should be considered in many situations. In some cases (eg, first-time mothers, extremely young mothers, and others at risk) it may be important to schedule a home visit to observe the mother-child unit. Additional instruction on care of the newborn, nutrition, and psychosocial issues should be customized to meet the needs of each woman. In addition, the home visit staff can assist the woman with other appropriate referrals (eg, housing, counseling). The scheduling of postpartum and initial pediatric visits is critical. The health care service system must impress on the woman the importance of postpartum care and renewed family planning services.

Unmet Need for Postpartum Care

Many women do not receive postpartum care for a variety of reasons.[56] However, no precise numbers from any sizable geographic region are readily available. NCHS, ACOG, the Centers for Disease Control's Pregnancy Risk Assessment Monitoring System, AGI, and a sample of states have been contacted directly, confirming the lack of concrete data on postpartum care contacts. NCHS is currently conducting a postdelivery follow-up survey that will provide the first nationally representative figures on postpartum care access rates. Data will not be available until early 1992.

A recent Texas in-hospital survey indicated that 23.4% of the women who did not plan to seek postpartum care (only 5% of the total) cited financial reasons; 54.6% of the women did not believe it was important or did not feel they needed the care.[57]

The interval between birth and (1) the formal postpartum visit (whether 10 days or 6 weeks after delivery) and (2) the first pediatric visit (typically 10 to 14 days after delivery with no complications) is a critical period, particularly for first-time mothers, during which virtually no contact occurs. During this time the new mother generally lacks health supervision, preventive education, and general contact with health care providers. In addition, the recent trend toward early discharge of mother and newborn increases the need for an early postpartum contact for both mother and infant.

Historically, relatives have gathered around to help with the many needs of the mother and child, particularly when no serious complications have surfaced. Times and family structures have changed, however, and these natural supports are no longer universally available. This point is often true for women living under at-risk physical and social conditions. Too often, new mothers have to deal with their altered circumstances without assistance from public or personal sources, and as a result they often experience considerable stress. Generally, provisions are made for emergency situations, but the new mother without serious complications is often left to her own devices. In the context of UMC, decisions based on in-hospital postpartum contacts should be made about a woman's potential need for increased assistance during the first weeks after delivery.

Summary

After delivery, parallel services are initiated for the mother and child. The first set of services focuses primarily on the mother and consists of postpartum care followed by renewed family planning care, as appropriate. Maternal postpartum care can be further clustered into two sets of services: those that occur after delivery and before hospital discharge and those that are typically scheduled approximately 6 weeks after delivery. The second set of services, infant care, focuses on the newborn. In both cases, the underlying goal is to monitor and facilitate the mother's stabilization and recovery and the infant's ability to thrive.

INFANT CARE

Protecting children's health is in large part what stimulated the creation and growth of the public health movement. Providing health care to infants and children involves both preventive and curative interventions (see chapters 3 and 7). Schorr asserts that

> whether present at birth (eg, low birthweight or congenital defects), or acquired later (eg, lead poisoning, anemia, or brain damage resulting from illness or injury), health problems become risk factors by interfering with development.[58(p87)]

Care of infants through the age of 18 months should generally include the following:

- Physical and anthropometric examinations (eg, monitoring height, weight, and head circumference).

- Screening (eg, PKU, hypothyroidism, galactosemias, development, hemoglobin and hematocrit, vision and hearing complications, and lead and sickle cell disease as indicated).

- Immunizations (diphtheria-pertussis-tetanus, poliovirus, measles-mumps-rubella, and *Haemophilus influenzae* type b, and careful monitoring of new trends with vaccines for chicken pox, hepatitis B, etc).

- Nutritional assessments (including counseling about breast-feeding and nutrient intake).

- Parental counseling on injury prevention (eg, car seats, stairways, pools, storage of toxic chemicals, hot water heater temperatures, smoke detectors), the effects of passive smoke, and dental care and fluoridation.

- Parenting education (normal child development, appropriate discipline, cognitive stimulation, etc).

- Psychosocial services (screening for risk of abuse and neglect).

- Referrals to Medicare's Early and Periodic Screening, Diagnosis, and Treatment program, WIC, or any other relevant federal or state programs for which the infant may qualify.

- The various complex services required to provide care for crippled, injured, or ill infants.

Good health care can help prevent adverse outcomes not only by improving health status but also by identifying and resolving problems that are not exclusively biologic. Alert health professionals can often spot subtle problems in a child's behavior or in intrafamilial relationships, which, when ignored, can become established and compounded and later contribute to adverse outcomes. Physical and emotional health are closely related at any age but particularly during early childhood.

Health conditions, too, can lead to later negative outcomes if they are not recognized and treated. Health conditions could include simple nutritional deficiencies (a target of the WIC program) or more complex health problems. Early detection of problems is imperative and is often easily accomplished by health professionals in a well-child clinic setting or during routine preventive checkups at a private physician's office. Some complications are completely preventable, such as neurologic complications that can occur as a result of pertussis or measles—both of which are preventable through immunizations.

Other conditions such as iron deficiency anemia are both preventable and treatable. When health professionals are familiar with the parent or parents, they can direct and guide them to better nutritional choices for their infant, thus directly preventing or averting such conditions, which can lead to slow development during infancy, attention problems in school, and behavior disorders in adolescence.

Infants With Special Needs

Although well-child health care drove much of the early growth of the public health movement, considerable resources are also spent on infants and children with special health care needs. State services for children with special health care needs range widely from advocacy efforts to diagnostic, treatment, and rehabilitative services for handicapped children. The Title V MCH Block Grant also contributes considerable resources to children with special needs. It is not, however, an entitlement program and has never been adequately funded to meet existing needs. A number of state-specific programs also target this population.

In the case of high-risk infants (ie, those who have existing complications, anomalies, or defects or are at risk of developing complications), the system must ensure access to the appropriate level of services, including level 3 neonatal intensive care. These facilities, staffed by specialized neonatologists and perinatologists, provide joint obstetric and pediatric care to those who are at risk beginning with the antepartum period through infancy.

Regionalizing intensive care is an attempt to minimize the fixed costs of such care by reducing duplication of effort. Thus, the system must allow for sufficient screening at all levels and adequate, rapid transportation and referral from lower level facilities to upper level facilities (see chapter 4).

Unmet Need for Infant Care

Early detection of any health or family problems and appropriate intervention during an infant's first few months of life result in enormous savings in human resources, prevention of long-term human suffering, and measurable financial benefits for our society. Yet despite commitments from our political leaders, only 82% of our minority 1-year-olds are fully immunized against polio, placing us 49th internationally.[9] Most newborns are healthy, yet each year nearly 20% (roughly 750 000) experience some complications, 10% experience major complications, and more than 31 000 die.[59]

Summary

Infant care includes services both to well children and to children with special needs. The two categories of care involve different system parts and different commitments of resources. Well children must be screened for complications and monitored closely as they grow and mature so that treatment of any conditions that develop can be implemented cost-effectively. Developmental expectations provide a worthwhile benchmark for such a monitoring process. At-risk infants, on the other hand, demand myriad services designed to prevent as much morbidity as possible. In some cases, as with PKU, extensive nutritional interventions can fully prevent serious mental retardation. In other cases, results are not as encouraging. Nevertheless, a UMC system must make the necessary contributions to both preventive and curative services.

ANCILLARY ISSUES

Thus far, we have presented a model of maternity and infant services that we feel should make up the universal access program espoused in this volume. A number of overarching issues are described in this section that do not lend themselves to a simple discussion within any of the clusters of services that have been described.

Facilities

Although we may appear to be advocating primarily clinic-based delivery of services, that is not the case. Services delivered from a single setting are more convenient for the patient, yet a variety of service settings may provide equally appropriate maternity and infant care. This point begs a discussion of two interrelated issues: provider types and the physical setting for care.

Maternal and infant care can be delivered in a number of settings, including hospital clinics, public clinics, HMOs, private group practices, single-practitioner settings, school- or employer-based clinics, and the home. There is no defensible reason for excluding smaller settings, but it is critical that services be comprehensive. That is, all parts of the service delivery system must be adequately linked to guarantee that the proper level of quality care is available when needed. It is also essential that service providers offer convenient hours of operation including evening and Saturday hours and that multilingual staff be available in many settings whenever possible.

Roughly 99% of all births occur in hospitals.[53] Regionalization has eliminated some duplication of effort; however, the system is primarily unidirectional (see chapter 4). That is, women and infants are referred to technically sophisticated facilities when complications arise, but they are not referred to less sophisticated facilities when all evidence suggests that a normal delivery is at hand. For reasons of efficiency and to alleviate simple shortages of some personnel and physical resources, the system should encourage effective use of all levels of facilities. To this end, low-technology birthing facilities could be made available in hospitals or nearby.

Providers

In our current health care system, existing medical care providers are either inaccessible or maldistributed and too compartmentalized and rigid in their delegation of responsibilities (see chapter 9). Many and varied health care providers play significant roles in the provision of services in a comprehensive maternity care system such as the one described here. Perinatologists, neonatologists, obstetricians, and pediatricians, all with extensive training and experience, are involved. These professionals are capable of providing various forms of care aimed at preventing and curing numerous complications during the course of pregnancy, delivery, and infancy.

None of these providers, however, could deliver even a small portion of that care without the various forms of "physician extenders" that play such a critical role in all service delivery environments, public or private. Nurses form the backbone of the health care delivery system. They often deliver the bulk of prenatal care under the supervision of physicians. Certified nurse-midwives (CNMs) are another type of registered nurse trained in midwifery. Although their ranks appear to be growing slowly (recent data indicate that 3% of deliveries are handled by midwives),[54] the trend is for fewer CNMs delivering outside hospital settings (see chapter 9). Adequate linkages to personnel and sites where more comprehensive, high-risk care can be accessed quickly are imperative.

> *If the system of care is inadequate, outreach only serves to further alienate women as well as providers by overloading the system.*

In addition, the role of a care coordinator or advocate is receiving increasing attention, and many pilot programs are in place across the country. These care coordinators may play a significant role in helping women to secure much-needed health care or social services and facilitating follow-through on the woman's part. By attending to details too frequently unaddressed in our current maternity care system (eg, outreach, follow-up, and general support), care coordinators could prove to be the backbone of a successful system of care that ensures widespread access. They may also assist in locating housing, baby-sitters capable of working with infants with complications, home nursing or hospital supplies, and welfare support.

Home Visits

A home visit is often an extremely valuable tool in a maternity care treatment plan.[60] Many routine pregnancies do not warrant such an addition to the assessment or treatment plan. However, when appropriate, at least one home visit by a nurse should be included to initiate contact with the spouse or significant others and to determine the nature of the home environment. In other instances, a series of ongoing home visits may be required to ensure adequate care. Home visits allow many contextual factors to be observed directly and other environmental needs to be determined. For example, it may be necessary to help the woman make preparations for the infant's arrival. Information garnered from home visits should be thoroughly integrated into the patient charts and the treatment plan.

Home visits also can provide community-focused, culturally sensitive, case-specific services to women who are otherwise unlikely to participate actively in care or who need more than can be provided in traditional venues.[61] Both educational (health promotion) and emotional support can be provided by means of home visits during critical periods of pregnancy. Home visits are a logical extension of the psychosocial and environmental components of care that improve the impact of the overall intervention program.

Although research findings on the effectiveness of home visits have been mixed, many studies have shown very strong effects linked to rates of participation in prenatal care and various environmental factors such as education, employment, and child development.[49,62] (See also chapters 3 and 5.) Home visits are less effective when communities do not have the necessary services to meet the needs of women or agencies involved do not communicate well among themselves.[61] However, evidence suggests that home visits by skilled nurses or trained indigenous workers can have a significant impact on the effectiveness of the overall treatment plan.[49,63]

Outreach

Awareness is an implied element of universal access. Outreach is a means of achieving awareness and, ultimately, access, but if the system of care is inadequate, outreach only serves to further alienate women as well as providers by overloading the system. Thus, outreach should focus on finding women only when the system of care is well established.

Ideally, all women should engage in preconception care or family planning practices or both before conception. Unfortunately, at least one third of expectant mothers do not receive first-trimester prenatal care, let alone any preconception care.[56,64] These women must be targeted by outreach programs that seek to ensure access to care during pregnancy. The full range of health promotion activities, media campaigns, and outreach strategies targeting would-be preconception candidates should also be aimed at the already pregnant population who have not yet participated in obstetric or preconception health care programs.

Unfortunately, a recent National Governors' Association-supported survey indicated that few state MCH program managers were aware of effective outreach programs already in place.[65] For outreach to be successful, incentives must be formally built into the infrastructure. These incentives must take into consideration the fee structures in place and the implications for motivation of health care providers for early outreach and enrollment.

Some areas in which health services have been underused will require special attention. For example, Brooks-Gunn et al recently reported on the effects of an outreach program that used indigenous workers in the community to identify and reach women who were otherwise not receiving any care.[66] These community-based caseworkers also provided support and referral services. The findings failed to detect a positive effect due to outreach, but they did identify several characteristics of women who do not receive services before outreach. The authors suggested several alternative outreach strategies, including the use of marketing strategies such as phone calls and bulk mail, then following up in person with those who are likely candidates for care. This emphasis on in-person contacts is supported by a large body of literature in mental health care diffusion research that has been in place for some time,[67] although such efforts increase program costs. Clearly, direct health care providers are not going to be supportive of outreach programs if they view as inadequate the reimbursement they receive for their eventual services. Because traditional market forces are guiding delivery of services, the reimbursement infrastructure must also be targeted for change.

... major weapons in our effort to reduce ... infant mortality and morbidity rates are the early initiation of care, the sharing of patient information among various providers, and continuity of care.

Referral and Follow-up

Once assessment and health education measures are undertaken, women should be referred to the most appropriate care setting in the private or public sector. Referral and follow-up are equally important for the preconception care patient being referred to prenatal care, the prenatal care patient being referred for additional nutritional or social counseling, and the new mother in the hospital scheduling the first postdischarge pediatric visit. All follow-ups should be pursued as vigorously as an abnormal Pap smear. The major weapons in our effort to reduce the numbers and devastating human and financial costs associated with our infant mortality and morbidity rates are the early initiation of care, the sharing of patient information among various providers, and continuity of care.

Research and Evaluation

Monitoring quality assurance in the proposed program is particularly important (see chapter 14). A universal access program for maternity care should be subject to the same sort of routine monitoring and auditing practices other federal programs undergo. However, such a program also affords us an opportunity to look carefully at the specific services delivered to a population of women with different characteristics. In 1985 the Institute of Medicine called for such a core component analysis when the authors wrote: "The appropriate goal now is to identify the components and combinations of prenatal services that are effective in preventing various poor pregnancy outcomes in well-defined groups of women."[6(p15)] Very little has happened on this front to date.

This unique opportunity to build research and evaluation into a new national service program could add immeasurably to our knowledge of critical components of maternity care programs. A national research agenda should be developed to take advantage of such a data base by building on our understanding of which maternity care services are most critical for ensuring the well-being of the nation's mothers and children.

For such a national system of data collection to be useful and truly unbiased, we must instill a sense of the value of such an undertaking in the vast numbers of health care delivery and support personnel who would be directly involved in data collection. One important step in this direction involves the infusion of additional policy analysis components to all health care-related training curricula. Without a doubt, such fundamental changes in the model of maternity care as are prescribed in this chapter and volume demand careful monitoring to ensure desired consequences.

IMPLICATIONS AND CONCLUSIONS

This volume has been developed because we firmly believe that our nation's women and children need and deserve better health care. The vitality of our citizenry, our best resource as a nation, depends on a reversal in the trends regarding the health of our women and children. Recent Medicaid expansion efforts have helped some women get care, particularly delivery services. However, there is a sore lack of evidence suggesting that women are getting into care earlier.

> The capacity to provide maternity services to the women who have become eligible under the expansions of Medicaid, or those who are still uninsured, is woefully inadequate. The government has ignored or underestimated the incentives required to ensure an adequate number of providers needed to serve poor women . . . Medicaid is so underfunded and so bureaucratically impaired that services cannot be delivered in a fashion that even approaches adequate.[68(p2)]

A program guaranteeing universal access to maternity care and primary health services for all infant health care needs (to 18 months) is the only long-term solution. The steps most critical to the success of UMC are to create linkages among a set of services that are now too separate, and to expand the goals of those services.

Implementing UMC requires consideration of many factors that will directly influence its success both in terms of services delivered and outcomes achieved. This chapter has provided an overview of the services that should be incorporated. Standards must be set for the content and quality of maternity services to be delivered. Services must include traditional medical care and risk assessment throughout the pregnancy. In addition, environmental, social, and psychological screening, referral, and related services must be widely available. More comprehensive educational services must be made available to women to ensure the best possible nutrition and health promotion counseling. Finally, there is a need for additional rigorous research to document adequately the impact of various components of the maternity care package. However, although universally available maternal and infant care will ensure both human and financial savings in the long run, nothing can be accomplished without an up-front commitment of resources for solving the maternity care crisis.

REFERENCES

1. Wallace HM, Gold EM, Oglesby A, eds. *Maternal and Child Health Practices.* 3rd ed. Oakland, Calif: Third Party Publishing Co; 1988.
2. Merkatz IR, Thompson JE, Mullen PD, Goldenberg RL, eds. *New Perspectives on Prenatal Care.* New York, NY: Elsevier; 1990.
3. US Public Health Service. Public Health Service Expert Panel on the Content of Prenatal Care. *Caring for Our Future: The Content of Prenatal Care.* Washington, DC: US Govt Printing Office; 1989.
4. American College of Obstetricians and Gynecologists. *Standards for Obstetric-Gynecologic Services.* 7th ed. Washington, DC: American College of Obstetricians and Gynecologists; 1989.
5. American Academy of Pediatrics and American College of Obstetricians and Gynecologists. *Guidelines for Perinatal Care.* 2nd ed. Elk Grove Village, Ill.; 1988.
6. Institute Of Medicine. *Preventing Low Birthweight.* Washington, DC: National Academy Press; 1985.
7. Peoples-Sheps MD. *The Content of Prenatal Care: Evidence of Effects and Recommendations for Essential Components.* Washington, DC: Bush Institute for Child and Family Policy, National Conference on Prenatal Care; May 1986.
8. Gordis L, Kleinman JC, Klerman LV, Mullen PD, Paneth N. Criteria for evaluating evidence regarding the effectiveness of prenatal interventions. In: Merkatz IR, Thompson JE, Mullen PD, Goldenberg RL, eds. *New Perspectives on Prenatal Care.* New York, NY: Elsevier; 1990.
9. Children's Defense Fund. *Children 1990: A Report Card, Briefing Book, and Action Primer.* Washington, DC: Children's Defense Fund; 1990.
10. Pear R. Vaccinate welfare children, US says. *New York Times,* Nov 29, 1990, A1, p. 1.
11. Harlap S, Kost K, Forrest JD. *Preventing Pregnancy, Protecting Health: A New Look at Birth Control Choices in the United States.* New York, NY: Alan Guttmacher Institute; 1991.
12. Forrest JD. Unintended pregnancy among American women. *Fam Plann Perspect.* 1987;19:2.
13. Grimes DA. Sexually transmitted diseases. In: Wallace HM, Ryan G, Oglesby AC, eds. *Maternal and Child Health Practices.* 3rd ed. Oakland, Calif: Third Party Publishing Co; 1988:347–356.
14. Rosenn B, Miodovnik M, Combs CA, Khoury J, Siddiqi TA. Preconception management of insulin-dependent diabetes: improvement of pregnancy outcome. *Obstet Gynecol.* 1991;77:844–845.
15. Plomin R, DeFries JC, McClearn GE. *Behavioral Genetics.* 2nd ed. New York, NY: WH Freeman and Company; 1990.
16. Chasnoff IJ, Landress HJ, Barrett ME. The prevalence of illicit-drug or alcohol use during pregnancy and discrepancies in mandatory reporting in Pinellas County, Florida. *N Engl J Med.* 1990;322:1202–1206.
17. Little BB, Snell LM, Klein VR, Gilstrap LC. Cocaine abuse during pregnancy: maternal and fetal implications. *Obstet Gynecol.* 1989;73: 157–160.
18. Little BB, Snell LM, Klein VR, Gilstrap LC, Knoll KA, Breckenridge JD. Maternal and fetal effects of heroin addiction during pregnancy. *J Reprod Med.* 1990;35:159–162.
19. Little BB, Snell LM, Gilstrap LC. Methamphetamine abuse during pregnancy: outcome and fetal effects. *Obstet Gynecol.* 1988;72:541–544.
20. Jones KL, Smith DW. Recognition of the fetal alcohol syndrome in early infancy. *Lancet.* 1973;2:999–1003.
21. Abel EL, Sokol RJ. Incidence of fetal alcohol syndrome and economic impact of FAS-related anomalies. *Drug Alcohol Depend.* 1987;19:51–70.

22. Hutchings DE, ed. Prenatal abuse of licit and illicit drugs. vol 562. New York, NY: Annals of the New York Academy of Sciences; 1989.
23. Fingerhut LA, Kleinman JC, Kendrick JS. Smoking before, during, and after pregnancy. *Am J Public Health*. 1990;80:541–544.
24. Sexton M, Hebel JR. A clinical trial of change in maternal smoking and its effect on birthweight. *JAMA*. 1984;251:911–915.
25. Ershoff D, Mullen P, Quinn V. Women who quit smoking at the beginning of pregnancy: clinical implications in identification and relapse prevention. Presented at the 114th Annual Meeting of the American Public Health Association; Oct 1, 1986; Las Vegas, Nev.
26. Ershoff D, Mullen P, Quinn V. A randomized trial of a serialized self-help smoking cessation program for pregnant women in an HMO. *Am J Public Health*. 1989;79:182–187.
27. Mayer JP, Newton JR, Knox EG. A randomized evaluation of smoking cessation interventions for pregnant women at a WIC clinic. *AM J Public Health*. 1990;80:76–78.
28. Ershoff DH, Quinn VP, Mullen PD, Lairson DR. Pregnancy and medical cost outcomes of a self-help prenatal smoking cessation program in a HMO. *Public Health Rep*. 1990;105:340–347.
29. Thompson JE. Maternal stress, anxiety, and social support during pregnancy: possible directions for prenatal intervention. In: Merkatz IR, Thompson JE, Mullen PD, Goldenberg RL, eds. *New Perspectives on Prenatal Care*. New York, NY: Elsevier; 1990;319–336.
30. Simpson JL. Surveillance for genetic disorders and congenital anomalies. In: Wallace HG, Ryan G, Oglesby AC, eds. *Maternal and Child Health Practices*. 3rd ed. Oakland, Calif: Third Party Publishing Co; 1990;371–400.
31. US Congress. Office of Technology Assessment. *Infertility: Medical and Social Choices*. Washington, DC: US Govt Printing Office; 1988. OTA-BA-358.
32. Mosher WD, Pratt WF. Fecundity and infertility in the United States, 1965–1988. *Advance Data from Vital and Health Statistics*. No 192. Hyattsville, Md: National Center for Health Statistics; 1990.
33. Mosher WD. Use of family planning services in the United States: 1982 and 1988. *Advance Data from Vital and Health Statistics*. No 184. Hyattsville, Md: National Center for Health Statistics; 1990.
34. Mosher W, Horn M. Source of service and visit rate for family planning services: United States, 1982. *Public Health Rep*. 1986;101:405–416.
35. Mosher WD, Pratt WF. Contraceptive use in the United States, 1973–1988. *Advance Data from Vital and Health Statistics*. No 182. Hyattsville, Md: National Center for Health Statistics, 1990.
36. Hatcher RA, Guest FJ, Stewart FH, et al. Methods of fertility control. In: Wallace HM, Ryan G, Oglesby AC, eds. *Maternal and Child Health Practices*. 3rd ed. Oakland, Calif: Third Party Publishing Co; 1988;325–346.
37. Sorenstein FL, Pittman KJ. The availability of sex education in large city school districts. *Fam Plann Perspect*. 1984;16:19–25.
38. Jack B, Culpepper L. Preconception care. In: Merkatz IR, Thompson JE, Mullen PD, Goldenberg RL, eds. *New Perspectives on Prenatal Care*. New York, NY: Elsevier; 1990;69–88.
39. David HP, Dytrych Z, Matejeck Z, Schuller V, eds. *Born Unwanted: Developmental Effects of Denied Abortion*. New York, NY: Springer; 1988.
40. US Public Health Service. Select Panel for the Promotion of Child Health. *Better Health for Our Children: A National Strategy*. Washington, DC: US Govt Printing Office; 1981.
41. Williams LB, Pratt WF. Wanted and unwanted children in the United States. *Advance Data from Vital and Health Statistics*. No 189. Hyattsville, Md: National Center for Health Statistics; 1990.
42. Blakely CH, Little BB, Eltinge J. The need for preventive services for pregnant substance abusers: a survey of the six largest public hospitals

in Texas. Presented at the annual meeting of the Southeastern Psychological Association; March 20, 1991; New Orleans, La.

43. Mastroianni L, Donaldson PJ, Kane TT, eds. *Developing New Contraceptives: Obstacles and Opportunities.* Washington, DC: National Academy Press; 1990.

44. Worthington-Roberts BS, Klerman LV. Maternal nutrition. In: Merkatz IR, Thompson JE, Mullen PD, Goldenberg RL, eds. *New Perspectives on Prenatal Care.* New York, NY: Elsevier; 1990:235–272.

45. Hann DM, Osofsky HJ. Psychosocial factors in the transition to parenthood. In: Merkatz IR, Thompson JE, Mullen PD, Goldenberg RL, eds. *New Perspectives on Prenatal Care.* New York, NY: Elsevier; 1990:347–362.

46. Thompson JE, Walsh LV, Merkatz IR. The history of prenatal care: cultural, social, and medical contexts. In: Merkatz IR, Thompson JE, Mullen PD, Goldenberg RL, eds. *New Perspectives on Prenatal Care.* New York, NY: Elsevier; 1990.

47. Torres A, Kenney AM. Expanding Medicaid coverage for pregnant women: estimates of the impact and cost. *Fam Plann Perspect.* 1989;21:19–24.

48. Mayer JP, Johnson CD, Condon JW, Bergquist CB. *Multi-state Prenatal Needs Determination Project. Final Report to the Bureau of Health Care Delivery and Assistance, US Public Health Service.* Lansing, Mich: University Associates; 1987.

49. Klerman LV. Home visiting during pregnancy. In: Merkatz IR, Thompson JE, Mullen PD, Goldenberg RL, eds. *New Perspectives on Prenatal Care.* New York, NY: Elsevier; 1990;593–602.

50. Paneth N, Kiely JL, Wallenstein S, Susser MW. The choice of place of delivery: effect of hospital level on mortality in all singleton births in New York City. *Am J Disabled Child.* 1987;141:60–64.

51. Paneth N, Kiely JL, Susser MW. Age at death used to assess the effect of interhospital transport on neonatal mortality. *Pediatrics.* 1984;66:854–861.

52. Marcus M, Paneth N, Kiely JL, Susser MW. Determinants of interhospital transfer of low birthweight newborns. *Med Care.* 1988;24:462–473.

53. American College of Obstetricians and Gynecologists. Trends in out-of-hospital births in the United States. In: *Manpower Planning in Obstetrics and Gynecology.* Washington, DC; 1985.

54. National Center for Health Statistics. Advance report of final natality statistics, 1988. *Monthly Vital Statistics Report.* vol 39, no 4 suppl. Hyattsville, Md: Public Health Service; 1990.

55. Warren CW, Keppel KG, Flock ML. Trends and variations in postpartum sterilization in the United States, 1972, 1980. *Monthly Vital Statistics Report.* vol 36, no 7. Hyattsville, Md: National Center for Health Statistics; 1987.

56. Institute of Medicine, National Academy of Sciences. *Prenatal Care: Reaching Mothers, Reaching Infants.* Washington, DC: National Academy Press; 1988.

57. Mayer JP, Johnson CD, Blakely CH. *The Texas OB Survey: Determining the Need for Maternity Services in Texas.* College Station, Tex: Public Policy Resources Laboratory; 1986.

58. Schorr LB. *Within Our Reach: Breaking the Cycle of Disadvantage.* New York, NY: Doubleday; 1989.

59. Alan Guttmacher Institute. *Blessed Events and the Bottom Line: Financing Maternity Care in the United States.* Washington, DC: Alan Guttmacher Institute; 1987.

60. Olds DL, Henderson CR, Tatelbaum R, Chamberlin R. Improving the delivery of prenatal care and outcomes of pregnancy: a randomized trial of nurse home visitation. *Pediatrics.* 1986;77:16–28.

61. National Commission to Prevent Infant Mortality. *Home Visiting: Opening Doors for America's Pregnant Women and Children.* Washington, DC: National Commission to Prevent Infant Mortality; 1989.

62. Mayer JP, Johnson CD. *Infant Health Initiatives Project: An Analysis of Services and Outcomes. Final Report Submitted to the Bureau of Community Services, Michigan Department of Public Health.* Lansing, Mich: University Associates, 1986.

63. US Congress. Office of Technology Assessment. *Healthy Children: Investing in the Future.* Washington, DC: US Govt Printing Office; 1988. OTA-H-345.

64. Singh S, Forrest JD, Torres A. *Prenatal Care in the United States: A State and County Inventory.* New York, NY: Alan Guttmacher Institute; 1989.

65. Hill IT, Breyel J. *Coordinating Prenatal Care.* Washington, DC: National Governors Association, 1989.

66. Brooks-Gunn J, McCormick MC, Gunn RW, Shorter T, Wallace CY, Heagarty MC. Outreach as case finding: the process of locating low-income pregnant women. *Med Care.* 1989;27:95–102.

67. Fairweather GW. *Methods for Experimental Social Innovation.* New York, NY: Wiley; 1968.

68. Davidson EC. Caring for new mothers: pressing problems, new solutions. Presented before the Select Committee on Children, Youth, and Families. US House of Representatives; October 24, 1989.

CHAPTER 14

Ensuring the Quality of Maternity Care

Arden S. Handler, DrPH
Janet D. Perloff, PhD
Joan F. Kennelly, BSN, MPH

By the end of the 1980s, a succession of changes in the Medicaid program had significantly expanded opportunities for an increasing number of low-income women and their infants to enjoy financial access to prenatal and infant care. Because this expansion in financial access has not kept up with increasing demand (see chapter 15), momentum for universal access to maternity and infant care continues to grow.

The public sector will undoubtedly play a major role in financing and implementing a universal maternity care (UMC) program. This chapter addresses lessons drawn from public sector experience and suggests strategies for ensuring the quality of care in a UMC program. Our observations are grounded in an exploration of the financing and delivery of prenatal care, but they also apply to ensuring the quality of the full range of reproductive services as well as infant and child health care. Rather than presume one particular vision of a UMC program, we address principles that should be the basis for ensuring quality in any system providing universal access to maternity care.

A FRAMEWORK FOR ENSURING THE QUALITY OF MATERNITY CARE

Donabedian's framework for assessing health care quality has gained wide recognition because of its universal applicability and intuitive appeal.[1] Assessment can be carried out in three ways:

1. Examining the structure of care (ie, characteristics of the providers of care, the physical and organizational settings in which they work, and the ways in which care is paid for).

2. Examining the process of care (ie, the set of activities engaged in by practitioners with other practitioners as well as patients in both the technical management and interpersonal process of care).

3. Examining the outcome of care ("a change in a patient's current and future health status that can be attributed to antecedent health care").[1(pp82-83)]

We have adapted Donabedian's framework to develop an approach for ensuring the quality of care that considers three interrelated strategies: structure, standards, and assessment.

Structure

Quality of care can be enhanced or diminished by alterations in the structure of care. One way to protect and promote the quality of care is to ensure both adequacy of resources and implementation of a well-designed system.[1] The General Accounting Office (GAO) has noted that "while it is important to have effective systems for monitoring the quality of care after it is provided, it is equally, if not more important to try to 'build it in' up front."[2(p8)]

Standards

The quality of care is also a function of the norms that govern the technical management and interpersonal process of care.[1] Modifying these norms as new information emerges and securing practitioner and institutional compliance with established norms through the application of standards are essential steps in ensuring quality.

Assessment

Developing and implementing effective assessment methods at both the micro (utilization review) and macro (monitoring and surveillance) levels is also crucial to ensuring quality care. Assessment efforts must focus on the adequacy of the health care delivery system and the extent to which practitioners and institutions comply with standards, as well as on health outcomes. Clearly, assessment will prove an ineffective tool for ensuring quality unless standards of care are universally applied and the delivery system is adequate to support these standards.

The following discussion examines lessons from the public sector that are applicable to ensuring the quality of care in a UMC program. Specifically, we examine public sector experience with respect to (1) the structural components necessary to ensure quality maternity care, (2) the development and implementation of maternity care standards, and (3) assessment methods necessary to examine and improve quality. We begin by presenting examples of standards for quality maternity care. These examples are a benchmark against which we review efforts to ensure quality through programs such as Title V and Title XIX (Medicaid) of the Social Security Act.

STANDARDS FOR QUALITY MATERNITY CARE

The quality of prenatal care is a direct manifestation of the norms that govern the technical management and interpersonal process of care and the degree of adherence to standards that reflect these norms. A profession's experts establish norms for the technical management of care based on the state of science and technology of the time. In contrast, norms governing the interpersonal process of care emerge from the country's health and social policies, the ethical values of the health professions, and the expectations and aspirations of patients.[1]

The standards we have chosen for high-quality technical management of care are based on the recommendations of the Public Health Service's Expert Panel on the Content of Prenatal Care.[3] Incorporating current best practice,[4] these recommendations emphasize health promotion and risk prevention, care during the preconception period, and care appropriate to the level and nature of a woman's risk for adverse pregnancy outcomes. Moving decisively beyond the medical model, these guidelines call for comprehensive care, including all necessary psychological, social, educational, and medical assessments and interventions.

Standards for the interpersonal process of care are generally less well developed and less explicit than those governing the technical management of care. Interpersonal process standards for prenatal care, however, are becoming increasingly explicit because of the growing recognition that adverse pregnancy outcomes may result from inferior interpersonal care during the prenatal period.

We have chosen the Institute of Medicine's (IOM)[5] recommendations for the organization and atmosphere of prenatal care as standards for high-quality care with respect to the interpersonal process of maternity care. The IOM regards high-quality prenatal care to be financially, physically, and psychologically accessible to clients. Attributes of the interpersonal process that foster quality prenatal care include those that:

- facilitate timely entry to care (eg, transportation, short waiting times for appointments);

- facilitate use of services (eg, minimal time in waiting room, bilingual staff or interpreters, cultural sensitivity, child care services);

- optimize continuity, comprehensiveness, and compliance (eg, co-ordination of prenatal appointments with other appointments, continuity of caregiver, case management services).

The standards we have selected to represent quality maternity care exemplify the current state of the art in prenatal care. They are a reference point as we review public sector experience in ensuring the quality of maternity care through structure, standards, and assessment.

Public sector experience offers lessons about four components of structure that are necessary to ensure quality maternity care: physician providers of care, payment for care, nonphysician providers of care, and the setting of care. **ENSURING QUALITY THROUGH STRUCTURE**

Physician Providers of Care

Maintaining an adequate supply of properly trained physicians is a key aspect of ensuring high-quality care in a UMC program. Experience with the Medicaid program has demonstrated that financial access does not guarantee that physicians will be available to deliver high-quality prenatal care. Problems in maintaining an adequate supply of maternity care physicians are discussed in chapter 9.

Whether the supply of physicians is "adequate" refers not only to absolute numbers but also to whether physicians are trained in state-of-the-art technical management and interpersonal process of care. Physicians' training has historically emphasized a medical model of patient care that gives scant attention to the development of interpersonal skills, ethnic and cultural sensitivity, and ability to function in multidisciplinary teams[6]—all critical aspects of quality care. In addition, requirements to update skills vary by state and specialty.[7,8] It is widely assumed that practitioners who are not university based have fewer opportunities for continuing education to keep abreast of changes in both technical management and interpersonal process of care.

Other factors that have a major impact on the adequacy of physician supply are demographics and geographic location, because both influence where maternity care physicians practice. Sparsely populated rural areas with aging populations do not attract maternity care physicians,[9] and although urban areas have a large young, childbearing population, many physicians (especially the most highly qualified) prefer to practice in higher income communities. Consequently, most inner-city women rely on hospital outpatient facilities, public and nonprofit clinics, and the practices of a small number of inner-city physicians who provide care almost exclusively to the poor.[10] Maldistribution and shortages of maternity care physicians are also caused by high maternity care practice costs, high obstetric malpractice premiums, fear of being sued for malpractice, and the unwillingness of obstetricians to participate in state Medicaid programs (see chapter 9).

To ensure access to the services of well-qualified physicians in a universal access program, training and continuing education programs will have to be implemented emphasizing comprehensive, multidisiciplinary, and interpersonally sensitive care. Public sector experience has also shown the necessity of substantially reducing reliance on market mechanisms to redistribute physician services. Various forms of direct government intervention will be essential.

Payment

Amount, method, and linkage of payment to specific expectations about service delivery all have important implications for quality of care in a UMC program.

Payment Level. Historically, many state Medicaid programs have paid very low fees to maternity care physicians in relation to other fees: for example, in 1986 the average Medicaid obstetric fee was approximately 44% of the average nationwide community charge.[11] Low payment levels have played a significant part in discouraging physicians from participating in state Medicaid programs[11,12,13] and have caused some physicians to limit the number of Medicaid patients they treat.[13] In many states, low Medicaid payment has also greatly limited the capacity of institutional providers such as hospital outpatient clinics, community and migrant health centers, and health departments to render maternity care to those in need.[10]

Some states have recently raised physician payment levels to encourage maternity care physicians to serve Medicaid eligibles.[11] Although this strategy holds promise, evidence suggests that it may not be effective, because exceedingly high payments may be required to encourage physicians to locate in underserved areas.[10]

Method of Payment. The method by which providers are paid (fee-for-service, prepaid capitation, salary) has important implications for the quality of maternity care. The primary payment methods, fee-for-service and prepaid capitation, offer somewhat different incentives that may affect both the costs and quality of care. Fee-for-service payment may lead to unnecessary care, because it offers no incentives to contain costs by providing health promotion and preventive services. By contrast, prepaid capitation payment methods give providers such as health maintenance organizations (HMOs) incentives to keep patients healthy, but these incentives may also lead to underservice.

Although state Medicaid programs are increasingly enrolling eligibles in HMOs, only a few studies have examined differential birth outcomes and the relative quality of maternity care rendered under the prepaid capitation form of payment.[14,15] Most available empirical literature suggests no cause for concern about the quality of care rendered in Medicaid HMOs.[16] However, it remains possible, as is suggested in the GAO's study of Medicaid HMOs in Chicago, that in some states these providers operate without sufficient safeguards against underservice.[17] If payment in a UMC program were fully or partially based on prepaid capitation, the use of standards could promote appropriate service delivery by specifying the content of services to be incorporated in the negotiated capitation agreement.

Linkage. Payment can be a powerful instrument in shaping aspects of the technical management and interpersonal process of care. An early example can be found in the delivery of maternity care through the Emergency Maternity and Infant Care (EMIC) program during World War II. The Children's Bureau required all agencies requesting payment for EMIC services to demonstrate that a certain minimum level of prenatal and postpartum care had been delivered. This requirement was seen as a way to improve quality through the use of administrative controls.[18]

A more recent innovation in Medicaid also exemplifies the use of payment to achieve improvements in the quality of care. The Consolidated Omnibus Budget Reconciliation Act of 1985[19] enables states to pay providers for an expanded package of prenatal care services including risk assessment, case management, nutrition counseling, and psychological support services. Some of these additional services can be rendered by providers other than physicians, such as nutritionists and social workers. Because providers are paid for specific components of a service package that focuses on both the technical management and interpersonal process of care, the likelihood that women receive comprehensive services is greatly increased.

Regardless of the amount and method of payment, establishing conditions for participation to obtain payment would be necessary to ensure quality maternity care.

Public sector experience has shown that in a UMC program with multiple payers, parity in payment for similar services by all payers, both public and private, would be essential so that providers would have little reason not to participate and little incentive to discriminate among patients on the basis of payer. Regardless of the amount and method of payment, establishing conditions for participation in order to obtain payment would also be necessary to ensure quality maternity care. These conditions could include evidence of licensure, admitting privileges, or ability to provide state-of-the-art maternity care. To maximize the interpersonal quality of care, additional fees for services such as transportation, bilingual providers, child care, or ability to provide night and weekend office hours or 24-hour coverage might also be provided.

Nonphysician Providers of Prenatal Care

An adequate supply of nonphysician providers of care, particularly certified nurse-midwives (CNMs) and nurse-practitioners (NPs), is also crucial to ensuring the quality of maternity care in a universal access program. Most NPs and CNMs practice in the public sector, where their effectiveness in delivering high-quality prenatal care has been demonstrated.

In 1986 there were 15 400 NPs and 2000 CNMs practicing in the United States.[20] From 1975 to 1988 the number of in-hospital births attended by CNMs increased 500%.[21] Numerous comparative studies evaluating the quality of care provided by NPs, CNMs, and physicians have been reviewed by the Office of Technology Assessment.[20] These studies demonstrate that NPs and CNMs practicing in their areas of training and expertise are "more adept than physicians at providing services that depend on communication with patients and preventive actions."[20(pp5,6)]

Although research demonstrates comparable birth outcomes for normal low-risk pregnant clients of CNMs and physicians, many studies also note the following to be characteristic of the care provided by CNMs: patient appointments are kept more regularly; less medication is used and more personal attention is provided during the intrapartum period; fewer forceps deliveries are performed; and low-risk clients have shorter in-patient stays than low-risk clients of physicians.[22-25] Research has also shown NPs and CNMs to be "particularly effective in managing the care of pregnant women who are at high risk of low birthweight because of social and economic factors."[26(p9)]

Despite their demonstrated ability to deliver high-quality, cost-effective prenatal care, NPs and CNMs are greatly underutilized. Barriers to increasing the supply and use of CNMs and NPs include the following:

- Limited third-party coverage and lack of direct payment as well as varying payment for services provided.[20]

- Restrictive state statutes and regulations and varying interpretation of states' legislation on nurse practice.[20]

- Inadequate malpractice insurance coverage.[20]

- Inability to obtain admitting privileges at local hospitals.[20]

- Physicians' attitudes.[20]

- Prohibitive tuition and related educational costs that preclude expansion of educational facilities and graduate programs (K. Fennel, ACNM, personal communication, December 1990).

The public sector has attempted to overcome some of these barriers. In the early 1980s, the federal government opened the door for third-party payment by authorizing coverage for services provided by CNMs directly and by physician-supervised NPs through its Medicaid and Medicare programs,[27] and by providing payment for these services through Title V. Medicaid and Medicare payment is, however, limited to the maternity cycle and does not cover family planning and other reproductive health services. In addition, Medicare has set a precedent by paying only 65% of an obstetrician's fee to CNMs (K. Fennel, December 1990).

The Omnibus Budget Reconciliation Act of 1989 (OBRA 1989)[28] made some improvements in the coverage of nonphysician practitioners through the Medicaid program. Since April 1, 1990, state Medicaid programs have been required to directly pay family and pediatric NPs for services they provide within the scope of their professional training and licensure and without the supervision of a physician. Realizing the benefits of this provision, however, will depend on state compliance. OBRA 1989 did not address the issues of differential payments for providers or payment for services beyond the maternity cycle.

A UMC program must consider strategies for increased use of NPs and CNMs, including employment based on national standards of education and clinical experience; coverage and direct payment by all payers to CNMs and NPs; parity in payment across provider types for services rendered; adequate malpractice insurance; affordable and accessible training programs; and increased public and physician education about these essential care providers.

Setting of Care

The site of care delivery is another factor that affects quality of care. Health care settings affect what type of medical personnel provide care, the availability and accessibility of nonmedical personnel, and the atmosphere in which care is delivered. A review of public sector experience in the delivery and financing of maternity care in three settings— private physicians' offices, health departments, and community and migrant health centers (CHCs-MHCs)—is informative with respect to the potential to provide quality care in a universal access program.

Private Physicians' Offices. Public sector experience with physicians' offices as a setting for the delivery of maternity care is based primarily on the Medicaid program. Thirty-five percent of women whose delivery is paid for by Medicaid obtain their prenatal care in the offices of private physicians.[29] Little is known about the quality of care provided in these offices, except for information available through the informal peer appraisal process that takes place among physicians, and through malpractice suits. Few, if any, state Medicaid statutes require physicians to follow established guidelines or standards of care in order to participate in Medicaid. Although some state Medicaid manuals or plans refer to "best practice" and "use of acceptable standards" for delivering prenatal care, in general all a licensed physician must do to participate in the Medicaid program is possess a billing identification number.

In many locales, provision of care through Medicaid "mills" is considered a major, although not well-documented, problem. Nearly 60% of all Medicaid patients treated in private practices are seen in large Medicaid practices,[30] where the technical management of care is suspected to be lower than in mainstream practices.[10,30,31] Medicaid program experience has also demonstrated that private practice physicians are less likely to be linked to a network of ancillary services and are more likely to adhere to a medical model of care delivery than is true in multidisciplinary, comprehensive settings.[5]

Data concerning the interpersonal process of care offered in the offices of private physicians who participate in the Medicaid program are equally scarce. In large Medicaid practices, women often have shorter waiting times than in public clinics and are less likely to be given block appointments.[5,32] However, a high volume of patients and short visits offering little preventive care and anticipatory guidance decrease personal interaction and lessen the opportunity for both the woman and the provider to gather information about the progress of the pregnancy.[10]

Health Departments. A recent survey of local health department officials and state Maternal and Child Health (MCH) directors[33] identified 2306 prenatal care sites funded by state MCH (Title V) agencies. Of these sites, 2017 were operated directly by health departments and 289 were operated by other agencies. Health departments are the largest clinic providers of prenatal care, accounting for approximately 37% of all clinic sites.[33]

Evaluations of maternity care services provided in local health departments have not been extensive. In a study to determine whether the type of sponsoring agency affected the productivity of Maternity and Infant Care (MIC) projects and Children and Youth (C and Y) projects before the MCH Block Grant was implemented, projects sponsored by health departments were found to be more likely to follow a nonmedical care provision model. These projects had a greater number of education and social work staff for a given level of expenditures than was true in nonhealth department projects.[34]

Data from Kentucky and North Carolina (N. Ward, P. Buescher, unpublished data, 1989) indicate that the low birthweight rate for Medicaid recipients who obtain care at local health departments is significantly lower than for Medicaid patients who obtain care in other settings. In an earlier study of one North Carolina county,[35] Buescher et al suggest that better perinatal outcomes for health department patients versus Medicaid-eligible patients who received care from private practitioners was more likely due to the health department setting than to unmeasured differences between the two groups of women. The health department studied employed NPs for care; used phone and home visit follow-up for patients who missed visits; provided health education, counseling, and nutrition services; and referred high-risk women for prenatal care at a nearby tertiary care center.

Despite the many positive aspects of the care delivered in public health departments, when financial resources are limited these settings are less able to provide the full array of ancillary services necessary for quality prenatal care. As a consequence, aspects of the interpersonal process of care may be neglected. The IOM points out that in publicly financed clinics (health departments as well as other sites including hospitals), women often have substantial on-site waiting times, primarily because of block appointments rather than integrated appointments.[5] In Chicago, waiting times to obtain prenatal care appointments at the city's MCH clinics averaged 53.25 days in 1989 because of cutbacks and personnel shortages.[36] Communication problems prompted by social and cultural differences, rude staff, language barriers, and dreary waiting rooms with no play areas for children are also common in prenatal clinics for low-income women.[5]

Community and Migrant Health Centers. Lessons regarding the potential of various settings to deliver quality care can also be gleaned from CHCs and MHCs, which are community-based comprehensive primary care providers. In 1987, CHCs and MHCs provided maternity care to between 150 000 and 225 000 women.[37] These health centers are generally well regarded by the public health community because of their attention to the interpersonal process of care (exemplified by their convenient locations and sensitivity to the communities they serve), accessible clinic hours (including nights and weekends), multilingual staff, and commitment to providing a broad spectrum of medical and supportive services. Using a comprehensive community-based model, CHCs and MHCs have demonstrated success in achieving community acceptance, reducing reliance on emergency rooms, improving the health status of the patients they serve, and being cost-effective.[38] However, like public health departments, when CHCs and MHCs are under financial stress, their ability to provide high-quality care is greatly diminished.

Public sector experience in the financing and delivery of maternity care in various settings suggests that comprehensive, multidisciplinary care in a universal access program may be most easily provided in adequately funded, organized settings such as public health departments or CHCs-MHCs. Although organized settings may be more likely than private physicians' offices to provide comprehensive care, without sufficient resources they too are apt to fall short in providing quality care. Increased emphasis on the interpersonal process of care will be necessary in whatever settings women seek care in a UMC program.

ENSURING QUALITY THROUGH STANDARDS

Establishing standards for both the technical management and the interpersonal process of care is an essential aspect of ensuring the quality of care in a UMC program. The development and implementation of care standards through the Title V program have set important precedents in this regard.

Since the 1940s, MCH services funded by Title V of the Social Security Act have operated under federal guidelines that stress comprehensive, multidisciplinary care. This point was first evident in the policy guidelines prepared by the Children's Bureau for the EMIC program during World War II, in which referrals for home nursing care before, during, and after delivery and referrals to the state or local welfare agency for "personal problems" were encouraged.[18]

The use of comprehensive maternity care standards was also an important feature of the MIC program of Title V (1963). In the Children's Bureau's 1964 guidance for the MIC program,[39] the federal government delineated its expectations regarding content of care. MIC programs were to make available a broad spectrum of diagnostic and specialist consultation services and to provide public health nursing, nurse-midwifery, medical social services, nutrition, and dental services.

Expectations regarding the interpersonal process of care were just as explicit. Services were to be available with "respect for the dignity of the individual regardless of the patient's social circumstances or ability to pay; with efficient administrative procedures for registering patients, avoiding prolonged waiting and multiple visits for registration; and, at times when patients most conveniently can come to clinics."[39(p5)]

In 1976 the Bureau of Community Health Services prepared additional guidance material to standardize the quality of care provided to mothers and children served through its programs. Detailed descriptions of the content of maternity and newborn care, including preconceptional care, were provided along with comprehensive job descriptions for nursing, medical, social work, and nutrition services and personnel.[40]

The 1976 program guidance also gave specific attention to the interpersonal process of care. Providers were encouraged to respond to factors that might prevent women from seeking care, including lack of child care or transportation and low self-esteem. They were instructed to treat women with dignity and respect, answer their questions, respond to their complaints, and pay attention to each woman's special needs during pregnancy.[40]

While no penalties were imposed for failure to comply with any aspects of the 1964 and 1976 guidance, technical assistance was provided and conditions were placed on specific line items in project budgets to ensure that the quality of care provided at the community level met the standards of care established at the national level (A. Koontz, DHHS, personal communication, April 1990).

In 1981, President Reagan's new federalism and policy of deregulation led to the creation of block grants to the states. Title V was subsequently amended to create the MCH Block Grant.[41] Under the amended statute, states were no longer required to maintain projects such as the MIC program, and written national guidance for care delivery was no longer provided to state agencies that received Title V funds. When guidance was requested, the Office of Maternal and Child Health continued to emphasize a comprehensive approach to prenatal care (A. Koontz, 1990).

The OBRA 1989 amendments to Title V marked the federal government's return to a more direct role in shaping the content of health services for pregnant women and children at the community level. State administration of MCH funds is now linked to the national health objectives for the year 2000. Providing services to federally designated target populations has been mandated.[28] The guidance provided by the federal Office of Maternal and Child Health for the preparation of state applications calls for the provision of family centered, community based, and coordinated care for pregnant women, mothers and infants up to age 1, as well as children and adolescents and children with special health care needs.[42]

The history of maternity care standards and guidance to programs funded through Title V establishes important precedents for a UMC program. Under Title V, standards for quality maternity care that were developed at the national level have been linked to the delivery of care at the local level, providing a model for such linkage in a universal access program.

MCH services funded by Title V have operated under federal guidelines that stress comprehensive, multi-disciplinary care.

ENSURING QUALITY THROUGH ASSESSMENT

In this section, we return to Donabedian's original framework[1] to review the public sector's approach to ensuring quality through assessment. The majority of our comments center on macrolevel monitoring and surveillance of the structure, process and outcomes of care, rather than microlevel activities such as utilization review.

The use of assessment as a tool to ensure the quality of care in public sector programs has not been consistent. Miller et al[43] noted that the extent to which data are collected, needs are assessed, or health status monitored reflects prevailing health policies. The public sector's categorical approach to program implementation has also meant a categorical approach to monitoring and surveillance activities.

With the creation of the Children's Bureau in 1912, the role of the government, particularly the federal government, as a collector of information about "all matters pertaining to the welfare of children and child life among all classes of our people . . . " was established.[44(p591)] Early efforts by the Children's Bureau led to the establishment of state vital statistics registries, which have come to play a major role in our national surveillance and monitoring activities for maternal and infant health.[44]

Historically, Title V programs have used classic health outcome measures such as infant and maternal mortality as broad indicators of the need for and adequacy of services provided for women and children. Later, the MCH Block Grant also required state agencies to submit reports of intended expenditures (RIEs) and statements of assurance that identified needs were being met equally within the state.[41]

Title V monitoring procedures were significantly altered by OBRA 1989, however. RIEs have been replaced by an application for block grant funds, a statewide needs assessment is required, and program plans and strategies to meet identified needs must be coordinated with the national health objectives for the year 2000. Each state must also prepare an annual report with specific information on health status measures, clients served, types of services and provider capacity. State applications for Title V allocations are reviewed, and failure to comply with requirements can lead to fiscal consequences.[28] Despite these more stringent reporting requirements, a mandate to examine the relationship between health outcomes and the delivery or content of services provided (eg, the number of infant deaths attributed to women who failed to receive prenatal care or comprehensive care) has yet to be established.

The monitoring activities that have been instituted through Medicaid have only minimally focused on quality of care provided. The Health Care Financing Administration's (HCFA's) requirement for standardized reporting by states on aggregate use and expenditures has encouraged the development of management information systems at the state level. However, few states have used their eligibility or claims data bases to summarize demographic or health status characteristics of the Medicaid population. States are required to employ some form of quality assurance and utilization review mechanism; some elect to use professional review organizations (PROs), a method that appears to give scant attention to the quality of care.[45] Medicaid monitoring activities have been aimed at reducing error rates and detecting fraud as well as underutilization and overutilization rather than at monitoring trends in the health status of the population served or evaluating the cost-effectiveness of the services provided.

Recently, some states have begun to link vital records to their Medicaid claim forms. This effort is supported by OBRA 1989, which requires the development of a national data system to link infant birth and death records with any claims submitted under Medicaid beginning in 1991. The legislation also acknowledges the sensitive relationship between payment and provider supply and requires state reporting of payment levels for review by HCFA.[28]

This recent shift in Medicaid's monitoring efforts is an important step toward the development of monitoring and surveillance systems in which health outcomes are linked to the structure of the delivery system (eg, how care is financed). However, this effort is limited by the extent to which state Medicaid management information systems include data on the process of care for each client (eg, the content of the visits reimbursed by Medicaid—risk assessment performed, referrals made, tests ordered, education provided).

Lessons from the public sector in the use of monitoring and surveillance to ensure the quality of care come not only from the service delivery and financing programs that have been the main focus of this chapter, but also from large-scale, ongoing surveillance and monitoring activities of the National Center for Health Statistics (NCHS). NCHS maintains both record-based (vital statistics, mortality, and natality follow-back surveys) and population-based data systems (eg, the National Health and Nutrition Examination Survey and the National Survey of Family Growth).[46]

Although vital statistics have become the foundation for monitoring the health status of mothers and infants, they have historically provided little information about the care received by the mother-infant pair during pregnancy or delivery. Although the revised 1989 US Standard Certificate of Live Birth includes more detailed information on obstetric procedures, implementation of the revised certificate by the states remains voluntary. Selected health status measures from national surveys have rarely been linked to information on availability and accessibility of health and social service programs, participation in these programs, the content of care, or socioeconomic status. Consequently, they do not contribute to our understanding of other system factors related to the health measures taken.

The public sector's categorical approach to program implementation has also meant a categorical approach to monitoring and surveillance activities.

245

Two recent efforts by the federal government provide examples of surveillance and monitoring activities that incorporate more than vital statistics in their assessment of maternity events. In the 1988 National Maternal and Infant Health Survey conducted by NCHS,[47] infant births, fetal deaths, and infant deaths (health outcomes) are linked to information collected from mothers, hospitals, and prenatal care providers on variables such as barriers to, charges for, and source of payment for prenatal care (structure) and the content of prenatal care (process), as well as variables related to the mothers' life style and work experiences. The Pregnancy Risk Assessment Monitoring System (PRAMS) initiated by the Centers for Disease Control (CDC) in 1988[48] is a state-specific, population-based survey of selected maternal behaviors, barriers to prenatal care, source and content of prenatal care, parenting behaviors, and source of and satisfaction with infant health care. When linked to vital statistics, the PRAMS data are expected to provide a rich data base for planning and evaluating maternity health programs designed to reduce adverse perinatal outcomes.

Ensuring the quality of care requires that we move beyond traditional quality assurance terminology...

Ensuring quality of care in a UMC program will require uniform methods for microlevel quality assurance as well as a standardized reporting system for surveying and analyzing trends at the local and national levels. The reporting system must incorporate a minimal set of common data elements and standard definitions throughout the nation as recommended in the year 2000 health objectives.[49] System data must generate information on the structure, process, and outcome of care, including measures of need, capacity, provider type, use, cost and setting of care, service content and practice, and health status. The system should be designed to ensure that service providers receive feedback in a timely manner and to indicate when standards of care are inadequate and must be updated. Client and provider satisfaction surveys could be used to enhance understanding of the factors related to the use and acceptability of services.

SUMMARY AND CONCLUSIONS

Because the United States has institutionalized a two-tier system of health care with more resources available to higher income individuals, universal access to maternity care is likely to increase the quality of care for a large group of middle and lower income women. Ensuring the quality of care in such a system however, requires that we move beyond traditional quality assurance terminology, which focuses on assessment and utilization review to emphasize mechanisms that ensure quality up front. Ensuring the quality of care in a UMC program will require the following:

1. Adoption of national standards for quality technical management and interpersonal process of care with compliance achieved through structural mechanisms supporting their implementation. Because norms change over time, monitoring and surveillance systems must include a mechanism to review these standards and permit timely revisions.

2. An adequate supply of physicians trained to deliver care that is high quality with respect to both technical management and the interpersonal process of care. Solutions to the problem of physicians who are either insufficiently or improperly trained to meet quality-of-care standards may lie largely outside the domain of a UMC program. Revising criteria for admission to medical schools to emphasize interpersonal capabilities or improving those capabilities in students during the course of undergraduate and graduate medical education (eg, requiring multidisciplinary training) may be required. A UMC program that articulates expectations for high quality in the interpersonal process of care and emphasizes care provided by a multidisciplinary team of providers may at least succeed in influencing the profession to move in this direction.

3. A significant reduction in reliance on market mechanisms to ensure the adequate supply and distribution of physician providers. Because a health care system based on full equity in the distribution and use of resources will take time to establish, several interim alternatives might be considered. One would be to lower obstetric practice costs, thus increasing the ability of physicians who participate in a UMC program to locate in underserved communities. Federal or state subsidies for obstetric malpractice premiums of physicians willing to locate in underserved communities could be provided; immunities offered by the Tort Claims Act could be extended to physicians practicing in government-financed settings;[50] or publicly funded health centers could be given subsidies to attract highly qualified physicians.

...past experience strongly suggests that a direct federal or state intervention in the health personnel supply will be needed to ensure an adequate supply of maternity care providers in high-risk underserved communities.

A second strategy would be to ensure parity in payment for similar services provided by all payers, public and private. Then private office-based physicians and private hospital outpatient clinics would have little reason to refuse to participate in a universal access program or to discriminate against patients on the basis of payer.

A third strategy involves directly investing resources in inner-city public sector institutions. Doing so would enable hospital outpatient facilities and public and nonprofit clinics located near urban high-risk populations to greatly expand their capacity.[10,51]

Finally, past experience strongly suggests that a fourth strategy—direct federal or state intervention in the health personnel supply—will also be needed to ensure an adequate supply of maternity care providers in high-risk underserved communities. Expansion of the National Health Service Corps scholarship program and similar state programs (eg, the Michigan Essential Health Provider Recruitment Strategy—a loan forgiveness program in exchange for service in an underserved area) would create incentives for health personnel to locate in underserved communities.

4. A commitment to full use of existing nonphysician providers as well as expansion of educational programs and opportunities to in-

crease the numbers of CNMs and NPs. This will require complete coverage by all payers, direct payment, adequate malpractice insurance, parity of payment across provider types for services rendered, and education of physicians and the general public about CNMs and NPs.

5. Linkage of standards for quality care established at the national level to the delivery of care at the community level. This linkage could be accomplished by establishing conditions of provider participation based on adherence to these standards in order to obtain payment. Payment could also be used to foster the interpersonal process of care if fees are provided for services such as transportation or child care. If documentation of provided services is required as a condition of payment, and timely audits are done to validate the accuracy of reporting, the actual delivery of high-quality services can be ensured. Documentation in a universal access program would be a requirement for all participating providers rather than the special burden of providers in a program for low-income individuals. Such documentation would be an important aspect of a standardized monitoring and surveillance system.

6. Emphasis on delivery of care in organized settings such as health departments and CHCs-MHCs, which have both the institutional capability and the experience in providing comprehensive, multidisciplinary care. Although a comprehensive array of services is most easily delivered in these settings, providing adequate resources to these providers will be essential to ensure that they can offer high-quality care.

Participation of private practice settings in a UMC program will require payment mechanisms that enable private physicians to provide a more comprehensive package of services and to link up with a multitude of other providers including nurses, nutritionists, health educators, and social workers. It will also require the development of case management services to help clients navigate myriad service providers.

Increased attention to the interpersonal process of care will be necessary in whatever settings women seek care under a UMC program.

7. Standardized methods for microlevel quality assurance as well as a standardized monitoring and surveillance system for the analysis of trends at the local and national level. A minimum data set with standard definitions should include structure (eg, provider type, setting, payer), process (eg, services provided, referrals made, use of ancillary personnel, waiting times, client satisfaction, etc), and outcome (eg, health status) measures.

The system should ensure that service providers receive feedback in a timely manner and are directly informed when standards of care are inadequate and must be updated. Finally, because some providers are likely not to participate in the delivery of care, it seems key that all providers, whether or not they participate in the UMC program, be required to contribute to a common data collection system.

Ensuring the quality of care in a universal access program will demand vigilant, up-front attention to the structure and standards of the care delivery system. Once universal access is fully realized, the contribution of health care services to further improvements in perinatal outcomes will ultimately depend on our ability to provide high-quality care that addresses the comprehensive needs of women and their infants. Without a major commitment by policymakers and planners to ensuring the quality of care, a UMC program will not realize its full potential to make a difference in the health and well-being of the women and children of this nation.

REFERENCES

1. Donabedian, A. Explorations in quality assessment and monitoring. vol 1. *The Definition of Quality and Approaches to Its Assessment.* Ann Arbor, Mich: Health Administration Press; 1980.
2. US General Accounting Office. *Quality Assurance: A Comprehensive National Strategy Is Needed.* Washington, DC: General Accounting Office; 1990.
3. US Public Health Service. Expert Panel on the Content of Prenatal Care. *Caring for Our Future: The Content of Prenatal Care.* Washington, DC: US Dept of Health and Human Services; 1989.
4. American College of Obstetricians and Gynecologists. *Standards for Obstetric/Gynecologic Services.* 7th ed. Washington, DC: American College of Obstetricians and Gynecologists; 1989.
5. Brown S, ed. *Prenatal Care: Reaching Mothers, Reaching Infants.* Washington, DC: National Academy Press; 1988.
6. Rezler AG, Flaherty JA. *The Interpersonal Dimension in Medical Education.* New York, NY: Springer Publishing Co; 1985.
7. American Board of Medical Specialties. *Annual Report and Reference Handbook, 1989.* Evanston, Ill; 1989.
8. Wentz D, Gannon M, Osteen A, Baldwin D. Continuing medical education. *JAMA.* 1989;262:1043–1047.
9. Fossett JW, Perloff JD, Kletke PR, Peterson JA. Medicaid patients' access to office-based obstetricians. *J Health Care Poor Underserved.* 1991;1(4):405–421.
10. Fossett JW, Perloff JD, Peterson JA, Kletke PR. Medicaid in the inner city: the case of maternity care in Chicago. *Milbank Q.* 1990;68:111–141.
11. Lewis-Idema D. *Increasing Provider Participation.* Washington, DC: National Governors Association; 1988.
12. Mitchell J, Shurman R. Access to private obstetrics/gynecology services under Medicaid. *Med Care.* 1984;22:1026–1037.
13. Perloff J, Kletke P, Neckerman K. Physicians' decisions to limit Medicaid participation: determinants and policy implications. *J Health Polit Policy Law.* 1987;12:221–235.
14. Research Triangle Institute. *Nationwide Evaluation of Medicaid Competition Demonstrations.* Baltimore, Md: Health Care Financing Administration; 1988.
15. Center for Health Administration Studies. *Medicaid Enrollees in HMOs:*

A Comparative Analysis of Perinatal Outcomes for Mothers and Newborns in a Large Chicago HMO. Chicago, Ill: Center for Health Administration Studies, University of Chicago; 1989.

16. Sullivan L. Report to Congress. *Incentive Arrangements Offered by Health Maintenance Organizations and Competitive Medical Plans to Physicians.* Washington, DC: US Dept of Health and Human Services; 1990.

17. US General Accounting Office. *Medicaid: Oversight of Health Maintenance Organizations in the Chicago Area.* Washington, DC: US General Accounting Office; 1990.

18. Sinai N, Anderson O. *EMIC (Emergency Maternity and Infant Care): A Study of Administrative Experience.* Ann Arbor, Mich: University of Michigan, 1948. Bureau of Public Health Economics, Research series No 3.

19. Public Law 99-272. Consolidated Omnibus Budget Reconciliation Act of 1985 (COBRA).

20. Office of Technology Assessment. *Nurse Practitioners, Physician Assistants, and Certified Nurse Midwives: A Policy Analysis.* Washington, DC: Office of Technology Assessment; 1986. Health Technology Case Study 37.

21. American College of Nurse Midwives. *American College of Nurse Midwives FACTS.* Washington, DC: American College of Nurse Midwives; 1990.

22. Slome C, Wetherbee H, Daly M et al. Effectiveness of certified nurse-midwives: a prospective evaluation study. *Am J Obstet Gynecol.* 1976;124:177–182.

23. Perry HB. Role of the nurse midwife in contemporary maternity care. In: Young D, Ernhardt A, eds. *Psychosomatic Obstetrics and Gynecology.* New York, NY: Appleton-Century Crofts; 1980.

24. Dickstein D. *Evaluation of the Group Health Cooperative Demonstration Midwifery Service: Report to the Kaiser Family Foundation.* Menlo Park, Calif.; 1983.

25. Riessman CK. The use of health services by the poor: are there any promising models? *Social Pol.* 1980;14(4):30–40.

26. Institute of Medicine. *Preventing Low Birthweight.* Washington, DC: National Academy Press; 1985.

27. Public Law 96-499. 1980.

28. Public Law 101-239. Omnibus Budget Reconciliation Act of 1989.

29. Gold RB, Kenney A, Singh S. *Blessed Events and the Bottom Line: Financing Maternity Care in the United States.* New York, NY: Alan Guttmacher Institute; 1987.

30. Mitchell JB, Cromwell J. Medicaid mills: fact or fiction? *Health Care Fin Rev.* 1980;2(1):37–49.

31. Mitchell JB, Cromwell J. Large Medicaid practices and Medicaid mills. *JAMA.* 1980;244:2433–2437.

32. Corcoran J, Hill N, Credle J et al. Improving the delivery of services in a local health department: integration versus block. *Public Health Nurs.* 1988;5(2):76–80.

33. Singh S, Forrest JD, Torres A. *Prenatal Care in the United States: A State and County Inventory.* vol 1. New York, NY: Alan Guttmacher Institute; 1989.

34. Kotch JB, Coulter ML, Porter CQ, Miller CA. Productivity and selected indicators of care in maternity and infant care and children and youth projects according to sponsorship. *J Med Syst.* 1988;12:285–294.

35. Buescher PA, Smith C, Holliday JL, Levine RH. Source of prenatal care and infant birth weight. The case of a North Carolina county. *Am J Obstet Gynecol.* 1987;156:204–210.

36. The Chicago Department of Health. *Clinics in Crisis—A Report on the Conditions and Capacity of the Chicago Department of Health's Clinic Facilities.* Chicago, Ill; 1989.

37. *Mothers, Infants, and Community and Migrant Health Centers: A Report on*

the First Year of the Comprehensive Perinatal Program. Washington, DC: National Association of Community Health Centers; 1989.

38. Rosenbaum S. *Community and Migrant Health Centers: Two Decades of Achievement.* Washington, DC: National Association of Community Health Centers; 1987.
39. US Dept of Health, Education, and Welfare. *Grants for Maternity and Infant Care Projects. Policies and Procedures.* 1964. MCH collection, document 1570.
40. US Public Health Service. Health Services Administration. Bureau of Community Health Services. *Program Guidance Material, Health Services for Mothers and Children.* 1976.
41. Public Law 97-35. Maternal and Child Health Block Grant. August 1981.
42. *Guidance on the New State Applications and Annual Report Requirements.* Bureau of Maternal and Child Health and Resource Development. 1990.
43. Miller CA, Fine A, Adams-Taylor S. *Monitoring Children's Health: Key Indicators.* 2nd ed. Washington, DC: American Public Health Association; 1989.
44. Lesser AJ. The origin and development of maternal and child health programs in the United States. *Am J Public Health.* 1985;75:590–598.
45. Lohr KN, Schroeder SA. A strategy for quality assurance in Medicare. *N Engl J Med.* 1990; 322:707–712.
46. Kovar MG. National data collection efforts in the US. In: Walker DK, Richmond J, eds. *Monitoring Children's Health in the United States.* Cambridge, Mass: Harvard University Press; 1984.
47. Sanderson M, Placek P. The 1988 maternal and infant health survey: design, content, and data availability. *Birth.* 1991;18(1):26–32.
48. Adams M, Shulman H. Follow-back methods for the prenancy risk assessment monitoring system. Presented at the annual meeting of the American Public Health Association; October 25, 1989; Chicago, Ill.
49. US Dept of Health and Human Services. Public Health Service. *Promoting Health/Preventing Disease: Year 2000 Objectives for the Nation.* Washington, DC: US Public Health Service; 1989.
50. Rostow VP, Osterweis M, Bulger RJ. Medical professional liability and the delivery of obstetrical care. *N Engl J Med.* 1989;321:1057–1060.
51. US General Accounting Office. *Prenatal Care: Medicaid Recipients and Uninsured Women Obtain Insufficient Care.* Washington, DC: General Accounting Office; 1987.

CHAPTER **15**

The Case for Universal Maternity Care

Jonathan B. Kotch, MD, MPH
Rosemary Barber-Madden, EdD

HEALTH STATUS OF WOMEN AND CHILDREN

The health status of women and children in the United States, once assumed to improve with each succeeding generation, can no longer be taken for granted. Although the majority of the 1990 health objectives for the nation, introduced in 1979, were related to the health of women and children, most of those concerning maternal and infant health were not achieved, including the following:

- That the infant mortality rate should be reduced to no more than 9 deaths per 1000 live births for the nation as a whole, and no more than 12 deaths per 1000 for any racial or ethnic subgroup.

- That low birthweight (LBW) should constitute no more than 5% of all live births for the nation and no more than 10.5% for any racial or ethnic subgroup.

- That virtually all women and infants should be served at levels of care appropriate to their needs by a regionalized system of primary, secondary, and tertiary care for prenatal, maternity, and perinatal health services.

- That the proportion of women in any county or racial or ethnic subgroup who obtain no prenatal care during the first trimester of pregnancy should not exceed 10%.

Although these objectives were promoted as a matter of national policy, no national plan or financing scheme has been described to assure their achievement. Indeed, the past decade has witnessed the subordination of health policy to the annual legislative review process for deficit reduction, established in 1981 with the passage of the Omnibus Budget Reconciliation Act. This step was a clear departure from the approach of the 1970s, when health policy was considered on its own merits and not in an atmosphere of increasing budget deficits that could not be attributed to the government's anemic response to the legitimate health care needs of women and children. These needs, documented in the preceding chapters, are summarized in the following sections. In addition, this chapter presents the Universal Maternity Care (UMC) proposal and compares it, by means of a policy analysis model, with two current examples of national health service (NHS) and national health insurance (NHI) proposals.

Maternal and Infant Health

The infant mortality statistic has long been the best single indicator of maternal and infant health status. Thus, in briefly discussing the current health status of pregnant women and children, we begin with this significant indicator.

Infant Health. The 1980s will be remembered as a decade in which the fortunes of pregnant women, mothers, and infants stagnated or deteriorated for the first time in 25 years. A measurable decline in infant mortality from 12.6 deaths per 1000 live births in 1980 to 10.1 in 1987 has been slowing until, in the past few years, consecutive annual rates of decline have been the lowest since the late 1960s.[1] The slight decline that has been achieved provides no cause for optimism, because other industrialized nations have improved their infant mortality rates faster than the United States, which slipped in the 1980s from 17th to 22nd place in the world.[2] This lower ranking occurred despite continued improvement in birthweight-specific infant mortality rates in the US in the early 1980s.[2]

The United States did not reach its 1990 goal of 9 deaths per 1000 live births, a rate that had been achieved by 15 nations 5 years earlier.[3] The underlying problem is still our excessive LBW rate, which, at 6.9% is higher now than at any time since 1979.[4] In addition, the Black-to-White infant mortality ratio and pregnancy rates among single women and women younger than 15 have increased.[5] In fact, nearly every measurable dimension of pregnancy outcome has stagnated or worsened, while drug abuse during pregnancy and acquired immunodeficiency syndrome have conspired to sabotage our feeble attempts to reverse declining maternal and infant health.

Maternal Health. The maternal health consequences of pregnancy in the United States are little better. High rates of cesarean section in the United States are associated with increased morbidity for pregnant women and with substantially increased cost. Increasing numbers of cesarean sections have failed to improve our infant mortality ranking relative to other developed countries with far lower cesarean section rates. If excess operative interventions resulted in improved outcomes for mothers and infants, perhaps the morbidity and expense associated with those interventions would be tolerable. Unfortunately, individual practice styles and fear of malpractice litigation are the primary motivations for performing cesarean sections in America today.[6]

Because maternal mortality is uncommon it is a frequently overlooked consequence of pregnancy, but the US maternal mortality rate remains unacceptably high. Among 26 countries with maternal mortality rates ranging from 2 per 100 000 (Norway) to 16 per 100 000 (Japan),[7] the

The 1980s will be remembered as a decade in which the fortunes of pregnant women, mothers, and infants stagnated or deteriorated for the first time in 25 years.

United States' rate from 1980 to 1987 tied with Australia's for 13th place at 8 deaths per 100 000.[7] Unfortunately, this figure may be conservative because of significant underreporting and misclassification of maternal mortality in the United States as well as other nations.

Child Health. Deficiencies in child health in the United States can be explained in part as the legacy of inadequate maternal and infant health care. Although children older than 1 year, and particularly those aged 5 to 14, are the healthiest group in the United States, our child mortality rates remain higher than those of most Western European nations. Recently, increasing prevalence of childhood chronic conditions has been described, and the incidence of intentional injuries involving children is rising.

Child Mortality. The mortality rate for children aged 1 to 14 has improved in the past decade, resulting in achieving the 1990 goal of 34 deaths per 100 000 population,[8] but this trend may be leveling off. Improvements have occurred in survival rates for children with conditions such as congenital anomalies, malignant neoplasms, and leukemia (the leading natural causes of death in this age group), but there has been less improvement, and very recently a slight deterioration, in childhood injury mortality.[9] US child mortality rates remain higher than those of most Western European nations principally because of our higher child injury mortality rates.[10]

Child Morbidity. Like the 1980s, the 1990s promise to be a period of small to no gains in child health status. The dramatic improvements in child health resulting from the prevention of most communicable diseases of childhood in the early to mid-1900s and from the increasing survival of LBW infants in the mid-1960s and 1970s appear to have peaked. Behavioral conditions, chronic illnesses, and injuries cause most health problems after infancy, and none of these factors is likely to be easily ameliorated in the near future. Ten years ago the Select Panel for the Promotion of Child Health recognized the increasing contribution of behavioral, social, and educational problems to the burden of childhood illness.[11] More recently, the increasing prevalence of childhood chronic conditions in the United States has come to light. From 10% to 20% of US children have some health impairment,[12] and 2.1% have an identified chronic illness.[13] In addition, the incidence of intentional injuries such as child abuse and other acts of violence against children is rising.[14] These complicated health problems can only add to the demand for already insufficient comprehensive health services for children.

ACCESS TO CARE AMONG WOMEN AND CHILDREN

At the same time women's and children's health status is deteriorating, their patterns of use of medical care are also changing. Access problems affect not only the uninsured but also the privately and publicly insured, because patterns of health care coverage are constantly shifting. Some of these changes in coverage, and the consequences for access to care, are discussed briefly in this section.

Insurance Coverage

Private Insurance. Medical care usage is heavily influenced by health insurance coverage. Conventional indemnity insurance does not adequately cover the population affected by the Title V Maternal and Child Health (MCH) Block Grant in this country (see chapter 10). Of the estimated 37 million Americans with no health insurance coverage (7 million more than in 1980), two thirds are in families with at least one working member and between 55% and 60% are women of childbearing age and children (approximately 12 million children). As a result, 19% of America's children and 17% of women of childbearing age have no health insurance coverage.[2] An additional 60 million Americans are underinsured.

Public Insurance. Public insurance, specifically Medicaid, liberalized eligibility requirements for pregnant women and young children in the second half of the 1980s (see chapter 11), but it has not kept pace with the increasing need created by unconscionable levels of poverty and homelessness and the erosion of employment-related health benefits among young families. Medicaid, which currently covers 16.3% of all children, in fact covers only 50% of all poor children.[2] Medicaid eligibility levels and requirements vary by state. As long as Medicaid remains a means of reimbursement for services and not a direct provider of services, Medicaid dollars will continue to flow disproportionately into long-term and tertiary care to the detriment of preventive care and ambulatory care for the acute illnesses of childhood.

Efforts largely focused on filling gaps in access to health services for vulnerable groups of women and children include Medicaid enhancements, innovative demonstrations that tap other sources of public funds to supplement Medicaid coverage, improvements in employee health benefit coverage in more enlightened sectors of industry, and innovative public-private partnership schemes. Yet new gaps are constantly appearing, and our ability to make real progress toward achieving the health objectives for the year 2000, let alone the unfulfilled 1990 objectives, may actually be hampered by this incremental approach. Despite Medicaid enhancements, the negative effect of inadequate insurance coverage can be seen in immunization rates, that most sensitive indicator of access to preventive care. As of 1985, 40% of children between the ages of 1 and 4 years were unimmunized for measles, a decrease in coverage since 1976.[2] Reported measles rates increased 423% in the United States from 1988 to 1989.[15] The absence of adequate access to reimbursement for health care affects children more than any other age group in the population.

Availability of Private Health Care Providers and Demand for Public Services

Private Providers. The insufficiency of health care providers in both rural areas and inner cities compounds the problems caused by inadequate rates of insurance coverage. Traditionally underserved areas, already hard hit by the loss of National Health Service Corps (NHSC) professionals (see chapter 11), are now faced with the withdrawal of private physicians from the practice of obstetrics due to malpractice insurance premium increases.[16] Even where private physicians are available, they are not necessarily accessible to the indigent and to those with Medicaid cards. Pediatricians are among the physicians most likely to see Medicaid patients. Forty-four percent of obstetrician-gynecologists refuse to accept Medicaid, the highest refusal rate among primary care physicians.[17]

For poor women who do have access to private, office-based care, pregnancy outcomes are not always salutary. Studies in North Carolina[18] and Michigan[19] have documented that indigent women have better pregnancy outcomes in comprehensive public prenatal care than they do in private care. This difference may be accounted for by the fact that public sources of primary prenatal care often have multiple professional disciplines available to deal with the variety of complex social and medical factors that face poor families. Enabling more indigent women to use their Medicaid cards for private care might paradoxically result in poorer pregnancy outcomes.

Public Providers. There appears to be a significant increase in the use of public sources of health care by the MCH population,[20] a fact that is not surprising in view of the high rates of childhood poverty, insufficient health insurance, and the decreasing availability of private physicians. Increasing use of public sources of care by poor women and children, whether or not they have Medicaid, would be a positive trend if sufficient public health resources were available to meet their needs.

Changing Demand for Maternal and Infant Health Services

Although it is clear that increasing numbers of children, continuing high LBW rates, and increasing prevalence of chronic illness and handicapping conditions will all contribute to increasing demand for health services, the response of the delivery system and of society is unpredictable. Loss of private insurance coverage and increasing copayments and deductibles for those who have health insurance will inevitably result in decreasing use of preventive services, which may in turn increase the demand for acute care.

The withdrawal of private physicians from the indigent care market is likely to increase demand for services offered by public providers. The full participation of certified nurse-midwives (CNMs), nurse-practitioners (NPs), and physician's assistants in both public and private settings can partially respond to the needs of poor and working-class families, but continuing pressure on health providers and policymakers to "do something" about deteriorating maternal and infant health status will lead to greater willingness to consider innovations in maternal and infant health care services. The most comprehensive solution to the access-to-care crisis for women and infants is UMC.

Faced with the deteriorating situation that has been described, an increasing number of organizations—for example, the National Commission to Prevent Infant Mortality, the Institute of Medicine (IOM), the American Public Health Association, and the American Academy of Pediatrics (AAP)—have called for a national effort to ensure access to prenatal care for all pregnant women in the United States. The first comprehensive proposal for guaranteeing services throughout the reproductive health cycle was proposed by the Council on Maternal and Child Health of the National Association for Public Health Policy (NAPHP) and is described in the following section.[21]

UNIVERSAL MATERNITY CARE

Definition. UMC is defined as guaranteed prenatal, intrapartum, postpartum, and infant care for all residents (legal or otherwise) in the United States, at no out-of-pocket cost to the recipient. The plan would have the following features:[22]

1. Publicly guaranteed access to comprehensive maternity and infant care services for every pregnant woman in the United States.

2. A full range of services, among which would be medical, laboratory, psychosocial, nutritional, educational, postpartum family planning, and neonatal services, and well-child care up to 18 months of age.

3. Free choice of providers, including both physicians and CNMs, public health departments and community health centers (CHCs), health maintenance organizations, and other organized health care settings, provided that they offer, or arrange to offer, the full range of comprehensive services.

4. Delivery in the setting most appropriate to the needs of the pregnant woman, including but not limited to hospitals and licensed birthing centers.

5. Financing through a single maternity care trust fund in every state, with funds from the following sources:

   - A federalized successor to the present Medicaid program, with minimum income eligibility across the nation of at least 185% of the federal poverty income guidelines regardless of family structure, assets or means.

- A per capita contribution from existing insurers (and self-insuring employers) based on the number of women of reproductive age in their respective plans. The trust would assume the risk of extraordinary medical expenses that can severely deplete reserves, thus providing an incentive to contribute to the trust for employers who are self-insured or those who participate in a group insurance plan.

- A payroll tax on employers who neither contribute to an employer-employee insurance fund nor self-insure.

- Premiums from uninsured individuals between approximately 185% and 250% of poverty, based on ability to pay.

- Public sources such as Title V of the Social Security Act (the MCH Block Grant) and state uncompensated care funds for those who remain uncovered despite the above-mentioned opportunities.

6. Negotiated per capita reimbursement for all maternity care providers without bonuses for operative deliveries.

7. Per diem (rather than per service or per procedure) reimbursement for hospitals and birthing centers based on documented costs of care for the average woman and newborn.

8. Federal administration through the Bureau of Maternal and Child Health.

9. State health department responsibility for certifying providers, enforcing standards, maintaining systems for collection and timely reporting of vital data, and providing technical assistance, consultation, and training.

10. Federal guarantees (through Title V, the CHCs and migrant health centers, NHSC, etc) of the availability of services in medically underserved areas.

11. Establishment of a fund, similar to the Immunization Compensation Fund, for compensating victims of adverse perinatal events, with allocation of such funds through mediation. As agents of states, providers would be protected from being individually liable except in the case of negligence or incompetence.

Policy Analysis

Policy analysis is a process for evaluating proposed public policies against general and specific policy criteria.[23] Six general criteria that may be applied to most policy proposals include equity, stigma, efficiency, cost, preference satisfaction, and political feasibility. To analyze proposals addressing the maternity care crisis, we have selected five additional criteria: comprehensiveness, availability, barriers, health status, and education and research. For comparison, we have applied these general and specific criteria to current examples of proposals to restructure the US health care system for the entire population.

The Physicians for a National Health Program (PNHP) proposal,[24] like the Canadian Medicare system after which it is modeled, is an NHI plan. The proposal that most resembles a pure NHS plan, according to the definition of Terris et al,[25] is the one proposed by California representative Ronald Dellums.[26] Table 15-1 presents the results of our analysis of these three proposals, along with the alternative of doing nothing, in relation to the general and specific criteria.

Equity. Equity in social policy demands that equals be treated equally and that unequals be treated unequally until the inequality is reduced. UMC specifically addresses equity by federalizing eligibility so that equals (according to income) are equally eligible to participate across states. Our present system and proposals for filling the gaps in existing reimbursement systems offer no guarantees that interstate inequities, and inequities between participants and nonparticipants in employee benefit plans who are at the same income level, will be reduced. To reduce inequities among people with widely differing incomes, UMC imposes a single source of payment for all, without the invidious

---

TABLE 15-1
**Decision Matrix for Guaranteeing Access to Care
for Women and Children**

Analysis Criteria	Policy Alternatives			
	Do Nothing	NHI	NHS	UMC
General				
Equity	−	0	0	+
Stigma	−	0	+	+
Efficiency	−	+	+	+
Cost	+	0	+	+
Preference satisfaction	0	+	−	+
Political feasibility	+	0	−	+
Specific				
Comprehensiveness	−	−	+	+
Availability	−	−	+	+
Barriers	−	0	+	+
Health status	−	0	+	+
Education and research	−	−	−	+

Note: + = satisfies criterion. 0 = equivocal or no effect. − = fails to satisfy criterion.

discrimination inherent in proposals that mandate minimum benefits but permit the purchase of premium supplements. All infants therefore start out with equal opportunity for appropriate, comprehensive maternity and infant care. Even the comprehensive PNHP and Dellums proposals do not completely eliminate existing inequities. For example, the PNHP proposal—like any reimbursement plan, no matter how generous—does not directly address the issue of availability of services in underserved areas.[24] In Quebec, Canada, providers apparently withdrew services from some children immediately after the introduction of first-dollar (ie, no deductibles or co-insurance), public health insurance coverage, because children's use of services declined in relation to use by adults aged 17 to 64.[27] And although an NHS proposal such as the Dellums proposal would directly address the maldistribution of services, it does not address the inevitable disadvantage faced by poor women and children who are competing with more advantaged adults and organized consumer groups for limited resources. For this reason, every Western European health system, be it NHS or NHI, makes special allowances for maternal and infant health services, and particularly perinatal services, to be well defined, universally available, and either free or available at negligible cost.[28]

Stigma. Stigma is a major consideration in designing a user-friendly maternity care system. No proposal that tolerates the welfare establishment's continuing involvement in health care can prevent the feeling of shame and embarrassment associated with Medicaid. UMC addresses stigma in two ways: first, by making maternity care exclusively a health program, and second, by eliminating the possibility that any provider can know the ultimate source of payment for any patient. There is no eligibility, no dehumanizing means or assets test, and providers are relieved of any anxiety over what percentage of their fees will be covered by the plan that covers any particular patient. No money passes between the provider and the client at any time.

Similarly, an NHS would eliminate stigma by creating a single system of health care services for all. A similar commitment to one class of care is possible under NHI, as appears to be the case in Canada,[29] but any NHI that establishes a minimum benefit package for all while tolerating purchase of supplements to provide elites with benefits or amenities that are out of the reach of the poor perpetuates the stigma associated with two classes of medical care.

Efficiency. Comprehensive care is efficient, if by efficiency we mean the maximizing of output for a given unit of input. One way of evaluating efficiency is to look at administrative costs. By this method, the US system is one of the least efficient in the world, because population-based outcomes for mothers and children (as measured by either use of care or health outcome) are unimpressive, whereas administrative costs are unacceptably high. The administrative cost for health care in the United States is estimated at 5.6% versus 1.3% in Canada.[30] Profit motives and the inefficiency of running multiple funding mechanisms and delivery systems without coordinated planning conspire to guarantee that US medical care costs more per unit of output (such as a healthy baby) than in any other country.

NHI and NHS plans also benefit from elimination of the unnecessary administrative costs associated with multiple purchasers of care, elimination of profit, and the creation of a single "prudent purchaser" of services. In a pure NHS, the government owns all the medical care facilities and employs all the providers, thereby acquiring absolute control over medical expenditures. This situation does not necessarily guarantee efficiency, but in terms of output per unit cost, infant mortality rates and life expectancies in the United States versus Canada and Great Britain suggest that NHI and NHS, respectively, are more efficient than the current medical care system in the United States.

Cost. Although a complete analysis of the cost of UMC is beyond the scope of this chapter, it is possible to estimate how much additional public and private funding would be necessary. To do so, we will assume that, of about 3.8 million deliveries in the United States per year, 555 000 will be totally without any public or private insurance, 333 000 will have private insurance that does not cover maternity care, and 630 000 will have Medicaid.[31] Of the 2.3 million with a private source of payment for maternity care, 40% or 920 000 of these will have to pay both prenatal and postnatal care charges out of pocket.[32] We further assume that a normal delivery costs $3200, a cesarean section (20% of all deliveries) costs $4800,[22] and prenatal care costs as little as $400.[33]

Using these figures, we calculate that maternity care for the totally uninsured and for the insured without any maternity care coverage would cost $3.126 billion. Prenatal and postnatal care for the privately insured without coverage for these outpatient charges would add $368 million to the $773 million it would cost to cover the estimated 10% in copayments that insured women currently must pay out of pocket for maternity care. The total new cost of UMC for maternity care alone would therefore by $4.267 billion, not all of which need be borne by government were private insurers required to cover the entire cost of maternity care for the employed and their dependents. Table 2 demonstrates the calculations, excluding Medicaid clients, whose maternity care is assumed for this purpose not to require additional funding.

Calculating the cost of infant and toddler care is more difficult. Sloan, Valvona, and Mullner reported that the average unpaid charges for nursery care for a newborn at Vanderbilt Hospital in 1982 was $6185.[34] The magnitude of these charges is undoubtedly due to the high cost of care in the neonatal intensive care unit for seriously ill newborns. Between 1982 and 1988, medical care costs for LBW newborns increased about 50%.[35] If we assume that those same 555 000 women without any insurance whatsoever incurred an average charge of $9278 for newborn care, UMC would pay another $5.15 billion.

UMC is defined as guaranteed prenatal, intrapartum, postpartum, and infant care for all U.S. residents at no out-of-pocket cost to the recipient.

TABLE 15-2
Cost of Uncovered Services To Be Assumed by Universal Maternity Care

	Number	Cost per person	Total cost (in thousands)	10% co-insurance (in thousands)	Cost to UMC* (in thousands)
NORMAL DELIVERIES					
1. Privately insured w/ outpatient care coverage	1,104,000	$3,200	$3,532,800	$353,280	$ 353,280
2. Privately insured w/o outpatient care coverage					
a. inpatient care	736,000	2,800	2,060,800	206,080	206,080
b. outpatient care	736,000	400	294,400		294,400
3. Uninsured or insured w/o maternity care coverage	710,400	3,200	2,273,280		2,273,280
C-SECTIONS					
1. Privately insured w/ outpatient care coverage	276,000	4,800	1,324,800	132,480	132,480
2. Privately insured w/o outpatient care coverage					
a. inpatient care	184,000	4,400	809,600	80,960	80,960
b. outpatient care	184,000	400	73,600		73,600
3. Uninsured or insured w/o maternity care coverage	177,600	4,800	852,480		852,480
TOTAL					$4,266,560

*The vast majority of these uncompensated costs are already being paid for through state and local tax support for public clinic and public hospital service and through cost-shifting.

The average cost of a year of a child's personal health care, according to the American Academy of Pediatrics and the National Association of Children's Hospitals and Related Institutions, is $745.[33] Recognizing that this is likely to be greater in the first year of life, but lacking an age-specific figure, we will multiply this figure by the number of children up to 18 months of age estimated to lack either public or private insurance. This figure, 1.08 million, is derived from 3.8 million live births per year and the most recent National Center for Health Statistics estimates of uninsured infants and toddlers from the National Health Interview Survey.[36] Personal health care (not including inpatient neonatal care) for children up to 18 months of age would therefore cost UMC $804.6 million per year.

These costs, however, should not be considered entirely new, because most of the uncompensated hospital charges for maternity and neonatal care are currently being paid for through cost shifting. In reality, the total cost of UMC, including all public and private sources combined, is likely to be less than the status quo or than any of the gap-filling proposals now being entertained. Savings can be anticipated through the following mechanisms:

- Use of nonphysician providers for most low-risk pregnancies.

- Reduction in the cost of care for LBW babies as a result of comprehensive care lowering the LBW rate.

- Use of less expensive alternatives to hospital delivery.

- Administrative savings realized by the creation of a single fiscal intermediary in each state.

- Increased use of free, postpartum family planning services.

- Reduction in cesarean rates resulting from the withdrawal of the financial incentive and the lower prematurity rate.

- Reduction of "defensive medicine."

Others (eg, the National Perinatal Information Center[37]) have estimated that the $16 billion we currently spend on maternity and neonatal care could fund an organized maternity and infant health care system that would deliver early and continuous prenatal care, intrapartum care, and neonatal care to everyone in the United States, with money left over to pay for medical care for children born with handicapping conditions to the age of 5 years.[37]

An NHS has the potential for being the least costly system if all sources of payment for medical care, public and private, are considered together. Any insurance system, private or nationalized, that reimburses private providers on a fee-for-service basis is likely to be more costly than a system based on capitation.[30] Under the present US system, providers are not required to accept assignment under typical indemnity insurance systems, permitting physicians and others to bill consumers any amount over and above that which insurance will pay. Under both the PNHP proposal and UMC, assignment would be required.

Preference Satisfaction. UMC offers the maximum opportunity for pregnant women to choose among providers and delivery sites by guaranteeing reimbursement to all qualified providers. Unlike any reimbursement-only plan, UMC makes government the "residual guarantor" that maternity care will be available everywhere in the nation. UMC states unequivocally that every woman and newborn in the country is entitled to comprehensive care. The PNHP proposal also allows free choice of provider, although there should be some concern about the availability of nonphysician providers under any system that leaves physician hegemony essentially unchanged. The Dellums version of NHS, on the other hand, appears to limit preference satisfaction by essentially requiring consumers to use the comprehensive health service that serves the geographic area in which they reside.[26]

UMC has the potential of addressing the preference satisfaction of providers as well. First, it will establish fair fees for providers through a negotiated process that will be 100% guaranteed. Subsidized and uncompensated care for mothers and infants will be things of the past. Second, providers will be removed entirely from any responsibility for determining eligibility, making a truly professional and helping relationship possible, unsullied by financial considerations. Patients will be motivated to return for follow-up appointments and to comply with medical regimens once financial barriers are removed. Providers will have to deal with only one payer, not dozens. Again, NHI would be similar, as physician satisfaction in Ontario demonstrates.[38] On the other hand, NHS provides little preference satisfaction for providers, all of whom would be civil servants. Only those exclusive enough to survive by practicing entirely out of the system would retain any autonomy. In addition, there would be little likelihood of newcomers being able to enter practice in desirable locations.

Similarly, hospitals and birthing centers that participate in UMC and NHS will no longer require a "wallet biopsy." Economic transfers will disappear, emergency rooms will not turn away pregnant women in labor, and deposits will no longer be required well in advance. In this environment it may not be farfetched to expect that malpractice litigation will decline, ultimately bringing more providers back into active maternity care. The role of hospitals and birthing centers in NHI is less clear. Unlike the situation in Canada, where most hospitals are run by community boards (although in fact the provincial ministers of health have almost absolute legal power over them),[39] the current heterogeneous mix of for-profit, private not-for-profit, and public hospitals in the United States is likely to remain, perpetuating opportunities for excess charges and for consigning poorer clients to poorer hospitals.

Political Feasibility. It is clear to any pragmatic observer that NHS is not likely to happen immediately in the United States. In fact, every western country that may be said today to have an NHS had some form of NHI first.[40] The issue, then, is which is more probable in the near term for the United States—some form of universal access for all, or UMC? The immediate and continuing criticism of the cost ($60 billion) of implementing all of the Pepper Commission's recommendations, and the apparent inability of Massachusetts to funds its own comprehensive health insurance plan, suggest that a less sweeping approach may be desirable.

One political advantage of UMC is that it is universal. Its objective is to serve all women and infants, not just the poor, the unemployed, and the less fortunate. Voters and taxpayers will be asked to finance the program, but they, their families, and people they know will benefit di-

UMC is universal. Its objective is to serve all women and infants, not just the poor, the unemployed, and the less fortunate.

rectly and almost immediately. NHI, being a financing innovation but not necessarily mandating a change in the organization of health services delivery, may not be perceived as an immediate benefit. Average people with health insurance will realize that what they currently pay in premiums is being collected by the government rather than by a private insurer, but the existing fee-for-service system and most existing client-provider relationships would remain intact. NHS, on the other hand, would introduce radical changes, undoubtedly requiring a transition phase during which consumers would experience some confusion and frustration and most providers would experience totally unfamiliar working conditions.

The potential health care cost savings that have been described may be realized sooner under UMC than under either NHI or NHS, and the savings achieved would reflect a higher proportion of start-up costs. Similarly, the efficiency and guaranteed payment to providers that a single fiscal intermediary with a very circumscribed responsibility within the health sector would offer is another advantage of UMC. Finally, UMC would be beneficial for small businesses or employers that are at a competitive disadvantage, because it removes one important recruitment advantage now held by large employers who offer health insurance that includes maternity coverage. Finally, UMC removes an important disincentive for families on welfare who now face the loss of Medicaid coverage for maternity and infant health services when they reenter the labor market. And it does so at a much lower cost than either NHI or NHS.

The United States has always advanced social policy incrementally, and in fact the Medicare program passed in 1965 was the result of a tactical retreat by health care strategists for whom NHI for all was still the ultimate goal.[41] There has not been a more propitious time since the Great Society for major policy innovation on behalf of mothers and children. Given the lower price tag and the political salience of maternal and infant health issues today, perhaps the most feasible medical care reform in the immediate future is in fact UMC, plus perhaps catastrophic coverage or long-term care for long-suffering middle-class adults.

Comprehensiveness. Among the specific criteria, comprehensive care is considered essential to ensure that maternity services are effective for that group of women (the young, the poor, and minority women) most likely to have LBW or otherwise compromised babies. Numerous studies have documented the success of comprehensive services in reducing LBW,[42] including their superiority over office-based, private physician care. UMC requires that all maternity care be comprehensive, providing women in need with access to the essential support services (nutritional, educational, and psychosocial) that are often lacking in private care. The Dellums proposal specifies that health care centers be comprehensive along the lines of neighborhood health centers and CHCs. The PNHP proposal, however, does little to change the configuration of the medical care delivery system. Therefore, it does

UMC requires that all maternity care be comprehensive, providing women in need with access to the essential support services that are often lacking in private care.

not address the issue of comprehensiveness and might in fact make it possible for socially at-risk pregnant women to choose more inappropriate, office-based private physician care over comprehensive care. Such care is believed to result in higher LBW rates for Medicaid women who, given more liberal eligibility requirements, choose (or are obliged to choose) private care.

The root cause of poor maternal and infant health in this country is a system of values that tolerates our youngest and most vulnerable citizens existing in poverty, discrimination, and neglect.

Availability. Conventional reimbursement systems, whether nationalized or not, fail to address directly the availability of services. The assumption has been that, given the demand created by universal access to financial resources to pay for care, services will become available. After 25 years of Medicaid, the availability of maternity care has deteriorated; it would continue to do so under any NHI that does not specifically address the availability of services. A distinct, deliberate strategy for providing services in rural and inner-city areas, as well as in more desirable areas where liability concerns have driven doctors from obstetrics, is called for. Such a strategy would be possible under both NHS and UMC. The NAPHP proposal for UMC requires governmental guarantee of the availability of maternity care. Between 1963 and 1980, Maternity and Infant Care projects demonstrated that such a guarantee was possible.

Barriers. The IOM report on prenatal care documents financial and nonfinancial barriers to maternity care experienced by pregnant women.[43] UMC wipes the financial barrier away completely. Gone are eligibility tests, deductibles, coinsurance, and the many onerous tasks associated with screening out potential beneficiaries and limiting benefits in the name of cost containment. Although the nonfinancial barriers are not directly addressed by UMC, the capitation fee approach would enable the most efficient providers to spend money on child care, transportation, translators, care coordination, or other services to make care more accessible. Similarly, an NHS such as that delineated by the Dellums bill would resurrect the community outreach services demonstrated by the neighborhood health center and CHC movement to be effective in reducing cultural and transportation barriers to access. On the other hand, an NHI system, although reducing or eliminating financial barriers, offers little potential for reimbursing services that are not medical in nature.

Health status. Which of the discussed proposals would most likely improve the health outcomes of pregnant women and children? Without the special programs targeted specifically for pregnant women and infants that every Western European nation provides in addition to national health, neither NHI nor NHS could guarantee improved access to care for those very women and children who are least likely to obtain appropriate care today. NHS, based on a comprehensive health care model, is admittedly more likely to result in improved health outcomes than an NHI plan that does little more than nationalize the existing reimbursement scheme.

UMC would not entirely alleviate the need for the kind of NHS with special health programs for pregnant women and children that most industrialized nations already have in place. It would, however, reduce financial barriers and stigma. By increasing equity, availability, preference satisfaction, and efficiency, and by mandating comprehensive care, UMC would make possible early, continuous, and coordinated care.

An organized system of care with a single payer in each state would make regionalization of perinatal services a reality without compromising access according to ability to pay. Intrapartum care tailored to levels of risk, reduced cesarean section rates, and free postpartum services including family planning promise to reduce maternal morbidity and increase the potential for subsequent healthy pregnancies. Finally, infants would benefit from free newborn care and free well-child care including immunizations for at least the first 18 months of life. If these innovations do not improve the health status of women and children, it is unlikely that any medical service would do so.

UMC is a substantial first step toward a comprehensive approach to our children's future.

Evaluation and Research. Each of the foregoing criteria is worthy of research and evaluation efforts. Therefore, any proposal to improve the delivery of services to pregnant women and their children must include enough financial support to permit both program evaluation and epidemiologic health services research. The kinds of issues that would lend themselves to the applied research contemplated here include the extent to which the program reduces stigma and inequities in access, provides comprehensive services efficiently and at reasonable cost, improves client and provider satisfaction, increases availability and appropriate use of services, and reduces maternal and infant morbidity and mortality.

A universal system of maternal and infant health services should be designed to generate a data base tailored to addressing questions such as, "What components of comprehensive prenatal care are associated with improved maternal and infant health outcomes?" Until a customized data base is created, researchers will have to rely on disparate data bases that are the consequence of the disorganized state of current maternity care financing and delivery. The same data that, linked with the processing of reimbursement claims, can document quality can also be linked with service statistics and health outcome data to provide a rich source of information for health services researchers (see chapter 14). The output of such research would be used to improve the efficacy and the efficiency of the maternity and infant health service.

CONCLUSION

The root cause of poor maternal and infant health in this country is a system of values that tolerates our youngest and most vulnerable citizens existing in poverty, discrimination, and neglect. Social change, not medical care, will ultimately reverse the circumstances leading to poor pregnancy outcomes in the United States. Medical care, in itself only a component of a comprehensive health care system for women and children, should be part and parcel of a series of social policies necessary to reverse two decades of redistribution of resources from the poor to the rich and from children to adults. Needed policies and programs include paid parental leave, subsidized day care, children's allowances, Head Start, nutrition programs and services, and the best possible education for every child in the country. If established historical patterns are followed, the United States will adopt new social policies affecting women and children gradually. In the meantime, UMC is a substantial first step toward a comprehensive approach to our children's future.

REFERENCES

1. US Congress. Office of Technology Assessment. *Healthy Children: Investing in the Future.* Washington, DC: US Govt Printing Office; 1988. OTA-H-345.
2. Office of Maternal and Child Health. Bureau of Maternal and Child Health and Resources Development. *Child Health USA '89.* Washington, DC: US Govt Printing Office; 1989. HRS-M-CH8915.
3. National Center for Health Statistics. Births, marriages, divorces, and deaths for 1990. *Monthly Vital Statistics Report.* vol 39, no 12. Hyattsville, Md: Public Health Service; 1991.
4. National Center for Health Statistics. Advance report of final natality statistics, 1987. *Monthly Vital Statistics Report,* vol 38, no 3 suppl. Hyattsville, Md: Public Health Service; 1989.
5. Miller CA, Fine S, Adams-Taylor S. *Monitoring Children's Health. Key Indicators.* 2nd ed. Washington, DC: American Public Health Association; 1989.
6. DeMott RK, Sandmire HF. The physician factor as a determinant of cesarean section rates. *Am J Obstet Gynecol,* 1990;162:1593–1599.
7. Grant JP. *The State of the World's Children.* Oxford: Oxford University Press and UNICEF; 1990.
8. US Public Health Service. Office of Disease Prevention and Health Promotion. *The 1990 Health Objectives for the Nation: A Mid-course Review.* Washington, DC: US Govt Printing Office; 1986.
9. National Center for Health Statistics, Fingerhut L. Trends and current status in childhood mortality, United States, 1900-85. *Vital and Health Statistics.* series 3, no 26. Washington, DC: US Govt Printing Office, 1989. US Dept of Health and Human Services publication (PHS) 89-1410.
10. Williams BC, Kotch JB. Excess injury mortality among children in the United States: comparison of recent international statistics. *Pediatrics.* 1990;86(6, part 2):1067–1073.
11. Select Panel for the Promotion of Child Health. *Better Health for Our Children: A National Strategy.* Washington, DC: US Govt Printing Office; 1981. US Dept of Health and Human Services publication (PHS) 79-55071.
12. Gortmaker SL. Demography of chronic childhood illnesses. In: Hobbs N, Perrin J, eds. *Issues in the Care of Children with Chronic Illness.* San Francisco, Calif: Jossey-Bass, Inc; 1985:135–154.
13. Gortmaker SL, Sappenfield W. Prevalence of childhood chronic illnesses in America. *Pediatr Clin North Am.* 1984;31:3–18.
14. US Centers for Disease Control. Division of Injury Control. Childhood injuries in the United States. *Am J Dis Child.* 1990;144:627–646.

15. Centers for Disease Control. Measles—United States, 1989 and first 20 weeks 1990. *MMWR.* 1990;39(21):353–356, 361–363.
16. Institute of Medicine. *Medical Professional Liability and the Delivery of Obstetrical Care.* Washington, DC: National Academy Press; 1989.
17. Orr MT, Forrest JD. The availability of reproductive health services from US private physicians. *Fam Plann Perspect.* 1985;17:63–69.
18. Buescher PA, Smith C, Holliday JL, Levine RH. Source of prenatal care and infant birth weight: the case of a North Carolina county. *Am J Obstet Gynecol.* 1987;156:204–210.
19. Schwethelm B, Margolis LH, Miller C, Smith S. Risk status and pregnancy outcome among Medicaid recipients. *Am J Prev Med.* 1989;5:157–163.
20. Williams BC. Recent performance of North Carolina public health departments: provision of key clinical services to women in poverty. Raleigh, NC: North Carolina Poverty Project; 1989.
21. Council on Maternal and Child Health. Background paper on universal maternity care. *J Public Health Policy.* 1986;7:105–123.
22. Barber-Madden R, Kotch JB. Maternity care financing: universal access or universal care? *J Health Polit Policy Law.* 1990;15:797–814.
23. Haskins R, Gallagher JJ, eds. *Models for Social Policy Analysis: An Introduction.* Norwood, NJ: Ablex; 1981.
24. Himmelstein DU, Woolhandler S. A national health program for the United States. *N Engl J Med.* 1989;320:102–108.
25. Terris M, Cornely PB, Daniels HC, Kerr LE. The case for a national health service. *Am J Public Health.* 1977;67:1183–1185.
26. American Public Health Association. Eight national health proposals compared to APHA principles for national health care. *Nation's Health.* March 1990:10–11.
27. Enterline PE, McDonald AD, McDonald JC. Some effects of Quebec health insurance. Hyattsville, Md: National Center for Health Statistics; 1979. US Dept of Health, Education, and Welfare publication (PHS) 79-3238.
28. Miller CA. *Maternal Health and Infant Survival.* Washington, DC: National Center for Clinical Infant Programs; 1987.
29. Iglehart JK. Canada's health care system faces its problems. *N Engl J Med.* 1990;332:562–568.
30. Terris M. Lessons from Canada's health program. *Technol Rev.* 1990;93(2):28–33.
31. Alan Guttmacher Institute. *Financing Maternity Care in the U.S.* New York, NY: Alan Guttmacher Institute; 1987.
32. Kovar MG, Klerman L. Who pays how much for prenatal care? Presented at American Public Health Association Annual Meeting; Nov. 13, 1984; Dallas, Tex.
33. National Association of Children's Hospitals and Related Institutions. *Questions for Candidates.* Alexandria, Va: Author; 1990.
34. Sloan FA, Valvona J, and Mullner R. Identifying the issues: a statistical profile. In: Sloan FA, Blumstein JF, Perrin JM, eds. *Uncompensated Hospital Care. Rights and Responsibilities.* Baltimore, Md: Johns Hopkins University Press; 1986:16-53.
35. Hughes D, Johnson K, Rosenbaum S, Liu J. *The Health of America's Children.* Washington, DC: Children's Defense Fund; 1989.
36. Bloom B. Health insurance and medical care: health of our nation's children, US, 1988. *Advance Data from Vital and Health Statistics.* No 188. Hyattsville, Md: National Center for Health Statistics; 1990.
37. Gagnon D. Long-term solutions to the maternity care crisis. Presented at the 14th annual Regional Conference in Maternal and Child Health, Family Planning, and Crippled Children's Services; April 6, 1987; Chapel Hill, NC.
38. Kravitz RL, Linn LS, Shapiro MF. Physician satisfaction under the Ontario health insurance plan. *Med Care.* 1990;28:502–512.

39. Sutherland R, Fulton J. *Health Care in Canada*. Ottawa, Ontario: The Health Group; 1988.
40. Roemer MI, Axelrod SJ. A national health service and social security. *Am J Public Health*. 1977;67:462–465.
41. Falk IS. Proposals for national health insurance in the USA: origins, evolution and some perceptions for the future. *Milbank Q*. 1977;55(2):161–191.
42. Institute of Medicine. Committee to Study the Prevention of Low Birthweight. *Preventing Low Birthweight*. Washington, DC: National Academy Press; 1985.
43. Institute of Medicine. Committee to Study Outreach for Prenatal Care. *Prenatal Care: Reaching Mothers, Reaching Infants*. Washington, DC: National Academy Press; 1988.

INDEX

Michigan Essential Health Provider Re-
cruitment Strategy, 247
Michigan, insurance initiative, 190-99
Michigan obstetric survey, 99
Model Standards for Preventive Health
Services, xviii
Mortality rates. See Infant mortality
rates or Maternal mortality rates.
Mumps, outbreaks of in 1980s, xiii, 114

N

NAPHP. See National Association for
Public Health Policy.
NCHS. See National Center for Health
Statistics.
National Academy of Sciences, 127
National Association of Children's Hos-
pitals and Related Institutions, 262
National Association for Public Health
Policy (NAPHP), 5, 6, 257
National Center for Health Statistics
(NCHS), 211, 220, 245, 262
National Council on Alcoholism and
Drug Dependence, 70
National Commission to Prevent Infant
Mortality, 6, 257
National Forum on the Future of Chil-
dren and Families, 133
National Governors Association (NGA),
74, 93, 151, 179, 226
National Health and Nutrition Exami-
nation Survey, 245
National Health Interview Survey, 262
National Health Service Corps (NHSC),
149, 154, 177, 247, 256, 258
National Hospital Discharge Survey, 67-
68
National Institutes of Health (NIH), 34
National Maternal and Infant Health
Survey, 246
National Leadership Commission on
Health Care, 136
National Medical Care Utilization and
Expenditure Survey, 143, 161
National Natality Surveys, 64, 91
National Perinatal Epidemiology Re-
search Unit, Oxford University, 51
National Perinatal Information Center,
263
National Survey of Family Growth,
211, 245
National WIC Evaluation (NWE), 71-
72, 74
Native Americans, 175
Needs assessment methods, prenatal
care
comparative need estimates, 101-102
direct survey techniques, 96-102
Michigan obstetric survey, 99

obstetric surveys, hospital-based,
99
Pregnancy Risk Assessment Monitoring System (PRAMS), 98-99
Special Project of Regional and National Significance (SPRANS),
100-102
strengths and weaknesses of, 97
estimate of unmet need, 101-02, 103
estimate of consequences of Medicaid expansion, 93-96
secondary data analysis, 89-96
absence of care, 91
late entry into care, 92
problems in using combined
datasets, 90, 91
proxy variables, 90-91
social area analysis, 91
social indicators, 89-90
Torres and Kenney study, 93-96,
101-02
surveillance systems, state-based
need for, 103-105
cost of proposed, 105
Neonatal intensive care
access to, 57-58
assessing effectiveness of, 51-60
benefits of, 52, 60, 87
components of, 51
costs of, 56
early setbacks, 50
evolution of, 49-51
mechanical ventilation of infants, 50
neonatal mortality, 37-38, 51-57
neurodevelopmental outcome, 59-60
levels of care, 51, 56-57
reduction in LBW mortality, 52
regionalization of services, 51, 56-58
VLBW births, as indicator of effectiveness of regionalization, 58
Neoplasms, 116
New York, insurance initiatives, 190-99
NHI (National Health Insurance). See
Health care proposals, analysis of.
NHS (National Health Service). See
Health care proposals, analysis of.
NHSC. See National Health Service
Corps.
NIH. See National Institutes of Health.
NPs. See Nurse-practitioners.
Nurse-practitioners, 140, 241
importance to Universal Maternity
Care, 238-239, 248, 257
underutilization of, 239
Nutrition. See also Special Supplemen-
tal Food program for Women, In-
fants, and Children (WIC).
community-based services, 73
factors influencing need for, 70-71
NWE. See National WIC Evaluation.

ORDER FORM *(Please print)*

Please send me ___ copies of **A Pound of Prevention: The Case for Universal Maternity Care in the U.S.** (ISBN 0-87553-206-3, 275 pages, softcover, Stock No. 014K) at $30.00 each for nonmembers and $21.00 for APHA members.

U.S.—Add $5.00 per book for shipping and handling. Non-U.S. Add $7.50 per book for shipping and handling. For orders over $200.00, call (202) 789-5667 for shipping and handling charges.

_____ Total dollars including shipping and handling.

___ Payment enclosed (make check payable to APHA). All checks and money orders must be in US dollars and drawn on US banks.

___ Visa   ___ Mastercard

Credit card no. _____ Expiration Date _____

Cardholder's signature _____

Name _____

Member No. _____

Organization _____

Address _____

City/State/Zip _____

Country _____

Phone ( ) _____

Is this a business address?   ___ Yes   ___ No

___ Send me your publications catalog

___ Send me membership information

Mail order form and payment to:
American Public Health Association
Publication Sales
Department 5037
Washington, DC 20061-5037

To charge by phone, call (202) 789-5636.
Prices subject to change without notice.